STUDY GUIDE

to accompany

EGAN'S

FUNDAMENTALS
OF
RESPIRATORY CARE

STUDY GUIDE

to accompany

EGAN'S
FUNDAMENTALS
OF
RESPIRATORY CARE

SEVENTH EDITION

STEPHEN F. WEHRMAN, RRT, RPFT

Professor/Program Director
Respiratory Care Program
Kapi'olani Community College
University of Hawaii
Honolulu, Hawaii

M Mosby

St. Louis Baltimore Boston Carlsbad Chicago Naples New York Philadelphia Portland
London Madrid Mexico City Singapore Sydney Tokyo Toronto Wiesbaden

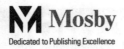
Mosby
Dedicated to Publishing Excellence

A Times Mirror
Company

Publisher: Don E Ladig
Editor: Janet Russell
Developmental Editor: Dina Shourd
Project Manager: Gayle May Morris
Manufacturing Manager: Karen Boehme
Cover Design: Theresa Breckwoldt

Printed in the United States of America

Composition by Black Dot Group
Printing and binding by Plus Communications

Mosby-Year Book, Inc.
11830 Westline Industrial Drive
St. Louis, Missouri 64146

International Standard Book Number: 0-8151-2891-6

98 99 00 01 / 9 8 7 6 5 4 3 2 1

Student Preface

The year was 1977. I had just started school to become a respiratory technician. My first textbook was *Egan's Fundamentals of Respiratory Therapy*. I have to confess, that I had to read everything three times to completely understand it—there was just so much in that book! When I began teaching, there was *Egan's* waiting for me—a new edition and a new challenge. Fifteen years and four editions later, I once again began to apply myself to the question of how to learn everything in *Egan's*. I knew it was a good book, full of almost all the information my students would need to know as they prepared for their careers in respiratory care. But how would I help them to read it and use it to its best advantage, allowing them to fully make sense of the information?

My students gave me the answer! They said, "You know how to make it easy to understand. You know what to emphasize. Why don't you write us a guide. . ." The rest is history. The problem for all students of health care is information overload. This is just as true for teachers as it is for anyone else. It is just as true for you as it was for me 21 years ago. This study guide will help you learn and sort out the important information you will need to succeed in practice and to pass your board exams.

If you want to get the most out of the study guide and *Egan's*, here's what you should do. First, read the assigned chapter in *Egan's*. Read lightly, using a highlighter to mark important points that jump out at you. Next, open the study guide and *Egan's* together. Complete the workbook as you review the material in *Egan's*. I suggest you note the page numbers where you found the answers. I've been careful to look up those answers in the text and have provided your instructors with a key. Sometimes you will come to problems where you have to really think and answer on your own. There are also experiments you can do at home or in the lab to help you understand concepts. At the end of each chapter you will find questions written in the same style the NBRC uses on the entry-level and written registry examinations. When you graduate and are preparing for your boards, you'll find that *Egan's Fundamentals* and this study guide will help you prepare.

Learning how to be a respiratory care practitioner is a challenging, fun, difficult, and sometimes painful experience. Don't ever give up along the way. Your instructors, textbooks, and clinical faculty are all there to help you succeed. You've chosen a dynamic and exciting field that will always keep you on your toes!

Aloha,

Steve Wehrman

P.S. I'd like to acknowledge some of the wonderful people who made this book possible. My wife Cathy and son James who supported; Colleagues Ken Mito and Aaron Koseki who suggested; editor Dina Shourd who encouraged; and most of all, my students who inspired.

P.P.S. Want to talk? Your feedback, questions, or comments are welcome at
wehrman@hawaii.edu

This book is dedicated to my dad, Robert Wehrman, who taught me how to think, and my mom, Susan Wehrman, who taught me that it is what you do with your mind that matters.

Contents

Quality Respiratory Care

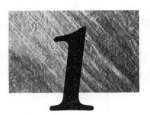

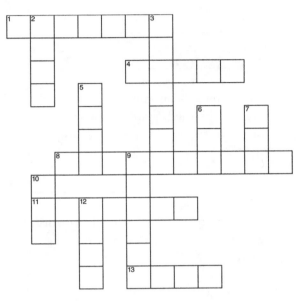

Everyone expects quality, from the goods we buy to the services we receive. Healthcare is no different. You want to work for a quality-oriented organization. You try to deliver quality care to your patients. The patients expect to be treated by qualified providers, and to get the best care at all times! In Chapter 1 we're going to look at what quality means in the healthcare setting and specific ways that we can monitor and achieve quality in the respiratory care profession.

ACROSS

1. _____ director. The physician who helps manage your department
4. Body that reviews health care companies such as hospitals
8. Recognition
11. Characteristic reflecting excellence
13. Credentializing organization for respiratory care

DOWN

2. Original author of your textbook
3. Permission to practice
5. Someone like you...
6. Informal training in the workplace
7. Agency that regulates drugs
9. Therapist _____ protocols
10. Improvement that is ongoing in nature
12. College of chest doctors

Word Wizard

Before you can understand quality care, you need to know the specific terms that are used to describe quality. Once you've read the first chapter of Egan, try your hand at completing this crossword puzzle!

Meet the Objectives

Chapter 1 presented three main objectives for learning. How well do you understand these important ideas about delivering the best care?

1. Providing quality care to the patient involves many dimensions. Name at least three elements that are part of quality respiratory care.
   A. _____
   B. _____
   C. _____

2. Quality must be monitored to ensure that it is being obtained. State the two basic monitoring strategies and give one example of each.
   A. _____
   B. _____

3. How can protocols enhance the quality of respiratory care services? Support your answer with evidence from the text.

Chapter Highlights

Fill in the blanks to identify eight key points from Chapter 1.

4. An energetic and competent _____ director is crucial to quality respiratory care.

5. Ordering too many respiratory care services is called _____ , and hinders delivery of quality care.

6. Specific guidelines for delivering appropriate respiratory care services are called _____ .

7. The _____ Respiratory Therapist is the highest credential in the profession.

8. Respiratory Care credentialing examinations are administered by the _____ .

9. _____ -_____ Care organizes staff and services around the needs of the patient, and is one approach to hospital redesign.

10. An ongoing form of quality assurance that puts emphasis on quality and cost-effectiveness is called _____ Quality _____ .

11. The two major forms of credentialing in health fields are state _____ and voluntary _____ .

Case Studies

Case One

Mary Young, a 25-year-old female, has returned to a medical/surgical nursing unit following an appendectomy. She has no history of lung disease and is wearing a nasal cannula at 3 L/min. Ms. Young is alert and oriented, with a respiratory rate of 18 and a heart rate of 82 beats/min. Her SpO_2 (pulse oximetry reading) is 99% on the nasal cannula. Her physician orders "Respiratory Therapy Protocol" and you are asked to assess this patient.

 Use the protocol found on Page 8 (Fig. 1-2) in Egan to help you answer the following questions.

12. What are the clinical signs of hypoxia/hypoxemia? Name at least three.
   A. _____
   B. _____
   C. _____

13. Using the oxygen therapy protocol, determine if the oxygen therapy is appropriate for this patient. Support your answer with information from the textbook.

14. What action would you recommend at this time?

Case Two

Mr. Parker Day, a 54-year-old male with a history of asthma and cigarette smoking, was admitted to the hospital for a hernia repair. Following the procedure, his chest radiograph shows an elevated diaphragm with bilateral atelectasis. The SpO_2 reading is 95% on room air. His heart rate is 84, blood pressure 110/78, respiratory rate 20, and temperature 36.8 degrees Celsius. Breath sounds are decreased bilaterally with apical wheezes. He has a weak, nonproductive cough. Mr. Day is alert and oriented.

15. Develop a specific respiratory care plan for this patient. Write your plan in the space below.

Respiratory care practitioners routinely plan, deliver, and assess the effects of care.

Board Exam Business

The National Board for Respiratory Care expects you to be able to participate in the development of care plans. You might expect to see five questions on this area in the Entry-Level Examination. I've written some questions that are similar in style to the ones on the boards for you to try on for size. If you're a beginner, you will need to look up the therapeutic interventions and disease management options in other parts of your text.

16. A patient with chronic obstructive pulmonary disease complains of difficulty breathing when he is ambulating. His SpO_2 is 88% at rest. Which of the following would you recommend?
   A. Oxygen therapy
   B. PEEP therapy
   C. Antibiotic therapy
   D. Aerosolized bronchodilator therapy

17. An alert 18-year-old patient is admitted with difficulty breathing. A diagnosis of asthma is determined, and you are asked to instruct the patient in the use of an MDI. An MDI is a device used for
   A. Oxygen therapy
   B. PEEP therapy
   C. Antibiotic therapy
   D. Aerosolized bronchodilator therapy

18. A patient with pneumonia is receiving oxygen via nasal cannula at 2 L/min. The SpO_2 is 89%. Heart rate is 110, and respiratory rate is 24. Which of the following would you recommend?
   A. Increase the liter flow to the cannula
   B. Intubate and begin mechanical ventilation
   C. Initiate aerosolized bronchodilator therapy
   D. Initiate postural drainage

19. Incentive breathing devices are primarily used in the treatment of
    A. Patients with emphysema
    B. Postoperative patients
    C. Adult respiratory distress syndrome
    D. Pulmonary fibrosis

Food for Thought

20. Protocol-based therapy and quality assurance efforts don't always work. Discuss some of the reasons you think these two strategies might fail.

21. Respiratory care practitioners (RCPs) don't just work in acute care hospitals. They work in pulmonary labs, sleep labs, home care, skilled nursing facilities, and physician offices. What do you think might be different about delivery and assessment of quality care in these settings? What would be similar to acute care?

Patient Safety, Communication, and Recordkeeping

Safety first. How many times have we heard that one?
Say the right thing at the right time. How do you do that?
Nobody loves paperwork, but the hospital environment is swimming in it.

Chapter 2 combines a huge amount of information that can be hard to swallow all at once. I'm going to break the information down into bite-sized pieces so that you can more easily digest the material.

Word Power

Read Chapter 2 in your textbook and then fill in the missing words below.

You'll Get a Charge Out of This

The medical center is filled with electrical equipment. Everything has a three-pronged plug. The third prong is the neutral wire, or _____ , which helps prevent elec-trocution. For this reason, no outside electrical devices are allowed in the hospital unless they are checked out by the biomedical staff. Electrocution can occur in the form of a _____ shock. This might happen if you were standing on a wet floor and a power cord fell onto the floor. Many of the power cords are detachable, so this is a potential hazard. Always clean up spills. A small shock, or _____ shock, is a hazard to patients who have pacemakers, ECG leads, and indwelling heart catheters. This may result in ventricular _____ and death. This could happen if the ground wire is broken, so don't ever roll beds or other equipment over the electrical power cords. Report frayed cords and take suspect equipment out of use.

Burn, Baby, Burn

Oxygen is necessary for fires to exist. Since high oxygen concentrations are used in respiratory care, fire is a real hazard. Even though oxygen is _____ and does not burn, it greatly speeds up an existing fire. For a fire to start you also need _____ material and heat. Remove any of these three and the fire will go out. You must make sure that ignition sources such as _____ are not allowed when oxygen is in use. Most hospitals will call a "Code Red" if a fire exists and you must respond. One of the RCPs responsibilities in a fire is to shut off the zone valve to the affected area if the fire is near a patient using

oxygen. (See Chapter 33: Storage and Delivery of Medical Gases.)

Keep it Moving!

Anyone who stays immobile in a bed for too long will suffer consequences. You need to ambulate patients as soon as they are stable.

Here are some guidelines for safe ambulation. Number them 1 through 7 in the right order.

_____ Dangle the patient.

_____ Sit the patient up.

_____ Assist to a standing position.

_____ Encourage slow, easy breathing.

_____ Lower the bed and lock the wheels.

_____ Move the IV pole close to the patient.

_____ Provide support while walking.

I Can't Hear You

Communication plays a big part in your ability to gain patient cooperation, evaluate progress, and make recommendations for care. What you do (nonverbal) is just as important as what you say (verbal). Communication will also play a role in your satisfaction on the job. Exchanging information and working out problems with other members of the health care team are an everyday part of hospital life.

Meet the Objectives

Chapter 2 presented 14 objectives for learning. We've already covered some of them. How well do you understand safety and communication? To find the answers, just read the book!

1. Name at least three risks that are common among patients receiving respiratory care.

   A. _____

   B. _____

   C. _____

2. Describe one way to minimize risk for each of the three common hazard areas named in question 1.

   A. _____

   B. _____

   C. _____

3. What is the main reason you should use good body mechanics?

4. State two factors you should monitor during patient ambulation.

   A. _____

   B. _____

5. Name at least four of the many factors that influence the communication process.

   A. _____

   B. _____

   C. _____

   D. _____

6. The text lists five ways to improve your effectiveness as a sender of messages. Describe two of these that apply to you. Give examples of situations where you communicated well (or not!).

7. Name four sources of conflict in interpersonal communication. Give an example of each.
   A. _____
   B. _____
   C. _____
   D. _____

8. What is a medical record? Who does it belong to? Who is allowed to read it?

9. State one legal and one practical essential of record keeping.
   A. _____
   B. _____

10. One of the most common formats that RCPs (and others) use in charting is the SOAP format. What does SOAP mean? Give examples of information you would chart for each category.

Chapter Highlights

Fill in the blanks to identify eight key points from Chapter 2.

11. You should begin _____ as soon as a patient is stable.

12. A _____ is a small current that enters the body through external catheters and may cause ventricular fibrillation.

13. Avoid electrical shocks by always _____ your equipment.

14. You can minimize fire hazards by removing flammable materials and ignition sources from areas where _____ is in use.

15. _____ skills play a key role in your ability to achieve desired patient outcomes.

16. Accommodating, avoiding, collaborating, competing, and compromising are basic strategies for handling _____ .

17. A medical record is a _____ document.

18. You must _____ each treatment you provide.

Case Studies

Case 1

The physician orders ambulation for Mr. C. Lunger, who is wearing oxygen. The nurse asks you to assist. Mr. Lunger is wearing a nasal cannula, running at 2 L/min. After 5 minutes of walking, you notice that he is breathing at a rate of 24, and using his accessory muscles of ventilation. His skin appears sweaty, and he is exhaling through pursed lips.

19. What equipment will you need *before* you try to walk this patient?

20. What observations are important to note in this situation? What action would you take?

Case 2

You are caring for a patient who is on a mechanical ventilator. You need to transport the patient to radiology for a CT scan. The nurse unplugs the IV pump and pulse oximeter from the *back* of each unit. The pumps and the pulse oximeter are now running on their battery systems. As you prepare to leave, you notice that the power cords are still plugged into the wall outlets. The doctor and the nurse are anxious to get the transport underway.

21. Describe the actions you would take if you encountered this situation.

22. What potential conflict/communication problems exist? How will you deal with them?

Board Exam Business

By now you should be asking the question, "Does any of this apply to my board examinations?" The answer is yes! The *CRTT Study Guide*, published by the National Board for Respiratory Care, state, in the examination matrix: "In any patient care setting, the respiratory care practitioner maintains patient records and communicates relevant information to members of the healthcare team . . ." More specifically, you should be able to:

1. *Explain* therapy to patients in terms they can understand
2. *Document* a treatment correctly
3. *Note responses* to therapy—this includes not only vital signs, adverse reactions, and so on

but also includes interpreting subjective and attitudinal response to therapy!

4. *Verify computations* and correct errors
5. *Communicate clinical information* to other healthcare practitioners
6. *Communicate to avoid conflicts*, maintain scheduling and sequencing of treatments

Wow! That must mean they really care about this stuff! You will probably see 2 or 3 questions on this specific material. (More on this subject in Chapter 14!) Try a few problems, in the good old board exam style.

23. A respiratory care practitioner has completed SOAP charting in the progress notes following a bronchodilator treatment. While signing the chart form, she notices that the wrong amount of medication has been entered. Which of the following actions should be taken at this time?
    I. Draw one line through the error
    II. Notify the physician of the error
    III. Write "Error" and initial
    IV. Recopy the progress notes
    A. I only
    B. I and II only
    C. I and III only
    D. IV only

24. An asthmatic has orders for albuterol by medication nebulizer every 2 hours. During the shift the patient improves, and the order is changed to every 4 hours. In regard to the new frequency, what action should you take?
    I. Note the new order in your charting
    II. Inform the RN of the order
    III. Notify the respiratory care supervisor
    A. I only
    B. I and II only
    C. I and III only
    D. I, II, and III

Food for Thought

Every year people die in work-related fires and electrocutions. The hospital can be a busy, stressful environment, and it is really easy to skip some of the steps in the safety process. That's one of the reasons the Occupational Safety and Health Administration (OSHA) requires health care institutions to train workers in fire, electrical, blood-borne pathogen, back, and other safety areas *every year!* We all know friends, patients, and co-workers who have been injured on the job. I hope you're not going to be one of them.

25. What do you think is the most common type of injury in health care?

26. On what shift do most injuries, accidents, and patient incidents occur?

Principles of Infection Control

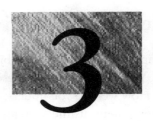

"The doctor is to be feared
more than the disease."
Latin Proverb

Nobody comes to the hospital to get sick! But let's face it, 5% to 10% of all the patients who enter a hospital get an infection while they are there. To make matters worse, up to 40% of these infections involve the respiratory system. It costs billions to treat hospital-acquired illness, and even more to pay for lost work time. Patients aren't the only ones who get sick. Each year, thousands of health-care practitioners are exposed to infectious organisms such as hepatitis, HIV, and tuberculosis, and some of them will be infected. Fortunately, there are plenty of simple, easy ways you can protect both yourself and the patients. (Personally, I think the freeway is more dangerous than the hospital!)

Slam the Door on Infections

Chapter 3 introduces a lot of new terms that you should know if you want to be able to beat bacteria and viruses. After you read about this timely topic you will be able to solve this puzzle.

ACROSS

1. Drug resistant, abbrev.
5. Type of acid found in vinegar
7. Watch out or you'll get punctured by this
9. Mosquito, for example
13. Presence of microorganisms in a host
14. Type of plastic
15. Wear this around TB patients
17. Sodium hypochlorite
19. Safety agency
20. Most important and frequent route of transmission

DOWN

2. Clean
3. Type of filter
4. These nebulizers are culprits
6. Center that studies disease
8. Sterilizing gas
9. Water or food are examples of this route of transmission
10. Wear these around body fluids
11. Wash them like your mother told you!
12. Dirty surfaces or equipment
16. Respiratory professional group
17. Put dirty equipment in this before transporting
18. Humidifier that does not use water

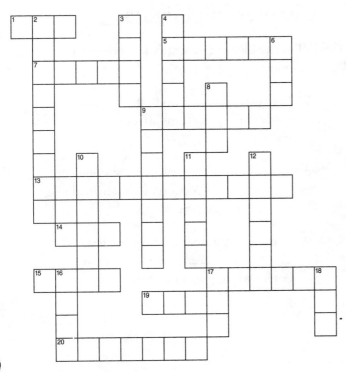

Meet the Objectives

Chapter 3 presented nine objectives for learning. We'll cover some of these later in this chapter. How well do you understand the principles of equipment disinfection and sterilization?

1. What is the first step in selecting a method for processing reusable equipment?

2. Describe the pasteurization process and give one limitation to this method of cleaning equipment.

3. Give an example of a high-level chemical disinfectant used in respiratory care. Describe a situation in which you would use this chemical.

4. State the six methods of sterilization. For each method, give an example of applicable equipment to be sterilized.

Method	Equipment
A. _____	_____
B. _____	_____
C. _____	_____
D. _____	_____
E. _____	_____
F. _____	_____

5. State the two types of processing indicators used with sterilization. Give an example of each.

Indicator	Example
A. _____	_____
B. _____	_____

6. List the three general barrier methods used to prevent exposure to organisms. Which one is considered the single best way to prevent the spread of infection?

   A. _____
   B. _____
   C. _____

Chapter Highlights

Fill in the blanks to identify key points from Chapter 3.

7. Between _____ and _____ of all nosocomial infections affect the respiratory system.

8. _____ is the best choice for high-level disinfection of semicritical respiratory care equipment.

9. Among respiratory care equipment, _____ have the greatest potential to spread infection.

10. Always use _____ fluids for tracheal suctioning and to fill nebulizers and humidifiers.

11. Thoroughly _____ your _____ after any patient contact, even when gloves are used.

12. Use standard (universal) precautions in caring for _____ patients, regardless of their diagnosis or infection status.

13. Wear _____ and _____ during any procedure that can generate splashes or sprays of body fluids.

14. _____ items should be bagged before removal from a patient's room.

15. Exercise extreme caution when handling or disposing of all "_____."

Case Studies

Case 1

You work in the surgical intensive care unit of a large urban hospital. Over the last two days, a number of patients in the unit have developed serious *Staphylococcus aureus* infections.

16. Why do postoperative patients have an increased risk of infection?

17. What is the most common source of *Staphylococcus aureus* organisms?

18. Identify three ways to disrupt the route of transmission in this situation.
    A. _____
    B. _____
    C. _____

Case 2

During your third day of clinical, you are assigned to go with a therapist who has an extremely heavy workload on a medical floor of the hospital. The therapist puts on gloves for each patient contact, and asks you to do so also. When you go to wash your hands after the first treatment, the therapist tells you "We don't have time for that, and besides the gloves will keep our hands clean."

19. Explain the role of gloves in protecting practitioners and preventing the spread of infection.

20. What other concerns does this situation raise?

Case 3

A serious tuberculosis outbreak occurs in a local prison facility. You are called to the emergency department as four of the sickest patients are being admitted together to your hospital for treatment.

21. By what route does tuberculosis spread?

22. When transporting these patients out of the emergency department, what action should you take?

23. What kind of precautions should be taken to prevent the spread of infection once these patients are admitted?

24. What special guidelines exist in regard to cough-inducing and aerosol-generating procedures for patients with active tuberculosis?

25. What other concerns do you have in working with these patients?

What does the NBRC Say?

You'd be right if you thought your board exams would place an emphasis on infection control. The Entry-Level Examination Matrix has this to say:

"In any patient care setting, the respiratory care practitioner . . . assures cleanliness of all equipment used in providing respiratory care."
More specifically, you should:

1. Choose the right method or agent for disinfection and sterilization
2. Perform disinfection and sterilization procedures
3. Monitor sterilization effectiveness
4. Protect the patient from nosocomial infection
5. Follow infection control policies and procedures

Here are some questions like the ones you might see on the test. I have put them in the form of a single case, but they will normally be spread throughout the exam. You can expect at least three questions on infection control in your entry-level boards.

Questions 26 through 28 refer to the following situation:

Mrs. Ima Marsa is a 72-year-old patient with COPD who has a tracheostomy tube following prolonged intubation and mechanical ventilation. She is currently in the medical intensive care unit. After you take her off the ventilator, you will need to set up a heated aerosol system with an FIO_2 of 40%.

26. What type of water should be placed in the nebulizer?
    A. Distilled water
    B. Tap water
    C. Normal saline solution
    D. Sterile distilled water

27. To help lower the risk of a nosocomial infection when using heated aerosol systems, the RCP should do which of the following?
    I. Label the equipment with the date and time it is started
    II. Avoid draining condensate into the nebulizer
    III. Remove the capillary tube to reduce the volume of water particles
    IV. Use aseptic technique during the initial set-up
    A. I and II only

B. I, II, and IV only

C. I, III, and IV only

D. I, II, III, and IV

28. The best way to prevent the spread of infection in the ICU is to
    A. Ensure that sterilized equipment is used
    B. Wash your hands after every patient contact
    C. Wear gloves when you come in contact with body fluids
    D. Isolate infected patients

Food for Thought

Many hospitalized patients acquire respiratory infections, so the RCP is really under a microscope at work. We have to maintain the highest standards of behavior to protect ourselves, our patients, and our loved ones.

29. One of your fellow students comes to clinical with a cold. He asks you not to tell your clinical instructor, since missed clinical days are hard to make up. What is your reaction to this situation? What are the potential problems with this scenario?

30. The college recommends that you get immunized against hepatitis B prior to attending clinical. The consent form lists a number of possible side effects of the vaccine, and the vaccination is expensive. What are the pros and cons of vaccines? What will you choose?

Ethical and Legal Implications of Practice

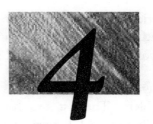

Malpractice. A word that strikes fear into the hearts of physicians. A word that could strike fear into your heart! Let's face it, we live in a society where lawsuits are commonplace. You hear about them every day. Do RCPs ever get sued? You bet they do. To make matters worse, the ethical issues that are always present in healthcare are crossing into the legal arena more and more. Should we terminate life support? How can health services be rationed? What if the patient cannot afford the care? Your two safeguards are knowledge and good defensive recordkeeping. Chapter 4 will provide you with the tools you need to provide care with confidence.

Word Power

Law, like medicine, has a language of its own that most people do not understand. (As Shakespeare said, "It was Greek to me.") You will need clear comprehension of some basic legal terminology to avoid ending up in court.

The two basic types of law in the United States are public and civil law. Public law is further divided into administrative law and _____ law. Healthcare facilities operate under a mountain of regulations set by government agencies. Private, or _____ law protects citizens who feel they have been harmed. The individual who brings a complaint is called the _____ and those accused of wrongdoing are known as _____. A _____ is a civil wrong. These cases could easily involve a healthcare practitioner. There are three types. _____ is the failure to perform your duties competently. Cases in which the patient falls, is given the wrong medication, or is harmed by equipment revolve around a provider's duty to anticipate harm and prevent it from happening.

Expert testimony, professional guidelines, or even circumstantial evidence can determine what a reasonable and _____ RCP would have done in a given situation. The Latin term _____ _____ _____ (the thing speaks for itself) is sometimes invoked to show that harm occurred because of inappropriate care. When a professional fails to act skillfully, breaches ethics, or falls below a reasonable standard, it is called _____. Wrongdoing may be considered intentional or unintentional. Intentional acts include _____, or placing another person in fear of bodily harm, _____, or physical contact without consent. Other common intentional harm occurs through _____, which is verbal defamation of character, and _____, which is written defamation of character. Finally, infor-

mation about patients is considered private, or _____, and cannot be shared with anyone who is not involved in their care.

There are two good defenses against all of these problems. The first is to show that actions were not intentional. For example, fainting during a procedure is not a voluntary act. The second defense is to obtain consent from the patient. Consent, whether verbal or written, should be obtained from the patient for most procedures. Of course you have to explain the risks and the procedure in clear language the patient can understand.

Case Studies

Case 1
You get a chance to meet with your fellow students for lunch in the hospital cafeteria during a busy clinical day. One of your classmates is bursting with excitement as you sit down to eat. "You won't believe what I got to do today! I was taking care of Mr. Tucker in the ICU, and he started to go bad and we had to intubate. Then he coded and I got to do CPR! It was so cool!"

1. What's the problem with this picture? What violation has your classmate committed?

2. What are the possible consequences of this scenario?

3. What action should you take?

Case 2
You receive an order to administer a bronchodilator to Daniel Rush, a 27-year-old asthmatic. Mr. Rush refuses the therapy, stating "I just can't take any more of this today." He appears alert and oriented.

4. Does the patient have a legal right to refuse in this case? Cite evidence from the text to justify your answer.

5. How would you respond to this situation?

6. What other action should you take at this time?

Case 3

After finishing with Mr. Rush, you receive a stat call to the orthopedic floor.

The RN informs you they are having problems with Marie Harme, a 76-year-old woman who recently had surgical repair of a broken hip. As you enter the room, you notice that Ms. Harme has removed her oxygen. She is breathing rapidly, and her color is not good. The pulse oximeter shows a saturation of 84%. When you try to get the patient to wear the oxygen, she screams at you to get out of the room.

7. Does the patient have a legal right to refuse in this case? Cite evidence from the text to justify your answer.

8. How would you respond to this situation?

9. Would physical restraints be an option or a possible case of battery?

What about Ethics?

No, I haven't forgotten about ethics (although this subject *is* less clearcut than the legal one). The law sets minimum standards that we all must try to follow. Ethics, on the other hand, are a set of guidelines for doing your job in a way that is morally defensible. The problem is not that there are a lot of people out working in healthcare who are immoral but rather the presence of ethical dilemmas that no one can avoid.

Start at the Beginning

The most famous ethical code in medicine is the Hippocratic Oath. We RCPs have our own code of ethics that was developed by the AARC. You can find it on p. 65 in Egan. Ethical codes seek to set general guidelines for behavior within a given professional group. What the codes don't do, however, is to help with the really difficult decisions.

Do No Harm vs Save Lives

When two or more "right" choices are in direct conflict, an ethical dilemma exists. A hot topic in medicine and government right now involves how we end our lives, or "assisted suicide." On one hand, we don't want people to suffer needlessly. Watching a terminally ill patient suffer is a sad and demoralizing experience for RCPs. On the other hand, taking someone's life is an equally difficult decision with far-ranging consequences (some of which could be legal consequences!). Reducing these issues to simple rules and formulas is not easy, perhaps not even possible. Every ethical principle involves two parts: professional duty, and patient rights.

Case Studies

Case 1

Oscar Miller, a 17-year old male, is admitted for pneumonia. This young man is depressed and has expressed thoughts of ending his life if "my worst fears are true about this illness." Laboratory studies reveal that Mr. Miller is HIV-positive. His physician expresses concern to the other caregivers about revealing Mr. M's diagnosis to him.

10. Under what circumstances can you lie (or not tell the truth) to patients?

11. What are your feelings about telling the truth to patients?

12. What would you do if Mr. Mild asked you if he has AIDS?

Francouer's Ethical Decision-Making Model

Let's apply Francouer's model to Case 1 (see p. 70 in Egan).

13. What is the problem or issue in this case?

14. Who are the individuals involved?

15. What ethical principle(s) apply here?

16. Who should make the decision to tell Mr. Miller?

17. What is your role as an RCP who is giving this patient treatments?

18. Are there short-term consequences to either decision? Long-term?

19. Make the decision! (What would you do?)

20. How would you proceed after you made your choice?

Case 2

Johnny M., a respiratory care practitioner, is a deeply religious individual who has strong feelings about homosexuality. When Johnny is assigned to provide therapy for Oscar Miller, he objects to the supervisor, saying "I do not want to take care of him. It is against my religious principles. Assign someone else."

21. What are some of the possible problems for the Respiratory Department that could arise out of this situation?

22. Patients are allowed to refuse even life-sustaining treatment for religious reasons. What about professional caregivers?

23. What would you do if you were the supervisor?

"I would rather be the man who bought the Brooklyn Bridge than the man who sold it."
Will Rogers

Chapter Highlights

Fill in the blanks to identify key points from Chapter 4.

24. Ethical _____ occur when there are two equally desirable or undesirable outcomes.

25. Professional codes of ethics are general guidelines to identify _____ behavior.

26. The two basic ethical theories are _____ and _____.

27. _____ law deals with the relationships of private parties and the government.

28. Professional _____ is negligence in which a professional has failed to provide the _____ expected, resulting in _____ to someone.

29. Practitioners must carry out their duties with an eye toward _____ themselves in the case of _____ action.

What About Those Board Exams?

Sorry, but ethics and legal issues aren't really a part of your examinations to obtain a license to practice respiratory care. Considering the case of a respiratory care practitioner in California accused of so-called "mercy killings," perhaps these areas should be on the test!

Food for Thought

When I go home from work, I usually feel pretty good about what I do for a living, but sometimes I have issues I need to work out.

30. When you have been involved in an ethical dilemma where you felt the wrong choice was made, how do you resolve the way you feel afterward?

Physical Principles in Respiratory Care

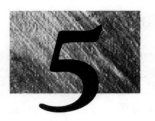

Physics is a subject that everyone struggles to understand. The purpose of this chapter is to help you figure out what's important and how to apply the information. You don't have to be a rocket scientist to understand physical principles of respiratory care.

Unlock Your Brain

Words are the keys that open up your mind so you can start to learn a difficult subject. After you read Egan, you will be able to put the right words into the blanks.

Yes, But It's a Dry Heat . . .

Without humidity, our airways become irritated and mucous gets thick. The actual amount, or weight, of water vapor in a gas is called _____ humidity. As RCPs, we compare the weight of water vapor with the amount it could hold if the gas was fully saturated. This ratio of content to capacity is known as _____ humidity. You hear about this on the weather report every day. I'm more interested in how much vapor gas can hold inside the airways. This amount is called percent _____ humidity. When inspired gas has less than 100% of its capacity, a humidity _____ exists. Humidifiers are used to make up the difference. When you get a can of icy soda on a hot day, water droplets begin to form on the outside of the can. That's because the air around the can is cooling (cold air does not hold as much water vapor as warm air). When air cools, and gaseous water returns to a liquid form, we say that _____ has occurred. The opposite effect occurs when the drink sits out. Water molecules escape from the liquid into the air. This process is called _____ and adds to the humidity in the air.

Some Like It Hot

Heat moves in mysterious ways—four of them to be precise. Newborn babies are especially sensitive to heat loss. Keeping a preemie warm can make the difference between life and death! When a baby is born, we dry them off to prevent loss through _____. Then the little one is wrapped in cloth to prevent _____, or loss that occurs when you are touching a cooler object. Finally, we put the newborn in an incubator. The incubator provides warmth in two ways. First, a special light _____ heat toward the baby. Second, warm air blows into the incubator. Transfer of heat through movement of fluids (or gas) is called _____.

 Now that you know some of the important terms, you need to . . .

Obey the Laws

Remember the bumper sticker: "Gravity, it's not just a good idea, it's the law!"? Gases have to follow the laws of physics, too. Since RCPs work with different gases, such as oxygen, nitrogen, carbon dioxide, and helium, it's important that you know the laws and how gases behave. In this section, I'll give you some real examples of gas laws in action, and you tell me which law is being demonstrated.

Example 1

A registered pulmonary function technologist (RPFT) is performing lung testing on a patient. The patient inhales 1.5 L from the spirometer.

1. What will happen to the volume of gas inside the patient's lungs?

2. Gas law: _____

Example 2

A home care therapist places an oxygen cylinder in the van so that she can take it to a client's house. The sun is shining through the window on the cylinder.

3. What will happen to the pressure inside the cylinder as it gets warmer?

4. Gas law: _____

Example 3

When you inhale, your diaphragm drops and your chest expands. In other words, you increase the size, or volume, of your chest.

5. What happens to the pressure inside your chest?

6. Gas law: _____

Try It, You'll Like It

Here are some safe, easy experiments you can perform in the lab at school or at home.

Experiment 1

Place a dry, empty glass soda bottle in the freezer for at least 15 minutes. Take the bottle out and immediately cover the mouth of the bottle with a balloon. Wait a few minutes and watch!

7. What happens to the balloon?

8. What gas law is responsible for the result?

Experiment 2

Cut a 1-inch by 5-inch strip of notebook paper. Hold one end of the paper to your chin, just below your lip. Blow steadily across the top of the paper.

9. What happened to the paper?

10. What principle is responsible?

Another experiment showing this same principle can be demonstrated with balloons. Blow up two round balloons and tie them off. Attach about 1 foot of string to each balloon. Tape the string to a stick (such as a ruler or yardstick) so the balloons are about 6 to 8 inches apart. Blow between the balloons.

11. What happened to the balloons?

Experiment 3

Get a coffee stirrer, an ordinary straw, and a big straw (the kind you use for a milkshake). Now get a couple of cups. Put some water in one cup,

and some honey in the other. Suck the water up through each straw. Now try the honey. To make this more interesting, get a 6-foot length of oxygen connecting tubing. Try the two fluids again.

12. Which tube is easier to suck through?

13. Which fluids are easier to suck up?

14. What hard to pronounce, French-sounding law explains all this?

Since gases and liquid are both fluids, the same rules apply to inhaling.

Case Studies

Case 1

A respiratory therapist decides to attend the AARC International Congress. To get there, the therapist must travel by air. Before taking off, the flight attendant explains about the oxygen system. The therapist pays attention (unlike everyone else) when he sees the partial rebreathing mask. He also knows that something interesting happens to oxygenation at 30,000 feet.

15. What is the barometric pressure and inspired (P_IO_2) partial pressure of oxygen at this altitude?

P_B _____

P_IO_2 _____

16. A properly fitting oxygen mask can deliver about 70% oxygen to passengers. What would the P_IO_2 be while wearing the mask?

17. What gas law did you use to make these conclusions?

Case 2

Respiratory care practitioners frequently draw arterial blood samples to measure the partial pressures of oxygen and carbon dioxide in the blood. Many patients have elevated or decreased body temperatures.

18. What effect does a fever have on these partial pressure readings?

19. A normal arterial carbon dioxide pressure ($PaCO_2$) is 40 torr at a body temperature of 37° Celsius. Estimate the new $PaCO_2$ if body temperature was 40° Celsius.

20. Why is temperature correction of arterial blood gas readings controversial?

Mathemagic

You must be able to perform calculations in the clinical setting and on board examinations. Chapter 5 gave several examples of problems found in both settings. Write the formula, then solve the following problems without using a calculator. (Since your board examinations do not allow use of electronic calculators, use a calculator to check your work only.) I always write the formula out first, then plug in the numbers to avoid mistakes. If you're good at math, just skip this step.

21. Convert 30° Celsius to degrees Kelvin.
    Formula: _____
    Solution: _____
    Answer: _____

22. Convert 68° Fahrenheit to degrees Celsius.
    Formula: _____
    Solution: _____
    Answer: _____

23. Convert 40° degrees Celsius to degrees Fahrenheit.

    Formula: _____

    Solution: _____

    Answer: _____

24. At body temperature, gas has a saturated capacity of about 44mg of water vapor per liter. If a gas has an absolute humidity of 22 mg/L, what is the relative humidity?

    Formula: _____

    Solution: _____

    Answer: _____

25. What is the humidity deficit in question 24?

    Formula: _____

    Solution: _____

    Answer: _____

26. Convert a pressure reading of 10 millimeters of mercury (mm Hg) to centimeters of water (cm H_2O).

    Formula: _____

    Solution: _____

    Answer: _____

27. Convert a pressure reading of 10 centimeters of water (cm H_2O) to kilopascals (kPa). Hint: it's alright to round off.

    Formula: _____

    Solution: _____

    Answer: _____

28. Air is normally about 21% oxygen. Calculate the partial pressure of oxygen in air (P_IO_2) when the barometric pressure is 760 mm Hg.

    Formula: _____

    Solution: _____

    Answer: _____

29. Now calculate the new P_IO_2 that would result if the barometric pressure were 500 mm Hg.

    Formula: _____

    Solution: _____

    Answer: _____

Math may be difficult for some of us. Becoming proficient at it can make the difference between success and failure on the board exams!

Computer Applications in Respiratory Care

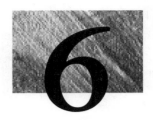

"The real danger is not that computers will begin to think like humans, but that humans will begin to think like computers."

Sydney Harris

Let's face it, we are living in the "Information Age." Microprocessor technology is part of everyday life, and healthcare practitioners use computers every day. (I used a computer to write this workbook!) If you can learn to use these tools effectively, you will be a more effective RCP.

Keys to the Highway

Most of the words that describe computers aren't even in the dictionary yet. If you want to travel the information highway, you will need to be able to talk the talk. Let's get started with a few key terms . . .

Computerese

The most common computers in use today are personal computers (PCs). Larger computers, called main frames, are also used (by big institutions such as colleges, medical centers, and the IRS) for large applications. Every computer needs _____ ware, such as the central processor, printer, keyboard, and mouse. You also need _____ware, or programs that are sets of instructions that tell the computer what to do. Information from a computer can be stored on floppy _____, magnetic drives, tapes, or optical memory systems such as _____-ROMs.

Talk to Me!

Computers can talk to each other through local networks inside the hospital, or they can go outside the institution. The global network of computer networks is called the _____. Your PC can talk to other computers via an analog-to-digital converter, which is designed to work with acoustic signals. This device can dial the phone, and is called a _____.

Computers in Healthcare

Clinicians use computers to help interpret data, reach a diagnosis, and to automate certain aspects of patient care. Now you need to open your textbook and look up some information about this subject.

1. Give five examples of how a modern hospital information system (HIS) is used by the institution and health care providers.
   A. _____
   B. _____
   C. _____
   D. _____
   E. _____

2. State one example of how computers are used to aid in patient monitoring and diagnostic testing.

3. Discuss the difference between open- and closed-loop control systems.

admitted to the emergency department with asthma and what happened to them. Mark wants to develop a report on the subject to present to administration. He plans to develop an asthma education program that will require a budget for equipment, personnel, and training materials.

6. What type of software program is most useful for gathering specific information on patient populations?

4. List four examples of clinical areas where a RCP might use a computer-assisted interpretation or diagnosis.
   A. _____
   _____
   B. _____
   _____
   C. _____
   _____
   D. _____
   _____

7. What program will Mark use to help prepare the budget for his project?

5. Identify the four main non-technical issues related to the use of computers in health care. Explain why these issues are concerns.
   A. _____
   _____
   B. _____
   _____
   C. _____
   _____
   D. _____
   _____

8. What kind of software will he use to prepare the written report for administration?

Case Studies

Case 1

Mark D. Sade, a technical director for a respiratory department in a large urban medical center, knows that asthma mortality is on the rise. He wants to find out information about patients

9. Students have to write reports, too! What specific program do you use for this task? What do you like about it? What are the limitations?

Case 2

A respiratory care student is asked by her instructor to locate the URL for the American Association for Respiratory Care (AARC) so she can access information on Clinical Practice Guidelines (CPGs).

10. What does the term URL mean?

11. What are the three major components of the URL?
    A. _____
    B. _____
    C. _____

12. Identify the three components of the URL for AARC.
    A. _____
    B. _____
    C. _____

13. What action can you take to avoid having to write down or remember the URL for sites you wish to revisit?

Practice Makes Perfect!

It isn't good enough to just talk the talk. Now you have to walk the walk! You will need a computer with access to the World Wide Web to practice some of the skills discussed in the text. Most colleges will provide a free e-mail account for stu-dents and have computers with Web access. If yours does not, you can try your local "Internet Café," a popular coffee shop with computers. Or go to the public library! (As a last resort, you might try a friend who has a computer.)

Activity 1: Information Search

14. Access an index: Yahoo! is a popular Internet index (http://www.yahoo.com).

You will need a computer that has a Web browser such as Netscape Navigator or Microsoft Explorer to get started. After you open the browser, enter Yahoo's URL. Select the top heading, "Health." Now select the category "Medicine." You should see a field in your computer that looks like Fig. 6-20 on page 132 in your textbook. Pick one of these topics that relates to Respiratory Care and spend some time browsing.

15. Conduct a search: Start up your browser and open Net Search," or go directly to the AltaVista search engine (http://www.altavista.digital.com). Now you can enter a keyword or phrase to look for information on a specific topic. Initially, it is alright to use natural language such as "asthma caused," or "what causes asthma" as a keyword. You may find too much information and need to narrow your search. Table 6-4 on page 133 in your text contains examples of Boolean operators or special words used in searches. For example, try "asthma AND causes."

When you find a site or article that looks worthwhile, bookmark the URL for future reference.

Activity 2: Evaluate!

Not all the information on the Internet is reliable. There is a lot of "junk science," too.

Find a web site now and answer these simple questions:

Site: _____

16. Is it clear who is sponsoring the page? Look at the URL. Does the address end in "edu" or "gov?" These sites tend to be reliable.

17. Can you verify the legitimacy of the sponsor? Look for a phone number or address for more information, not just an e-mail address.

18. Is it clear who wrote the material (and the author's qualifications)?

19. Is the information free of spelling, grammatical, and typographical errors?

20. Is the information free of advertising?

21. Are there dates on the page to indicate when the material was written or revised?

22. Is it clearly stated when data or statistical information was collected?

The more "YES" answers you have, the more reliable the information!

Activity 3: Respiratory Care

23. In this exercise, you will locate a specific document from the AARC's Web site. Open the AARC home page (http://ww.aarc.org/). Find the section on Clinical Practice Guidelines (CPGs). Open the guideline on pulse oximetry. Print this guideline and use it as a study reference. Why? One reason is the reliability of this material. Another good reason is that the National Board for Respiratory Care says in its newsletter: "CPGs are a valuable tool for preparing for board examinations."

Food for Thought

It is easy to learn how to use the computer for more than just games. Besides those listed above, you may want to try these activities:

24. Locate the home page for your college.

25. If your program has a Web site, locate it and print the home page or find some specific information from the page. If you don't have a page, find one from another program. These sites are easily accessed from AARC's web site. (You can find my program at keyword: Respiratory Care Hawaii, or at the URL: http://leahi.kcc.hawaii.edu/dept/resp/).

26. If you don't have a program web site, design one as a class project. Ask your media or learning center to provide skills and access to the campus server. With the new software available, *anyone* can learn to make a web site.

27. If your college offers e-mail accounts for students, get the entire class to sign up. Create an address list for the class, and send messages via e-mail. Ask your instructors to e-mail assignments, class syllabus, etc. (Save the trees!)

28. Search any of the web sites in Table 6-2 on page 132 in the textbook. Find a specific article, protocol, practice guideline, or other information that can be linked to a class activity or personal need. For example, the National Board for Respiratory Care site contains information related to the board exams. AARC's site has journals, protocols, and much more! You could use this to help write a report or complete a journal assignment.

29. Post a query on a Listserv like RCWorld. You can get opinions and information from practitioners all over the world. Try asking about hypoxic drive or the use of helium with obstructive disease, or continuous nebulization of bronchodilators. Anything interesting, unusual, or complex is fair game. Print the replies you get and share them with your fellow students or your instructors.

The Respiratory System

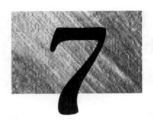

───── "Anatomy is destiny." ─────
Sigmund Freud

Structure and function have a lot to do with each other. Anatomy even has clinical applica-

tions! In this chapter, we'll be trying to bring anatomy back to life (sounds like Dr. Franken-stein?). Before we go there, I just want to check and see if you still remember some important terms that relate to the anatomy of the respiratory system.

ACROSS

2. Pectoralis _____
4. Cells that produce mucus
7. Type of cells that make up the structure of the alveoli
9. Lining of the airways
11. Chemical name for carbon monoxide
15. Small airways without cartilage
16. Alveolar cells that make surfactant
17. Lobes in the right lung
18. Chemical name for nitric oxide
19. Point where airways and vessels enter the lung
21. Warms, filters, humidifies

DOWN

1. Chemical name for helium
3. _____ apple
5. Pertaining to the mouth
6. Primary anatomical divisions of the lungs
8. Pertaining to the nose
10. _____ abdominus
11. Pertaining to the ribs
12. At the end of the breastbone
13. Opening to the lower airway
14. Nerves to the diaphragm
15. Large airways
20. Cells that store histamine

A Picture is Worth a Thousand . . .

Rather than talk about anatomy, there's something else I want you to do. Identify the structures I've labeled in the following figures.

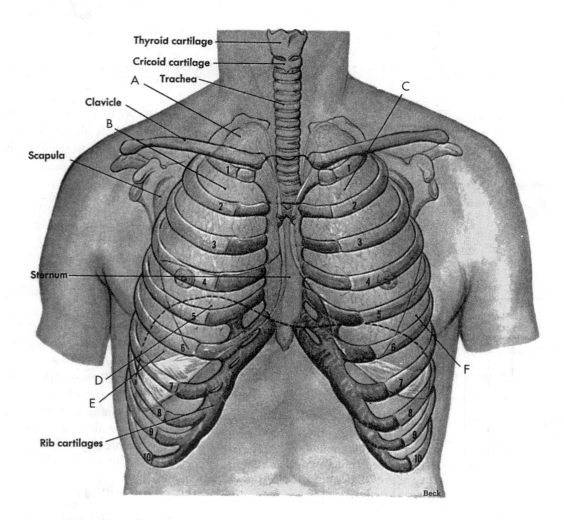

Projection of the lungs and trachea in relation to the rib cage and clavicles. (From Anthony CO, Thibodeau GA: *Textbook of anatomy and physiology*, ed 12, St Louis, 1987, Mosby.)

▶ 1. Where are your lungs?

A. _____
B. _____
C. _____
D. _____
E. _____
F. _____

Pneumopnuggets. When you put your stethoscope just below the clavicle you are listening over the upper lobes. You can also see that the lower lobes aren't really on the front of the chest at all. There's a little on the side, but mostly in the back. If you know your location of the apices, you will see they are above the clavicle. So if someone inserts a subclavian line, the lung could get punctured in the process!

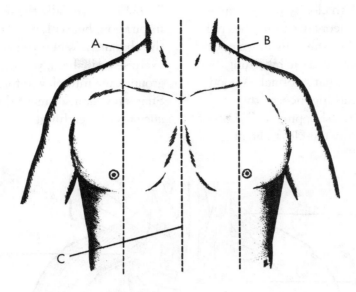

Imaginary lines on anterior chest wall.

▶ 2. Imagination 1

A. _____

B. _____

C. _____

▶ 3. Imagination 2

A. _____

B. _____

Pneumopnuggets. You could use these imaginary lines for a couple of things. First, when you perform a 12-lead ECG on a patient, you use the lines to line up the electrodes (plus counting the ribs). The lines are also useful if you notice something unusual (such as a scar or a lesion) and want to document where it is located.

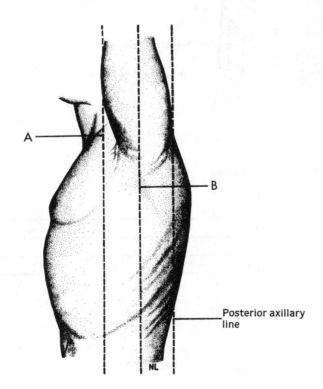

Imaginary lines on lateral chest wall.

Pneumopnuggets. Watch closely when someone breathes. Start with someone who breathes normally, such as a child. See the belly move out on inspiration. That's diaphragmatic breathing. See the relaxed exhalation. That's normal. A good place to see people breathing incorrectly (besides the hospital) is a shopping mall! Lots of people use their accessory muscles to breathe.

The chest, especially the upper chest, moves on inspiration, but with no outward excursion of the abdomen. When you get into distress or exercise really hard, you will see the abdominal group come into play to force exhalation. Sharpen your assessment skills by watching the *anatomy* of breathing!

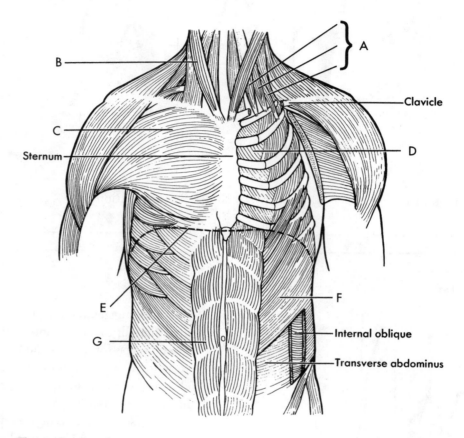

The muscles of ventilation.

4. Pump me up

A. _____

B. _____

C. _____

D. _____

E. _____

F. _____

G. _____

Pneumonuggets. Look at the nasopharynx. You'll be sticking tubes in there. It's fun if you know your anatomy. Notice that it goes straight back (a short distance) then drops down into the oropharynx. When you insert a catheter or airway, don't go straight back (very far): aim downward. Stay midline along the septum or you'll ram the turbinates (ouch!). In this cross-sectional view, it's easy to see how the tongue could block the airway if it falls back.

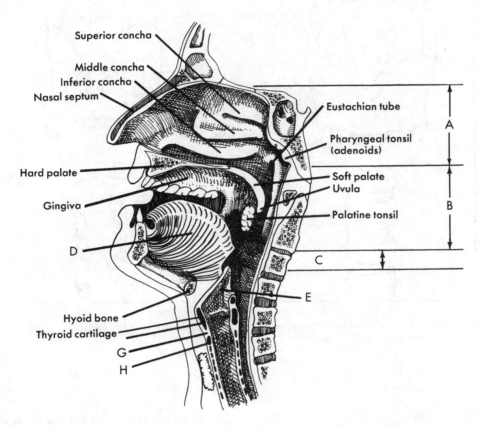

Structures of the upper airway and oral cavity. (From Ellis PD, Billings DM: Cardiopulmonary resuscitation: Procedures for basic and advanced life support, St Louis, 1980, Mosby.)

5. What's up, Doc?

A. _____
B. _____
C. _____
D. _____

E. _____
F. _____
G. _____
H. _____

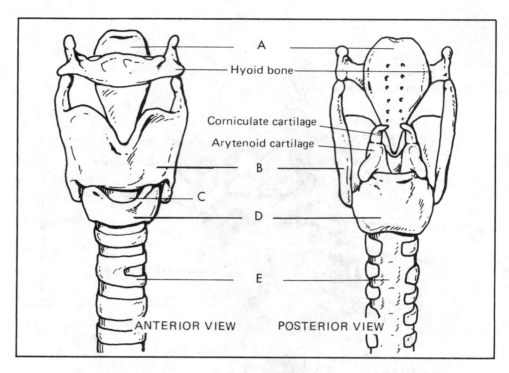

Anterior and posterior views of the laryngeal cartilages and trachea. (From Martin DE, Youtsey JW: *Respiratory anatomy and physiology*, St Louis, 1988, Mosby.)

▶ 6. "Adam's Apple"

A. _____
B. _____
C. _____
D. _____
E. _____

Pneumopnuggets. The thyroid cartilage sticks out on guys, so this will work best with a male partner. Palpate the thyroid cartilage. Feel the front and the sides. Now move your finger down (just a little) from the big bump on the front. Feel the soft spot? That's the cricothyroid membrane. (You might learn how to do a cricothyrotomy in school.) The cartilage just below that is the cricoid, the trachea's only complete ring. Keep going and feel the rings of the trachea. Gently (!) grasp the whole box in your fingers and wiggle back and forth. It's supposed to be mobile! Now ask your partner to swallow while you keep your fingers on the thyroid cartilage. What happened?

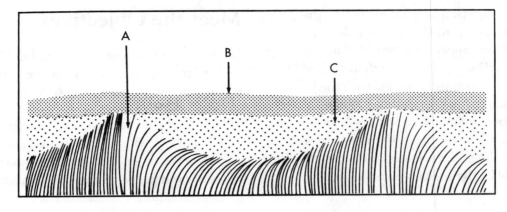

From Martin DE, Youtsey JW: *Respiratory anatomy and physiology*, St Louis, 1988, Mosby.

7. See Cilia

A. _____
B. _____
C. _____

Pneumopnuggets. Your airway makes more than 100 ml of mucus every day. Where does it all go? Without good ciliary function where would it go? Drugs (such as nicotine in cigarettes) can impair ciliary function. Hot or toxic gases (such as those resulting from smoking) can destroy cilia. There are also diseases that involve the cilia.

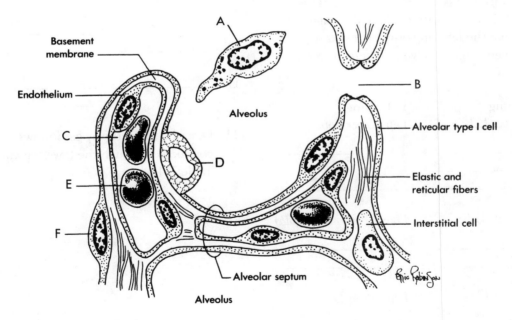

Very high-power view of alveolus.

8. You Can Call Me Al

A. _____
B. _____

C. _____
D. _____
E. _____
F. _____

Pneumopnuggets. These are small! The distance from alveoli to blood is only about 2.0 microns. (Remember, there are 1000 microns in a millimeter!) Oxygen has less than 1 second to cross this distance and combine with the RBC. So anything that increases this distance, such as the fluid from pulmonary edema, will impair gas exchange. There are about 300 million alveoli in an adult lung. If you flatten them out, the area would be the size of a tennis court!

Lobes and Segments

Students are always dismayed when they have to learn postural drainage and find out the lungs have five different lobes and 18 individual segments. It's not so hard when you know there are some duplicates and break the whole thing down into little pieces. Fill in the chart below. You can make your own version of this and fill it in until you get them memorized. This will really help you with postural drainage. Notice that the left lung only has eight segments, even though we've numbered them 1 through 10.

Right Lung

Right Upper Lobe

1. _____
2. _____
3. _____

Right Middle Lobe

4. _____
5. _____

Right Lower Lobe

6. _____
7. _____
8. _____
9. _____
10. _____

Left Lung

Left Upper Lobe

1 + 2. _____

3. _____

Lower Portion (Lingula)

4. _____
5. _____

Left Lower Lobe

6. _____
7 + 8. _____

9. _____
10. _____

Meet the Objectives

We've covered most of the material in Chapter 7. Here are a few more ideas that are important to know about the respiratory system.

9. Name the nerves that innervate the diaphragm, intercostal muscles, and larynx. State the origin of these nerves and describe what will happen if they are damaged.

   A. _____
   _____

   B. _____
   _____

   C. _____
   _____

List the four divisions of the upper airway and describe their main functions.

	Division	*Function*
A.	_____	_____
		_____
B.	_____	_____
		_____
C.	_____	_____
		_____
D.	_____	_____
		_____

11. Describe the pathway gas follows as it is conducted through the lower airway. Use Table 7-4 on page 166 of Egan as a guide.

Chapter Highlights

Fill in the blanks to identify six key points from Chapter 7.

12. The _____ houses and protects the lungs.

13. The _____ is the primary muscle of ventilation.

14. The upper respiratory tract _____ and _____ inspired air and protects lungs against _____ substances.

15. The lower respiratory tract _____ gases from the upper airway to the respiratory _____ of the lung.

16. The airways branch into _____, which are in turn made up of _____ in both the left and right lungs.

17. The respiratory bronchioles and _____ provide a large _____ area that facilitates gas exchange.

Case Studies

Case 1

A cruel respiratory instructor forces the students to learn the anatomy of the lung. Completely by coincidence, the instructor slips while running with scissors, and the sharp shears puncture his right chest. The students gather around their fallen facilitator to discuss the anatomical consequences of this tragedy.

18. What would happen to the lung on the affected side?

19. What would happen to the pleural space on the affected side?

20. What is this condition called?

21. What is the treatment for this condition?

Case 2

An RCP is working the night shift at a large urban medical center. As he makes his rounds, he hears loud snoring coming from a patient's room. Even though snoring is a commonly heard sound at night, the RCP stops to investigate.

22. What anatomical change results in snoring?

23. What is OSA, and how is it treated?

24. What is the similarity between snorers and unconscious victims who require resuscitation?

25. How would you approach management of the airway of an unconscious person?

Food for Thought

I hope you had fun with your lungs today. Lung function is pretty miraculous when you think about all the parts that have to be working together to make ventilation and respiration successful. What happens to these structures when disease is present?

26. What happens to the airways and alveoli when a patient is having an acute episode of asthma?

27. What changes to the airways and alveoli occur in emphysema?

What About Those Board Exams?

Respiratory anatomy is not on the boards, but the kinds of applications we've been using in this chapter are part of the test. For example, you'll probably see several questions about pneumothorax.

The Cardiovascular System

8

"We are all alike, on the inside."
Mark Twain

The Heartbeat of America

Your heart beats, on average, about 38 million times in one year! No matter how well the respiratory system works to exchange gas with the blood, it would be meaningless without the heart pushing that blood out to the organs via the vascular system. Those blood vessels are the best transportation network in the world, constantly reacting to the need for more or less flow of nutrients to the tissues.

Language of the Heart

Since the cardiovascular function is closely connected to the respiratory system, you will meet up with it again and again in the course of your training. The words you learn today will help you throughout your career. Match the terms to the definitions listed below as they apply to respiratory care.

Term

_____ 1. Afterload
_____ 2. Automaticity
_____ 3. Baroreceptors
_____ 4. Cardiac output
_____ 5. Chemoreceptors
_____ 6. Pericardium
_____ 7. Preload
_____ 8. Stenosis

Definition

A. Membranous sac that surrounds the heart
B. Stroke volume multiplied by heart rate
C. Ventricular stretch provided by end diastolic pressure
D. Biological sensors that monitor arterial blood pressure
E. Pathological narrowing or constriction
F. The force the ventricle pumps against
G. Biological sensors that monitor arterial blood oxygen
H. Ability to initiate a spontaneous electrical impulse

Meet the Objectives

Chapter 8 presented five objectives for learning. How well do you know your cardiovascular system?

9. We all know there are four valves in the heart. Patients commonly suffer disorders of the mitral valve. What is the effect of mitral stenosis on the lung?

10. Explain how specialized tissue allows the muscle cells in the ventricle to contract in a coordinated and efficient manner.

11. Compare and contrast local control of blood vessels with central control mechanisms.

12. Describe how the cardiovascular system responds to exercise and blood loss by balancing blood volume and vascular resistance.

13. Match the mechanical events to their corresponding electrical events in the normal cardiac cycle.

Electrical Event   *Mechanical Event*

A. _____   _____
B. _____   _____
C. _____   _____

Chapter Highlights

Fill in the blanks to identify six key points from Chapter Eight.

14. The _____ system consists of the heart and vascular network, which maintain _____ by regulating the distribution of blood flow in the body.

15. Cardiac _____ is primarily determined by preload, _____, contractility, and _____.

16. Central control of the vascular system is primarily maintained by the _____ division of the _____ nervous system.

17. The heart and vascular systems ensure that tissues receive sufficient blood to meet their _____ needs.

18. Just as faucets control the flow of water into a sink, the _____ control blood flow into the capillaries.

19. Specialized myocardial tissue, such as the _____ fibers, conduct impulses rapidly to ensure synchronous contraction of the ventricles.

Case Studies

Case 1

Cora Sone, a 57-year-old patient, is admitted to the Coronary Care Unit with a diagnosis of mitral stenosis. The patient is breathing rapidly and complains of shortness of breath. Her pulse oximetry readings reveal hypoxemia. Auscultation reveals inspiratory crackles in the posterior lower lobes.

20. What is mitral stenosis?

21. What mechanical events are occurring to cause pulmonary edema and stiffening of the lung tissue?

22. What action should the RCP take at this time?

Case 2

A respiratory care student is giving an aerosolized bronchodilator to Keith Kane, a 27 year-old patient with asthma. Breath sounds reveal bilateral wheezing. The pulse oximeter shows a 98% saturation on room air. The student notices the heart rate rising from 82 to 98 beats/min during the therapy.

23. What are the effects of sympathetic and parasympathetic stimulation on the sinus node in the heart?
    A. _____
    B. _____

24. Describe the two ways that drugs produce bronchodilation.
    A. _____
    B. _____

25. Based on this information, why would you expect increased heart rate to be a common side effect of drugs that cause bronchodilation? How much can the heart rate increase before you would consider terminating the treatment?

What does the NBRC Say?

Cardiac anatomy, like respiratory anatomy, does not have a particular place on the national exams. However, we use this material as a foundation for clinical applications such as hemodynamics and electrocardiography.

Food for Thought

26. What four mechanisms combine to aid in promoting venous return to the heart?
    A. _____
    B. _____
    C. _____
    D. _____

27. What is meant by the term *thoracic pump*? What effect does positive pressure ventilation, such as IPPB, have on venous return to the chest?

Just for Fun . . . ?

Find the words in this word search to help build your cardiovascular vocabulary.

L	N	A	V	C	H	O	R	D	A	E	E	Y	Y
A	A	Y	O	E	R	L	V	T	J	N	B	R	O
R	Y	R	T	R	I	G	O	H	D	A	E	U	T
T	R	H	T	I	T	N	J	O	R	T	T	T	R
E	A	G	Z	I	C	A	T	O	R	P	A	P	I
R	L	A	U	T	M	I	R	A	U	R	K	N	C
I	L	Y	F	K	O	E	T	T	C	G	W	K	U
O	I	U	O	W	C	C	D	A	V	A	H	I	S
L	P	E	O	E	A	C	M	I	M	A	Z	D	P
E	A	D	P	R	H	C	T	N	T	O	L	I	I
S	C	T	D	E	E	E	H	B	T	O	T	V	D
P	O	I	M	D	A	O	L	E	R	P	R	U	E
R	A	O	D	A	O	L	R	E	T	F	A	A	A
C	F	M	U	I	D	R	A	C	I	R	E	P	C

AFTERLOAD	CHORDAE
AORTA	ENDO
ARTERIOLES	MITRAL
ARTERY	OUTPUT
AUTOMATICITY	PERICARDIUM
BARORECEPTOR	PRELOAD
CAPILLARY	TRICUSPID
CARDIAC	VALVE
CAROTID	VEIN
CHEMO	

Ventilation

Chapter 9 is less than 20 pages long, but those 20 pages are loaded with important information. Our challenge will be to sort out what is important to remember, learn the basic principles, and make the knowledge connect to what is clinically important.

First Things First

I want to start off by emphasizing the difference between ventilation and respiration.

Remember that the primary purpose of the lung is to supply the body with oxygen and remove wastes in the form of carbon dioxide (CO_2). _____ is the process of moving air in and out of the lungs. When CO_2 builds up in the body the pH of blood decreases and a state of _____ results. We can measure the amount of air that moves in and out with a device called a _____. The pressure changes in the chest are measured using a body box, or _____. Finally, the actual rate of air flow is measured using a _____ Much of respiratory care is

aimed at reducing the _____ of breathing and restoring adequate ventilation. The process of _____, on the other hand, is the exchange of gas between blood and other tissues. This involves some complex chemical and physiological events at the cellular level. We'll dive into this subject more in Chapter 10.

A number of factors affect our ability to move air in and out at a reasonable oxygen cost. These could be factors outside the chest such as _____, a fluid build up in the abdomen, which impairs diaphragmatic movement. Or they could be the result of spinal disorders like _____, a twisted and curved spine, or _____ _____, a severe stiffening of the spine. Problems also arise inside the lung itself. Conditions like pulmonary fibrosis make the lung stiffer, or less _____.

Picture This . . .

Air moves in and out of the chest because of pressure gradients. Label the following diagram to help improve your understanding of these pressure changes. Write out the definition of each gradient.

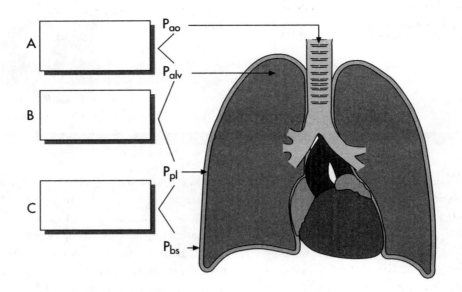

Pressures, volumes, and flows involved in ventilation. (From Martin L: *Pulmonary physiology in clinical practice: The essentials for patient care and evaluation*, St Louis, 1987, Mosby.)

▷ 1. Trans what?

A. _____
_____

B. _____
_____

C. _____
_____

Pneumopnuggets. Our ability to generate the necessary pressure changes requires muscle power. Muscles need glucose, oxygen, and nerve innervation (among other things) to work properly. Any clinical condition that requires bigger pressure gradients to move air (such as asthma) makes the muscles work harder. Just as when you work out, a pulmonary patient can experience muscle fatigue from increased work of breathing.

Can I have another . . .

Fill in the missing pressures for the apex and base of the lung.

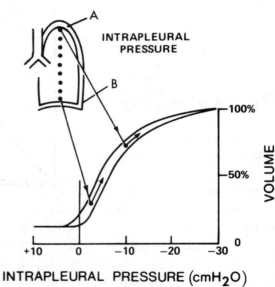

Causes of regional differences in ventilation down the lung. (From West JB: *Respiratory physiology: The essentials*, ed 4, Baltimore, 1990, Williams & Wilkins.)

▷ 2. Where has all the ventilation gone?

A. _____

B. _____

3. Where does the bulk of ventilation go during a normal breath in an upright person?

Pneumopnuggets. You can use this information clinically. When a patient has a serious unilateral, or one-sided, lung disease (like a bad pneumonia) he will have poor ventilation in the affected side. Positioning the patient so the good lung is dependent will preferentially increase the ventilation in that lung and away from the bad lung. *Remember: Down with the good lung!*

Work of Breathing

Work of breathing, or WOB, has a definite energy cost. We can measure the metabolic cost in terms of oxygen consumed, and we can reduce the work for patients through our interventions. A healthy person consumes about 250 ml of oxygen per minute. Only 5% of this oxygen is needed to power the muscles of ventilation. The cost goes up about 1 ml for each liter of additional ventilation. Look at what happens to this cost when a patient has emphysema.

There are four factors that contribute to WOB: compliance, resistance, active exhalation, and breathing pattern. Let's work at each of these separately and talk about strategies for improvement.

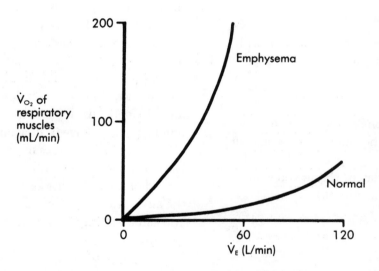

Relationship of oxygen cost of breathing to expiratory minute volume for a healthy subject and for a patient with emphysema. (From Slonim NB, Hamilton LH: *Respiratory physiology*, ed 5, St Louis, 1987, Mosby. After Campbell EJM, Westlake EK, Cherniack RM: *J Appl Physiol* 11:303, 1957.)

Compliance

Compliance is a measure of lung elasticity, or stretchability. It is defined as: Change in volume (liters) ÷ Change in pressure (cm H_2O). A healthy lung is pretty stretchy and compliance is 0.2 L for every cm H_2O of pressure you generate.

But, the lungs sit inside the heavy thorax, which has its own compliance. Completely coincidentally, the compliance of the chest wall is 0.2 L/cm H_2O also! You have to remember that the lung wants to recoil in and the chest wall wants to spring out, so they are pulling in opposite directions. Mathematically this is a cancellation, so the net result is a compliance of 0.1

L/cm H_2O for healthy lungs in a healthy chest. *But*, if the lungs are overinflated or underinflated, the balance changes. You can understand this by trying a simple experiment.

Experiment

Get an ordinary balloon. Blow it up a little bit. This is your underinflated lung. Blow it up some more. Hard to do, right? Now blow it up some more. Pretty easy. Now inflate the balloon until it is almost full. Blow in some more. Hard to do! Lungs are a little like this balloon. A patient who has a very low lung volume has to work harder to take a breath than a person with a normal amount of functional residual capacity (FRC). A person with air-trapping (as occurs in emphysema), is like the balloon that is overinflated. Try this for yourself: Take a deep breath. Don't exhale. Now try to breathe in. You get the idea.

Bottom line: You can move 500 ml of air with 5 cm H_2O pressure. Pretty good!

Questions

4. What interventions can we apply to the lung to increase the amount of residual air (and compliance) in a patient's lungs when they are underinflated? (Hint: you won't find this one in Chapter 9.)

5. What interventions can we apply to the lung to decrease the amount of residual air in a patient's lungs when they are overinflated?

Resistance

Resistance comes in two kinds: tissue and frictional. Tissues have to move when the chest expands. Obesity (outside the lung) and fibrosis (inside the lung) are examples of increased tissue resistance. The really big problem is the frictional resistance created when you move air through your pipes (80% of all resistance). Airway resistance (R_{aw}) is defined as: the driving pressure it takes to create a flow of gas. Or to put it mathematically: R_{aw} = Change in pressure (cm H_2O) ÷ Change in flow rate (liters/min). Your upper airway causes most of this resistance. Normal value is 0.5 to 2.5. Cm H_2O per liter per second of flow. Conditions like asthma narrow the airways and significantly increase resistance. You can understand this with another simple experiment.

Experiment

Get a straw and a coffee stirrer (the hollow kind). Breathe in fast through the stirrer. Now breathe in fast through the straw. Which one is easier? Now try putting your lips and sucking in the air really fast. Feel the work?

Bottom line: The inner diameter of the airway determines the amount of resistance. (Remember old what's his name's law?) If the bronchi decrease from 2 mm to 1 mm in diameter, the resistance increases 16 times! Your muscles will have to generate a much higher pressure to achieve ventilation if the airway is narrow.

Questions

6. What three changes occur in the airway of an asthmatic patient to increase resistance? (Hint: this one isn't in the chapter either!)

7. What kind of medications can RCPs use to reduce airway resistance in asthma?

Active Exhalation

Normal exhalation is passive. The power comes from energy you stored by stretching the lung and chest during inspiration. When you actively exhale, you have to use your abdominal muscles (and internal intercostals). Remember that additional muscle work takes additional energy. You can actually observe patients using their abdominal muscles when they are in distress and trying to get the air out more quickly, or through narrowed airways. You can try this for yourself.

Experiment

Place your hands on your belly. Breathe in. Exhale normally. Breathe in again. This time, push firmly in with our hands as you exhale. This air moves faster, right? Release your hands and breathe in again. This time, bear down with your abs and blow our hard and fast until your lungs are empty. It feels like work!

Bottom line: Actively exhaling has a price. When you see a patient doing this, they are either exercising or in distress.

Questions

8. What can you do about active exhalation?

9. What happens to a person with a spinal cord injury who can't use their abdominal muscles? (Hint: what other important respiratory activity uses these muscles?)

Ventilatory pattern

The way you breathe can change the amount of work. In healthy people, a deep breath increases the elastic part of WOB. Fast breathing increases the frictional work.

Healthy people adjust their tidal volume and respiratory rate to minimize the work of breathing during exercise. Our patients minimize the work of breathing patterns, too. Patients with fibrosis (loss of elasticity) breathe with a rapid shallow pattern to reduce the mechanical work of distending the lung. Patients with obstructive diseases such as asthma and emphysema need to reduce their rate to reduce work, because they have increased frictional resistance.

Experiment

Tie something tightly around your upper chest. I use a bathrobe tie. This will restrict chest movement. Try breathing faster with shallow breaths. Now try to breathe slowly and deeply. Which way feels better? Now, untie yourself and get out your straw or coffee stirrer. Breathe rapidly and shallowly through the tube. Now take slow deep breaths. Which way feels better? (This is as close as I could come to simulating these two conditions?)

Bottom line: You can learn a lot by observing someone's breathing pattern.

Questions

10. What is the optimal pattern of breathing for patients with obstructive airway diseases?

11. I don't have anymore questions, do you?

Dead Space

Dead space is, plainly put, wasted ventilation; gas that does not participate in exchange with the blood. You normally waste the first third of each breath, or about 1 ml per pound of ideal body weight. Alveolar dead space occurs when gas enters the alveoli, but no blood comes to pick up the oxygen. A pulmonary embolus (blood clot, fat clot, air bubble, and so on) blocks blood flow to alveoli and causes increased dead space. Too much dead space (50% to 60% of each breath) will result in the inability to maintain adequate ventilation through spontaneous breathing. The patient will need mechanical ventilation until the problem improves.

Could I See a Picture Please . . .

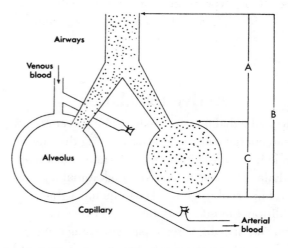

Three types of dead space.

▷ 12. Label the types of dead space in this diagram.

A. _____

B. _____

C. _____

Questions

13. What is the normal range for anatomical dead space?

14. What type of breathing pattern will be seen with significantly increased dead space?

15. What is the difference between *hyperventilation* and *hyperpnea*?

Mathemagic

In Chapter 5, I mentioned that math is part of our board examination process and a clinical reality. Don't use a calculator to solve these problems!

16. Calculate exhaled minute ventilation for a patient who has a tidal volume of 800 ml and a frequency of 8 breaths/min.

Formula: _____

Calculation: _____

Answer: _____

17. Calculate anatomical dead space for a patient who is 6 feet tall and weighs 180 pounds.

Formula: _____

Calculation: _____

Answer: _____

18. Calculate alveolar minute ventilation using the data from questions 16 and 17.

Formula: _____

Calculation: _____

Answer: _____

What About Those Board Exams?

The NBRC (and everyone else) will expect you to be able to calculate exhaled minute volume, alveolar minute volume, and apply the information. Here's a sample:

19. The minute volume for a 68 kg (150 lb) patient who has a respiratory rate of 12 and a tidal volume of 600 ml would be
    A. 4800 ml
    B. 5400 ml
    C. 6000 ml
    D. 7200 ml

20. The estimated alveolar minute ventilation for an 82 kg (180 lb) patient who has a respiratory rate of 10 and a tidal volume of 500 ml would be
    A. 3200 ml
    B. 3500 ml
    C. 4800 ml
    D. 5000 ml

21. Which of the following ventilator settings would provide the optimal alveolar ventilation?

Rate	Volume
A. 10	600
B. 12	500
C. 15	400
D. 20	300

Gas Exchange and Transport

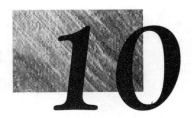

10

"To air is human,
to respire divine."
Paul Thackara, RRT

In Chapter 10 we're going to go for it and jump in the deep end (of physiology, that is). I know you'll find this challenging at first, but when you have mastered the basics of gas transport you're going to be exhilarated! It's going to feel good to get a grasp of how gas exchange works and how RCPs apply physiology to patient care.

All Aboard

Let's get on the hemoglobin-oxygen train and take a little ride. First you're going to learn the different names for all those forms that hemoglobin (Hb) takes when it combines. It's natural for this complex molecule to want to be in a relationship. Hemoglobin meets oxygen. When the get together, the new name is _____. Their newfound affinity is likely to end when they meet up with the _____ effect at the tissue level. So, hemoglobin takes up with CO_2 and we get _____. The fickle heme will drop CO_2 off at the lung when they run into the _____ effect. Life could go on like this, unless our conjugated protein meets up with a really unusual gas like carbon monoxide. This combination is called _____, and really lasts because hemoglobin's affinity for CO is _____ times greater than its affinity for oxygen.

I think we're in Kansas

Not all hemoglobins are created equal. Some are downright unnatural. Abnormal hemoglobins are given letter designations, often according to the geographic locale where they were first identified. Hb K is the designation for hemoglobin _____, a form that has a decreased affinity for oxygen. HB R, or _____, has an increased affinity. Sometimes heme is altered in other ways. When the iron compound is oxidized, we get _____, which causes the blood to turn a brownish color. Nitrite poisoning can cause this transformation of our gas-loving protein. Hb S, whose common name is _____ _____ hemoglobin, not only carries on poorly with oxygen, it can cause red blood cells to deform and clump together into thrombi.

Oxygen Transport

You can tell me Al

Before oxygen can go to the tissues, it has to get into the alveoli. There is a useful formula for calculating the partial pressure of oxygen (PAO_2) in those little grape-like clusters. True, this equation has never won any popularity contests with students, but it is clinically useful (and can show up on those board exams!). So, put on your thinking caps and we'll show them

who's in charge here! The fancy formula looks like this:

$$PaO_2 = FiO_2 (Pb\text{-}Ph_2O) - PaCO_2(FiO_2 + 1 - FiO_2/R)$$

We usually simplify this to read:

$$PaO_2 = FiO_2 (Pb\text{-}47) - PaCO_2/0.8$$

Or, in English . . .

The partial pressure of oxygen in the alveoli is equal to the inspired oxygen percent times the barometric pressure minus water vapor pressure.

Why? Dalton's law gives us the first part (partial pressure = concentration × total pressure). Because water vapor in the lung acts like a gas, it takes up space. That's space oxygen can't occupy.

Next: Subtract arterial CO_2 times a factor.

Why? What we want to know is how much CO_2 is in the alveoli. (CO_2 takes up space too.) This is hard to measure. Solution: Use a converted arterial value in its place. You don't really need to do this when the patient is breathing a high FiO_2 like 60% or more.

At this point my students usually ask:

Who Cares?

All of this would only be useful in the pulmonary laboratory, except for the fact that we can use this formula to find out how efficiently the lungs are transferring oxygen into the blood by comparing *Alveolar PO₂* with *Arterial PO₂*! This relationship is called the A-a gradient. A normal A-a gradient is about 5 to 10 mm Hg on room air, or about 10%.

Mathemagic

1. Calculate alveolar oxygen tension for a person breathing room air. Assume that baro-

metric pressure is 760 mm Hg. FiO_2 is 21%, and $PaCO_2$ is 40 mm Hg.

Formula: _____
Calculation: _____
Answer: _____

2. If the patient in problem 1 has an arterial PO_2 of 90, what is the A-a gradient?

Formula: _____
Calculation: _____
Answer: _____

3. Calculate alveolar oxygen tension for a person breathing 60% oxygen. (Pb is 760; CO_2 40.)

Formula: _____
Calculation: _____
Answer: _____

4. If the patient in problem 3 has an arterial PO_2 of 90, what is the A-a gradient?

Formula: _____
Calculation: _____
Answer: _____

Both patients have identical PaO_2s of 90 mm Hg. If you only look at PO_2, or only look at oxygen saturation, they would seem the same.

But, the A-a gradients are very different. The second patient is having serious problems getting oxygen from the lung into the blood. In fact, the patient breathing 60% oxygen should have a PaO_2 of 349! (PaO_2^-, 10 %.)

"By the pricking of my thumbs . . ."
Everyone loves a good rule of thumb. If you're in a big fat hurry and don't have a calculator at the bedside, you can try this shortcut. To estimate alveolar PO_2 for a patient breathing room air, multiply FiO_2 by 5 (5 × 20 = 100). For 40% or more, multiply by 6 (40 × 6 = 240). Remember: this only works when the CO_2 is normal. Besides, what RCP doesn't have a calculator at the bedside?

Kodak Moment

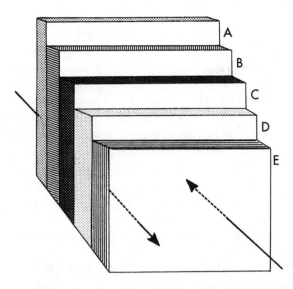

The five barriers through which O_2 and CO_2 pass at the alveolar-capillary membrane. (From McLaughlin AJ Jr: Essentials of physiology for advanced respiratory therapy, St Louis, 1977, Mosby.)

▶ 5. Do not pass go until you pass through . . . the five parts of this picture.

A. _____
B. _____
C. _____
D. _____
E. _____

Pneumopnuggets. The partial pressure of a gas is the main driving force across the A-C membrane. Respiratory care practitioners routinely increase the driving pressure of oxygen by increasing the PaO_2. CO_2 has a much lower driving pressure, but is about 20 times more soluble than O_2, so it has little difficulty in making the journey. In some cases time can limit diffusion due to increased blood flow. Fever and septic shock are clinical examples.

Let's get moving!

Once it gets into the blood, oxygen is transported in only two ways. First, it dissolves in the plasma. To calculate dissolved O_2, multiply by 0.003.

Dissolved O_2 = PaO_2 × 0.003   Easy!

The second way that oxygen is transported is as oxyhemoglobin. 1.34 ml of O_2 bind to each gram of hemoglobin (per 100ml of blood). If all the hemoglobin carried oxygen, this would be simple, but it doesn't. Remember the anatomical shunt? Hemoglobin saturation is usually less that 100%.

Combined O_2 = 1.34 × Hb × %Saturation

Put them together and what have you got?

O_2 content = PaO_2 × 0.003 + 1.34 × Hb × %Saturation

Mathemagic

While computers in the hospital will usually calculate content for you, the National Board for Respiratory Care thinks you should be able to do this yourself (and without a calculator!).

6. Calculate oxygen content for a patient with a Hb of 15 g, SaO_2 of 97%, PaO_2 of 100 mm Hg.

Formula: _____
Calculation: _____
Answer: _____

7. Calculate oxygen content for a patient with a Hb of 15 g, SaO_2 of 805, PaO_2 of 50 mm Hg.

Formula: _____
Calculation: _____
Answer: _____

8. Last one. Calculate oxygen content for a patient with a Hb of 10 g, SaO_2 of 97%, PaO_2 of 100 mm Hg.

Formula: _____
Calculation: _____
Answer: _____

Now compare the results. Patient 2 has pretty crummy values, but a good hemoglobin. Patient 3 has good values but a crummy hemoglobin. Who has better oxygenation?

The moral of the story

Looking at pulse oximetry values, or any other simple indices of oxygenation like PaO_2, doesn't tell the whole story. You always have to consider hemoglobin. A patient may need blood as a treatment for poor oxygen content. Remember that there may be enough hemoglobin, but it may not be able to combine with oxygen. Like carbon monoxide poisoning.

Throw Me a Curve

The last piece of the oxygenation puzzle (for now at least) is to look at the relationship of oxygen and hemoglobin. This relationship is described by the oxyhemoglobin dissociation curve. Look at the curve shown on p. 225 in Fig. 10-10. The flat upper part of the curve means that you can have a large drop in PaO_2 and only get a small drop in saturation. In fact, PaO_2 can drop from 600 mm Hg to 60 mm Hg and the saturation will only drop from 100% to 90%! The steep part of the curve is equally cool, physiologically speaking. A small increase in PaO_2 will give you a large increase in saturation. If you raise the PaO_2 from 27 mm Hg to 60 mm Hg, the saturation will rise from 50% all the way to 90%. Normally, a given PaO_2 will produce a predictable hemoglobin saturation (with a normal pH) on the chart below:

	PaO_2	SaO_2
9.	40 mm Hg	_____
10.	_____	_____
11.	60 mm Hg	_____
12.	_____	97%

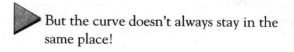 But the curve doesn't always stay in the same place!

Fill in the correct answers for how the curve will shift on the chart below:

Factor	Shift
13. Acidosis	_____
14. Hypothermia	_____
15. High 2.3 DPG	_____
16. Fever	_____
17. Hypercapnia	_____
18. Carboxyhemoglobin	_____

The shift of the curve to the right facilitates oxygen unloading to the tissues, but a given PaO_2 will have a lower hemoglobin saturation. A left shift does the opposite.

Carbon Dioxide Transport

CO_2 is transported three ways in the blood. Just like oxygen, it dissolves right into the plasma. This factor is more important than dissolved oxygen, since it transports a fair amount of CO_2. Just like oxygen, CO_2 is carried by hemoglobin. Unlike oxygen, this is a relatively small amount. The majority of the CO_2, about 80%, is transported in the form of bicarbonate. Sorry, no math problems for you to do right now. But do remember this equation:

$$CO_2 + H_2O = H_2CO_3 = HCO_3^- + H^+$$

This reaction is called hydrolysis, because it involves combining CO_2 with water. First carbonic acid is formed, but this quickly ionizes into bicarbonate and hydrogen ions. Remember, the reaction can move in both directions. Most of the hydrolysis occurs inside the red blood cell because of the presence of an enzyme (carbonic anhydrase) that speeds up the reaction rate.

Carbon dioxide levels are inversely proportional to alveolar ventilation. If you increase alveolar ventilation, the CO_2 will decrease. Normal $PaCO_2$ is 35 to 45 mm Hg. A high CO_2 level means that the patient is not ventilating adequately. We will draw arterial blood gases when we want to accurately assess ventilation. A high CO_2 level in the blood indicates hypoventilation. Because CO_2 has an acidifying effect on the blood, the pH of the blood will decrease when the carbon dioxide rises. The normal lower limit of pH is 7.35. The normal upper limit is 7.45. Low values reflect acidosis, while increased pH represents an alkaline state.

Bad Gas Exchange

Oxygen delivery and carbon dioxide removal are where it's at, physiologically speaking. The following questions will test your knowledge of the causes of poor gas exchange.

19. Inadequate delivery of oxygen to the tissues is known as _____.

20. _____ is the medical name for a low level of oxygen in the blood.

21. Physiological _____ occurs when blood passes through areas of the lung that have no ventilation.

22. Ventilation-_____ imbalances are the most common cause of low blood oxygen in patients with lung disease.

23. Patients with pulmonary fibrosis have a _____ and poor tissue oxygen delivery.

24. Low blood pressure results in _____ and poor tissue oxygen delivery.

25. Myocardial infarction is an example of _____, a localized reduction in blood flow to tissues that can result in tissue death.

26. Increased _____ space ventilation may result in increased levels of carbon dioxide in the blood.

27. Drug overdose may result in an inadequate _____ ventilation due to central nervous system depression.

28. Patients with severe COPD are unable to maintain adequate ventilation due to ventilation _____ imbalances.

Board Exams

The NBRC thinks you should be good at assessing gas exchange and treating abnormalities. Here are some examples:

29. A blood gas reveals the following results: pH, 7.50; $PaCO_2$, 30 mm Hg; PaO_2, 110 mm Hg. This data indicates the presence of
    A. Metabolic acidosis
    B. Acute hyperventilation
    C. Acute hypoventilation
    D. Chronic obstructive pulmonary disease

30. Calculate oxygen content for a patient with the following data: Hb, 10 g; PaO_2, 80 mm Hg; SaO_2, 95%.
    A. 12.73 ml 02/dl
    B. 12.97 ml 02/dl
    C. 13.40 ml 02/dl
    D. 13.64 ml 02/dl

31. Calculate PAO_2 for a patient with the following data: Pb, 747 mm Hg; FiO_2, 0.21; PaO_2, 95 mm Hg; $PaCO_2$, 40 mm Hg; SaO_2, 97%.
    A. 97 mm Hg
    B. 103 mm Hg
    C. 107 mm Hg
    D. 117 mm Hg

Case in Point

Case 1

Kelsey O. a 29-year-old housewife, is brought to the emergency department following exposure to smoke during a house fire. She is breathing at a rate of 30 per minute. Her heart rate is 110. Blood pressure is 160/110. The patient complains of headache and nausea. The pulse oximeter is reading a saturation of 99%.

32. Why are pulse oximetry readings unreliable in this setting?

33. What is wrong with this patient?

34. What action would you take at this time?

Case 2

James Westbrake is brought back to the unit following major surgery after a motorcycle accident. Mr. Westbrake was given a massive trans- fusion of blood to replace loss from both the trauma and the surgical procedure. The pulse oximeter is reading 96% on room air, but the nurse has requested you to evaluate due to the patient's clinical condition. You find him sitting up and breathing 32 times per minute. He has tachycardia, tachypnea, and complains of difficulty breathing. Breath sounds are clear on auscultation.

35. The patient's clinical signs are consistent with what gas exchange abnormality?

36. What is one of the potential problems with banked blood?

37. Name some of the other possible causes of Mr. Westbrake's distress.

38. What diagnostic procedure could you recommend?

41. What is absolute anemia, and how is it treated?

Case 4

Vern Yoga has been brought by paramedics to the emergency department after an accidental overdose of narcotics at a party. Mr. Yoga is unconscious and has a respiratory rate of 8. The pulse oximeter shows a saturation of 85%.

42. Why would CO_2 be elevated in this patient?

Case 3

Jeannie Corpus is admitted with a diagnosis of pneumonia. Arterial blood gases reveal a pH of 7.55, $PaCO_2$ of 25 mm Hg, PaO_2 of 75, and an SaO_2 of 94%. She complains of feeling short of breath.

39. Interpret this blood gas in terms of gas exchange.

43. Why is the oxygen saturation so low?

40. What other laboratory information plays a key role in helping determine oxygen content?

Food for Thought

Is your brain full yet? Dysoxia is a form of hypoxia where cells do not uptake oxygen properly.

44. What is the classic example of dysoxia?

45. When does tissue oxygen consumption become dependent on oxygen delivery?

46. Why does lactic acid form when tissues are hypoxic?

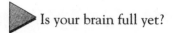 Is your brain full yet?

Solutions, Body Fluids, and Electrolytes

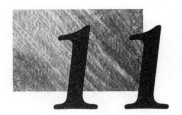

**"I am a prohibitionist.
What I propose to prohibit
is the reckless use of water."**
Bob Edwards

Imagine yourself swimming in a warm ocean lagoon. The salty water is filled with life. Currents move you and waves propel you through this complex ecology. Now think about the inside of your body. Warm, wet, and filled with salts. An intricate environment where life depends on the relationships of fluids and electrolytes. Chapter 11 reviews various types of solutions, the mechanisms that control fluid movement, acid-base basics, and the role of major electrolytes in body function.

Drowning in Words

You'll need to have some new vocabulary to keep you afloat in the sea of salts and solutions. It looks like a crossword puzzle is needed here! See the puzzle on p. 66.

Water, Water Everywhere . . .

The human body is mostly water. Water makes up as much as 80% of your weight. Since water is relatively heavy, the easiest way to track gain and loss is by weighing the patient. Clinicians also monitor intake and output (I and O) of water very closely.

Now you need to open your textbook and look up some information about this subject.

1. Rank the relative amount of water in the following individuals. Put "1" by the lowest amount of water, and "5" by the person with the largest percent of body water.

   _____ Males
   _____ Newborns
   _____ Children
   _____ Females
   _____ Obese individuals

2. Name the two major compartments for body water. List subdivisions and give the relative amount (%) of water in each area.

Compartment	% H$_2$O
A. _____	_____
B. _____	_____
1. _____	_____
2. _____	_____

Where Has All the Water Gone, Long Time Passing . . .

A lot of water leaves your body every day through sensible and insensible loss. Give examples of these water losses and an average daily amount.

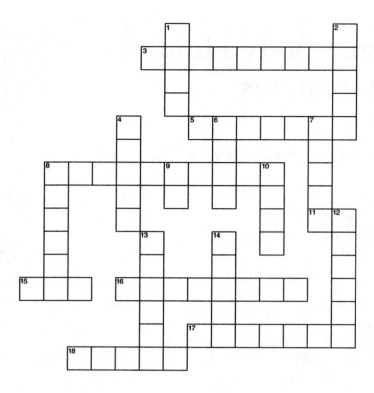

ACROSS

3. Solutions with maximum amount of solutes
5. Refers to potassium in the blood
8. Plasma is one example of this type of solution
11. Chemical name for calcium
15. Another name for colloid solution
16. Refers to sodium in the blood
17. Positively charged ions
18. _____ covalent solutions are produced by molecular compounds in water that produces ions

DOWN

1. Gives hydroxyl ions when placed in solution
2. Presence of abnormally large amount of fluid in the intercellular tissue space of the body
4. _____ tonic, a solution with more than 0.9% NaCl
6. Yields hydrogen ions when placed in solution
7. Electrovalent physiological solution
8. Substance dissolved in solvent
9. Chemical name for sodium
10. Table salt's chemical name
12. Negatively charged particles
13. Red bloods cells in _____, are an example of a suspension
14. Fluid in the interstitial spaces

Source	Amount
3. Sensible	_____
A. _____	_____
B. _____	_____
C. _____	_____
4. Insensible	_____
A. _____	_____
B. _____	_____

You can also lose water through additive losses such as sweating, diarrhea, and vomiting.

5. Describe the loss of water that occurs through fever.

6. Lost water is regained via two primary sources. List these sources and give amounts.

	Source	Amount
A.	_____	_____
1.	_____	_____
2.	_____	_____
B.	_____	_____

Acid-Base Basics

If your body was a playground, acids and bases would be the see-saw ride! You don't have to be a chemistry major to play. Acids are substances that release hydrogen ions (H^+) when placed in a watery solution. Another definition states that acids are substances that are proton donors. Bases release hydroxyl ions (OH^-) or accept protons. Pure water is the reference point for determining acidity or alkalinity. Any solution with more H^+ ions than water is considered an acid. A solution with less hydrogen ions is considered alkaline, or basic. A logarithmic scale, called the pH scale, is used to indicate the relative amount of acidity or alkalinity of a substance. Water is assigned a value of 7.0 on the pH scale. Since the scale is logarithmic, a pH of 6 is 10 times more acidic than water. The human body exists in a narrow range of pH values. Normally, our arterial blood has a pH of 7.35 to 7.45. A prolonged pH below 7.0 or above 7.60 is usually fatal! In Chapter 12 we'll get into clinical applications and interpretations of acid-base balance.

Electrifying Information

Electrolytes are chemicals that dissociate into ions when placed into solution, thus becoming capable of conducting electricity. Positively charged ions are called cations, and negative particles are called anions. There are seven major electrolytes in the body that are essential to life. Electrolytes are naturally regulated by the kidney (mostly), and can be manipulated by oral or intravenous intake in the healthcare setting. Let's see if you know your electrolytes.

7. List the seven major electrolytes and their primary purpose in the body.

	Electrolyte	Symbol	Purpose
A.	_____	_____	_____
B.	_____	_____	_____
C.	_____	_____	_____
D.	_____	_____	_____
E.	_____	_____	_____
F.	_____	_____	_____
G.	_____	_____	_____

You will also need to know the average normal plasma value for these babies. Match the value to the chemical in the list below.

Chemical

8. _____ Bicarbonate
9. _____ Calcium
10. _____ Chloride
11. _____ Magnesium
12. _____ Phosphorus
13. _____ Potassium
14. _____ Sodium

Value
A. 140 mEq/L
B. 24 mEq/L
C. 4.0 mEq/L
D. 5.0 mEq/L
E. 100 mEq/L
F. 1.2 mEq/L
G. 1.3 mEq/L

Electrolytes are so important that a patient will exhibit some pretty interesting signs and symptoms if these powerful substances become too high or low. Complete the chart below to match up disorders, causes, and symptoms of electrolyte disturbances.

Imbalance	Cause	Symptom
15. _____	Sweating	_____
16. Hypokalemia	_____	_____
17. _____	Starvation	Diaphragmatic weakness
18. Hypercalcemia	_____	_____
19. _____	Chronic renal disease	_____

Notice the similarities in the symptoms of many of these imbalances. . . what's a clinician to do? When you see muscle weakness, abnormal fatigue or ECG disturbances, or metabolic acid-base disorders, *take a look at the electrolytes!*

Case Studies

Case 1

John Dough, a 68-year-old with CHF, is being treated for this condition with a combination of diet and diuretics. Mr. Dough returns from a trip to New Orleans complaining of difficulty breathing and swollen ankles. He is admitted to the coronary care unit for observation and treatment. Auscultation reveals bilateral inspiratory crackles in the lung bases. His respiratory frequency is 28, heart rate 110 with dysrhythmias.

20. Patients with CHF are usually placed on what special type of diet? Why?

21. Diuretics commonly cause loss of what specific electrolyte that affects cardiac function? How will this electrolyte be replaced in the hospital? The home?

22. As an RCP, what action will you take to further assess cardiopulmonary status? What is likely to be your initial treatment of this patient?

23. What is the etiology of this patient's crackles?

Case 2

Andy Wilson is a 68-year-old, homeless alcoholic who is found in respiratory distress by the paramedics and brought to your emergency department. Mr. Wilson is malnourished. Auscultation reveals bilateral inspiratory crackles in the lung bases. His respiratory frequency is 28, heart rate 110.

24. What protein accounts for the high osmotic pressure of plasma? Why is Mr. Wilson lacking in this substance?

25. Explain why this patient has crackles.

26. As an RCP, what action will you take to further assess cardiopulmonary status? What is likely to be your initial treatment of this patient?

Mathemagic

Respiratory care practitioners frequently work with weight/volume solutions and perform dilution calculations. Dilution calculations are used in drug preparation and in the pulmonary laboratory. You will be expected to perform some of these calculations on your board examinations. Remember, no calculators!

27. Albuterol is prepared in a 5% solution (weight/volume). How many grams of albuterol are dissolved in 100 ml to make this solution?

Formula: _____
Solution: _____
Answer: _____

28. Respiratory care practitioners don't usually administer 100 ml of drugs to their patients. Instead, they give 1 ml or less. How many milligrams of albuterol would be found in 1 ml of the 5% solution in problem 20?

Formula: _____
Solution: _____
Answer: _____

29. After drawing up 1 ml a 5% solution of albuterol into a syringe, the RCP places the bronchodilator into a nebulizer along with 2 ml of saline for dilution. The total solution is now 3 ml in the nebulizer. What is the new concentration of the drug?

Formula: _____
Solution: _____
Answer: _____

What About Those Board Exams?

The National Board for Respiratory Care would give this chapter three gold stars for emphasis of important test material. Here are some sample questions in the same format as your tests.

23. A patient with severe hypokalemia is receiving an intravenous infusion of potassium to correct this serious disorder. What should you monitor?
   A. SpO_2
   B. Respiratory frequency
   C. Mental status
   D. ECG rhythm

31. Which of the following signs and symptoms would you expect to observe in a patient with hypokalemia?
    I. Metabolic acid-base disturbance
    II. Muscle twitching
    III. ECG abnormality
    A. I only
    B. I and II only
    C. I and III only
    D. I, II, III

32. All of the following would be consistent with administration of a large amount of intravenous saline *except*:
    A. Increased pulmonary vascular markings on the chest radiograph
    B. Presence of crackles on auscultation
    C. Increased urine output
    D. Increased hematocrit

33. A respiratory care practitioner delivers isotonic saline to a patient via nebulizer. What concentration of saline is the practitioner delivering?
    A. 0.0%
    B. 0.45%
    C. 0.90%
    D. 1.0%

34. What happens to cells in the presence of a hypertonic solution?

35. What happens to cells when a hypotonic solution is given?

36. What name is given for the movement of water across a semi-permeable membrane?

Food for Thought

Administration of fluids with varying tonicities by both IV and aerosol routes is common.

Acid-Base Balance

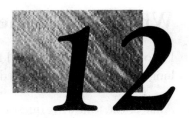

——— "There's so much pollution
in the air now that if it
weren't for our lungs there'd
be no place to put it all."
Robert Orben

If our bodies are factories that use oxygen and glucose to manufacture energy, then they are also producers of waste in the form of water, heat, and carbon dioxide. A respiratory care practitioner must understand the role the lung and the kidney play in removing waste, how buffering systems work, and how to interpret the results of arterial blood gases. Drawing, analyzing, and most of all interpreting blood gas findings is one of the hallmarks of our profession. Learning this skill will require some memorization and lots of practice!

Interpret what?

There's no point to building your knowledge without a foundation. Before you can learn to use acid-base information clinically, you will have to know your terminology.

Match the following terms to their definitions.

Term
1. _____ Acidemia
2. _____ Volatile acid
3. _____ Anion gap
4. _____ Hyperventilation
5. _____ Metabolic acidosis
6. _____ Alkalemia
7. _____ Kussmaul's breathing
8. _____ Hypoventilation
9. _____ Fixed acid
10. _____ Respiratory alkalosis
11. _____ Metabolic alkalosis
12. _____ Standard bicarbonate
13. _____ Base excess
14. _____ Respiratory acidosis
15. _____ Buffer

Definition
A. Acid that can be excreted in gaseous form
B. Decreased hydrogen ion concentration in the blood
C. Ventilation that results in decreased CO_2
D. Respiratory processes resulting in increased hydrogen ions
E. Acid that is excreted by the kidney
F. Abnormal ventilatory pattern in response to metabolic acidosis
G. Non-respiratory processes resulting in decreased hydrogen ions
H. Difference between electrolyte concentrations
I. Respiratory processes resulting in decreased hydrogen ions
J. Increased hydrogen ion concentration in the blood
K. Non-respiratory processes resulting in increased hydrogen ions
L. Chemical substance that minimizes fluctuations in pH
M. Plasma concentration of HCO_3^- corrected to a normal CO_2
N. Difference between normal and actual buffers available
O. Ventilation that results in increased CO_2

Where has all the acid gone?

I know I was surprised when I found out that the lung excretes more acid each day than the kidney!

Answer the following questions to find out if you understand the buffering process.

16. Draw a diagram of the process called isohydric buffering.

17. Explain how the lungs can compensate for increased production of fixed acids.

18. Buffers are composed of what two components?

    A. _____

    B. _____

19. What happens when you add the acid hydrogen chloride to sodium bicarbonate?

20. Describe the two general types of buffering systems in the body and give examples of each system and what they buffer in the body.

    A. _____

    B. _____

21. Does ventilation actually remove hydrogen ions from the body? Support your answer with information from the text.

22. Why are buffers in the kidney essential for the secretion of excess hydrogen ions?

Balancing Act

When you're healthy, the lungs, kidney, and buffers work together to keep your pH normal so that enzyme systems can function and homeostasis is maintained. The system responds pretty rapidly to local or systemic changes. As long as the ratio of bicarbonate buffer to dissolved CO_2 is 20:1, your pH will be about 7.40. A variety of conditions can cause the balance to shift. Increases in ventilation will result in respiratory alkalosis. Increases in bicarbonate (or other base buffers) will result in metabolic alkalosis. These changes are referred to as acute if they take place over a short period of time. If they become chronic, the body will try to compensate to bring the pH back to normal. Of course, the respiratory system responds rapidly to metabolic disturbances, but the kidney takes time to adjust the bicarbonate. Answer these questions to test your understanding of simple acid-base disturbances.

23. List the normal range of values for pH, $PaCO_2$, and HCO_3^-. (You have to memorize these values!!)

	Low Normal	to	High Normal
A. pH	_____		_____
B. $PaCO_2$	_____		_____
C. HCO_3^-	_____		_____

24. Write out the Henderson-Hasselbach equation.

25. Complete the primary acid-base and compensation chart below.

Disorder	Primary Defect	Compensation
A. Respiratory acidosis	_____	_____
B. Respiratory alkalosis	_____	_____
C. Metabolic acidosis	_____	_____
D. Metabolic alkalosis	_____	_____

26. What is the rule of thumb for determining the expected increase in bicarbonate for any acute increase in carbon dioxide?

27. How much will bicarbonate increase with a chronic increase in carbon dioxide?

A Method to the Madness

There is a simple, four-step method for interpreting blood gas values.

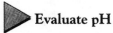 **Evaluate pH**

1. >7.45 = Alkalosis
2. <7.35 = Acidosis
3. 7.35-7.45 = Normal (or fully compensated)

 Evaluate respiratory status ($PaCO_2$)

1. <35 = Alkalosis
2. >45 = Acidosis

 Evaluate metabolic status (HCO_3^-)

1. >26 = Alkalosis
2. <22 = Acidosis

 Evaluate compensation

1. Complete: pH is normal with abnormal CO_2 and HCO_3^-

(Even with complete compensation, the pH will tend to be on the primary disorder's side of 7.40.)

2. Partial: pH is abnormal, but not as much as expected

Try It, You'll Like It!

Interpret the following blood gas results. I'll help you with the first one.

pH 7.26; $PaCO_2$ 60 mm Hg; HCO_3^- 26 mEq/L

The pH is below 7.35, so the overall state is acidosis. The $PaCO_2$ is above 45, which represents *acidosis*. The pH and the $PaCO_2$ agree! We have *respiratory acidosis*. The bicarbonate has risen 2 mEq/L above normal. This elevation is most likely due to the increased CO_2 (remember, bicarbonate goes up 1 for each 10 mm Hg acute increase in CO_2). So, we have **Acute (uncompensated) respiratory acidosis.**

Now it's your turn.

28. pH 7.34; $PaCO_2$ 60 mm Hg; HCO_3^- 31 mEq/L

29. pH 7.38; $PaCO_2$ 60 mm Hg; HCO_3^- 34 mEq/L

Stop right there! We're going to continue interpreting blood gas results in our case studies and board exam review questions.

Welcome to the Gap!

When a patient has a metabolic acidosis, it can be life threatening, so we need to try to establish the cause. One way to do this is through history. For example, we know the patient took an aspirin overdose. Another method for determining the type of metabolic acidosis is by looking at the difference between positive and negative ions. Of course, you need the electrolyte values to do this calculation. Here's how you do it:

Sodium (Na^+) − Chloride (Cl^-) + Bicarbonate (HCO_3^-) or $140 - (105 + 24) = 11$.

A normal range for the gap is 9 to 14 mEq/L. Usually, potassium is ignored.

When the body loses bicarbonate through diarrhea, chloride increases and the gap stays normal. When bicarbonate is used to buffer excess fixed acids, the gap will increase.

30. Name the three common causes of anion gap metabolic acidosis.
    A. _____
    B. _____
    C. _____

31. What are the signs of respiratory compensation for metabolic acidosis?

32. What are the neurological symptoms of severe acidosis?

Mathemagic

There have been several math calculations in this chapter. You will have to use a scientific calculator to solve some of them.

Bicarbonate Blues

33. Calculate the new bicarbonate (assume 24 as the starting point) level for an acutely elevated $PaCO_2$ of 50 mm Hg (assume it started at 40).

Formula: _____
Solution: _____
Answer: _____

34. Calculate the new bicarbonate (assume 24 as the starting point) level for an acutely elevated $PaCO_2$ of 70 mm Hg (assume it started at 40).

Formula: _____
Solution: _____
Answer: _____

35. Calculate the new bicarbonate (assume 24 as the starting point) level for a chronically elevated $PaCO_2$ of 70 mm Hg (assume it started at 40).

Formula: _____
Solution: _____
Answer: _____

Hassle?

36. Calculate pH if HCO_3^- is 30 mEq/L and $PaCO_2$ is 40 mm Hg.

Formula: _____
Solution: _____
Answer: _____

37. Calculate pH if HCO_3^- is 24 mEq/L and $PaCO_2$ is 40 mm Hg.

Formula: _____
Solution: _____
Answer: _____

38. Calculate pH if HCO_3^- is 24 mEq/L and $PaCO_2$ is 60 mm Hg.

Formula: _____
Solution: _____
Answer: _____

Gap?

39. Calculate anion gap if Na^- is 140, Cl^- is 105, and HCO_3^- is 24.

Formula: _____
Solution: _____
Answer: _____

40. Calculate anion gap if Na^+ is 140, Cl^- is 105, and HCO_3^- is 12.

Formula: _____
Solution: _____
Answer: _____

Case Studies

The following case studies will systematically take you through the major acid-base disorders. Let's start with some simple, acute states. Remember to evaluate using the four-step process.

Case 1

Mrs. Miller takes too much Valium and is found shortly thereafter in a coma breathing slowly and shallowly. ABG results reveal: pH 7.24, $PaCO_2$ 70 mm Hg, and HCO_3^- 29 mEq/L.

42. How would you interpret this ABG?

43. What is the primary cause of the disorder?

47. What is the primary cause of the disorder?

Case 2

Mr. Miller is really worried about Mrs. M's condition. She complains of dizziness and tingling in her hands. ABG results reveal: pH 7.66, $PaCO_2$ 20 mm Hg, and HCO_3^- 22 mEq/L.

44. How would you interpret this ABG?

Case 4

Debbie Miller, a teenager, has not been taking her insulin. ABG results reveal: pH 7.17, $PaCO_2$ 40 mm Hg, and HCO_3^- 14 mEq/L.

48. How would you interpret this ABG?

45. What is the primary cause of the disorder?

49. What is the primary cause of the disorder?

Case 3

Little Jimmy Miller has been sick with the stomach flu. ABG results reveal: pH 7.58, $PaCO_2$ 40 mm Hg, and HCO_3^- 36 mEq/L.

46. How would you interpret this ABG?

Of course, blood gases don't stay simple for long. Partial or complete compensation may occur.

Case 5

Grandpa Miller has smoked for years, and now he has COPD. ABG results reveal: pH 7.35, $PaCO_2$ 53 mm Hg, and HCO_3^- 29 mEq/L.

50. How would you interpret this ABG?

51. What is the source of compensation?

Case 6

As soon as Debbie Miller's brain realizes the acute nature of her illness, compensation begins. ABG results now reveal: pH 7.37, $PaCO_2$ 25 mm Hg, and HCO_3^- 14 mEq/L.

52. How would you interpret this ABG?

53. What is the source of compensation?

Case 7

Grandma Miller has CHF. She takes Lasix to reduce extra water in her body. ABG results now reveal: pH 7.48, $PaCO_2$ 45 mm Hg, and HCO_3^- 32 mEq/L.

54. How would you interpret this ABG?

55. What is a possible cause of the primary disorder?

What About those Board Exams?

Blood gas (acid-base) analysis is one of the largest areas in all of the exams. The Entry-Level Examination will focus on simple interpretations, while the Registry Examinations will ask you for higher order thinking. Here are some examples.

56. A 17-year-old woman is brought to the emergency department by paramedics. Her mother states she is a diabetic. Room air ABGs reveal:

pH	7.26
$PaCO_2$	16 mm Hg
HCO_3^-	8 mEq/L
PaO_2	110 mm Hg

This information indicates which of the following?
   I. Partly compensated metabolic acidosis
   II. This PaO_2 is not possible on room air
   III. Respiratory alkalosis is present
   A. I only
   B. III only
   C. I and II only
   D. I and III only

57. Interpret the following ABG results:

FIO_2	.21
pH	7.36
$PaCO_2$	37 mm Hg
HCO_3^-	22 mEq/L
PaO_2	95 mm Hg

   A. Acute respiratory alkalosis
   B. Acute metabolic alkalosis
   C. Compensated respiratory alkalosis
   D. Normal ABG

58. During CPR, blood gases are drawn. The results are as follows:

FIO_2	1.0
pH	7.15
$PaCO_2$	55 mm Hg
HCO_3^-	12 mEq/L
PaO_2	210 mm Hg

What action should be taken to correct the acid-base abnormality shown here?
   A. Increase the rate of ventilation
   B. Decrease the FIO_2
   C. Administer sodium bicarbonate intravenously
   D. Add positive end expiratory pressure (PEEP) to the ventilation system

59. The results of an arterial blood gas are below.

FIO_2	.21
pH	7.55
$PaCO_2$	25 mm Hg
HCO_3^-	24 mEq/L
PaO_2	105 mm Hg

These data indicate which of the following?
   A. Metabolic acidosis
   B. Metabolic alkalosis
   C. Uncompensated hyperventilation
   D. Uncompensated hypoventilation

60. A 72-year-old man with a history of renal failure is seen in the emergency department. The RCP notes that the patient is taking 28 very deep breaths per minute. Which of the following accurately describes this breathing pattern?
   A. Cheyne-Stokes breathing
   B. Ataxic breathing
   C. Kussmaul's breathing
   D. Eupnic breathing

Exercise your Mental Muscles

In later chapters you will be called on to use your newfound blood gas interpretation skills to make many clinical decisions about patient care. *If you are having difficulty interpreting the acid -base status, you should take time to solidify these skills now!* Here are some suggestions.

1. Get access to blood gas interpretation software. Your instructors probably have a program that will give you sample after sample to interpret.

2. Make flash cards. Take some 3 x 5 inch cards. Write high, normal, and low values for pH, $PaCO_2$, and HCO_3^-. Make two extra cards for pH that will represent compensation. Use 7.36 for compensated acidotic states and 7.44 for alkalotic states. On the back of each card write out the name of the state. For example, on the $PaCO_2$ 50 mm Hg card, write "respiratory acidosis." Now proceed to go through the combinations using the four-step method of interpretation. Pretty soon you will be an ace!

Drill, Drill, Drill until you have mastered basic blood gas interpretation!

Food for Thought

Blood gas disorders can get really complicated at times. Just like life in some cases, a patient will have one disorder superimposed on another. Take the continuing saga of Grandpa Miller. . .

Grandpa Miller has acquired a lung infection after visiting his daughter in the hospital. ABG results now reveal: pH 7.53, PaCO$_2$ 35 mm Hg, PaO$_2$ 57 mm Hg, and HCO$_3^-$ 28x mEq/L.

61. How would you interpret this ABG?

62. Why did the blood gas change from Case 5?

Regulation of Breathing

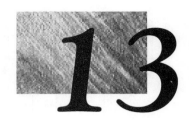

You are getting sleepy, very sleepy. . . you didn't stop breathing, did you? In just 1 year as an adult, you will breath more than *seven million times*! Most of those breaths will be automatically initiated by your brainstem. Just like clockwork. It makes sense that RCPs would need to know how this system works and what happens when it doesn't. Chapter 13 is a fitting end to the section on anatomy and physiology, because it summarizes the control mechanisms that regulate the respiratory system.

Reading, Writing, and Regulating

The brain and nervous system have a language all their own. Learning these terms will make it easier to understand concepts in this chapter. (And you can impress your friends with your linguistic abilities!) Fill in the crossword puzzle on p. 82.

Where's the Action

Input into how we breathe comes from many areas. Conscious thought, receptors throughout the body, and reflexes all play important roles. The medulla's job is to organize the information and send messages to the motor fibers that innervate the muscles of the airway and chest. (A sort of mental air-traffic controller.) The medulla is located in your brainstem just above your spinal cord. If you cut the brainstem below the medulla, all ventilatory effort ceases. Another structure, the pons, sits on top of the medulla.

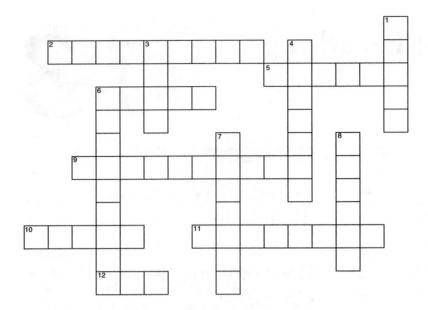

ACROSS

2. Chemo _____ , respond to changes in oxygen and pH to signal the need to breathe
5. + Breuer = parasympathetic inflation reflex
6. Absence of breathing
9. Receptors in the carotid bodies
10. 5 deep breaths...apnea...five deep breaths...apnea?
11. Coughing, sneezing, laryngospasm, bronchospasm, and more when you stimulate these receptors!
12. Fluid that bathes the brain instead of blood

DOWN

1. Important cranial nerve involved in sensory and motor reflexes
3. The other center in the brainstem
4. Big Boss of the brainstem
5. Breathing pattern characterized by prolonged inspiratory gasps
7. Primary chemoreceptors
8. + Stokes = gradually increasing, then decreasing volumes with apneic episodes

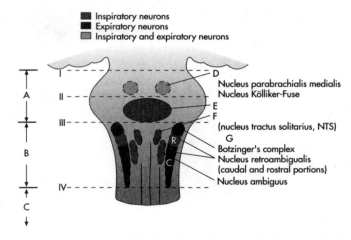

Dorsal view of the brainstem. Dashed lines I to IV refer to transections at different levels. (From Beachey W: Respiratory care anatomy and physiology: Foundations for clinical practice, St Louis, 1998, Mosby.)

1. Label the parts of the central controlling bodies illustrated on p. 82.
   A. _____
   B. _____
   C. _____
   D. _____
   E. _____
   F. _____
   G. _____

2. Briefly explain the role of the two primary respiratory groups in the medulla.
   A. _____
   _____
   B. _____
   _____

3. Compare and contrast the two primary centers in the pons.
   A. _____
   _____
   B. _____
   _____

4. What diseases or conditions might affect the performance of the brainstem's respiratory controllers?

Automatic Pilot

Respiratory reflexes are involuntary nervous responses located in airways, muscles, and tissues that influence breathing by sending information directly to the medulla (mostly via the vagus nerve). You'll need to be able to identify the most important reflexes, so here goes. Each reflex goes with a particular stimulus and has a response from receptors in a specific location.

Reflex	Stimulus	Response	Location
5. Hering-Breuer	_____	_____	_____
6. Deflation	_____	_____	_____
7. Head	_____	_____	_____
8. Vaso-vagal	_____	_____	_____
9. C fiber	_____	_____	_____
10. Proprioceptor	_____	_____	_____

Later on we'll apply some of these reflexes to the clinical setting and bring them to life.

Better Living through Chemistry

Regulating ventilation ensures that tissues are exposed to just the right amount of oxygen, carbon dioxide, and hydrogen ions. Blood carries these substances to specialized nerve structures called chemoreceptors that are strategically placed in the brainstem, carotid bodies, and arch of the aorta. All these chemoreceptors will respond in some way to decrease levels of oxygen and pH, or increased CO_2 in the blood (or vice versa).

Central Chemoreceptors

These are sitting in the medulla taking a bath in the cerebrospinal fluid. They are not in direct contact with the blood because of the blood-brain barrier, a semipermeable membrane that surrounds the brain.

11. Explain the process that allows CO_2 to stimulate the central receptors.

12. Describe the stimulating effects of CO_2 on the receptors in terms of the immediate and delayed responses.

15. How does altitude modify the receptor's response to hypoxemia?

16. Describe the peripheral receptor response to hypercapnia and acidemia. How is it different than the central response?

Peripheral Chemoreceptors

Somebody thought it would be a good idea to monitor the chemical composition of blood leaving the heart and heading toward the brain. Pretty smart!

13. Describe the peripheral receptor response to decreased arterial oxygen levels.

No One Understands Me!

I want to introduce you to one of the most misunderstood concepts in the pathophysiology of lung disease. When you understand this one, you'll really be able to amaze the doctors, nurses, and respiratory instructors (not to mention your mom and dad).

14. What specific range of PaO_2 values causes the greatest response?

Some patients, especially those with chronic obstructive pulmonary disease (COPD), become chronically hypoxic and hypercapnic. This happens when a high arterial CO_2 level persists over time. The kidneys compensate, which restores pH. Some of the bicarbonate diffuses into your head and corrects the pH in the CSF. The central receptors are fooled into thinking everything is fine. Since they are low on oxygen, the hypoxic stimulus drives their ventilation. When someone intervenes, and gives this special type of patient oxygen, they may experience an acute rise in arterial CO_2. The simple explanation is that they are no longer driven by the peripheral receptors to breathe because of low oxygen levels. While this is true, it is too simple of an explanation. Increased oxygen also worsens the ventilation/perfusion relationship in the lung by increasing blood flow to poorly ventilated areas and through absorption atelectasis. Ventilation is decreased in the low V/Q areas, and increased in the high V/Q regions. The result is an increased arterial PCO_2. (My students always ask "so what?" at this point!) *The point is* that CO_2 in high concentrations in the blood is bad for you. It further decreases the drive to breathe by depressing the central nervous system. So, don't give the patient too much oxygen, but ***never withhold oxygen from a hypoxic patient!***

17. What concentration of oxygen is usually given to chronically hypercapnic patients?

18. What is the best way to monitor oxygenation in these patients?

19. Why do low concentrations of oxygen usually result in adequate improvement?

Ouch!

Obviously, if the brain is physically or physiologically injured, abnormal breathing patterns will occur. When you observe these patterns, you know something is wrong with the controller.

20. Describe Cheyne-Stokes breathing (use words or draw a picture). State two important causes of this distinctive pattern.

21. How does Biot's breathing differ from Cheyne-Stokes in terms of pattern and origin?

22. Describe apneustic breathing. What does this pattern indicate?

23. What are the two central neurogenic breathing patterns? State three events that could cause these patterns.

Case Studies

Case 1

Bobby Donor rides his motorcycle without a helmet. He suffers a closed-head injury during an accident that results in a subdural hematoma. Bobby is intubated by the paramedics with an endotracheal tube.

24. What is the goal of ventilation during the early period following acute closed-head trauma?

25. Why would you limit the use of this technique after 24 hours?

Case 2

Grandpa Miller (Chapter 12) is back in the hospital. Grandpa became short of breath at home and his family increased his oxygen from 2 liters to 6 liters per minute. When he arrives at the hospital he is somnolent (sleepy) and difficult to arouse. ABG results reveal: pH 7.25, $PaCO_2$ 75 mm Hg, PaO_2 90 mm Hg, HCO_3^- 32 mEq/L on 6 L by nasal cannula.

26. What changes should you make in Grandpa's therapy? Why?

27. What target PaO_2 would be more appropriate for this patient? Why?

What About Those Board Exams?

The NBRC won't exactly ask you direct questions about the information in this chapter, but they do have related questions. For example, variations on this theme:

28. A patient who has had COPD for many years is admitted for an acute episode of dyspnea. An arterial blood gas is drawn on room air with these results:

pH	7.53
$PaCO_2$	48 mm Hg
PaO_2	44 mm Hg
HCO_3^-	36 mEq/L
SaO_2	84%

What therapy do you recommend at this time?
A. 28% venturi mask
B. 35% venturi mask
C. Nasal cannula delivering 5 L/min
D. Simple mask delivering 10 L/min

29. A cooperative elderly patient with chronic asthma presents at her pulmonologist's office. You observe the following findings:

Pulse 94
RR 28
Temp 36.5°C
BP 135/90
FIO_2 .21
pH 7.31
$PaCO_2$ 70
PaO_2 35
HCO_3^- 34 mEq/L

What action would you take at this time?
A. Administer bronchodilator therapy via MDI
B. Administer oxygen via 24% venturi mask
C. Administer oxygen via cannula at 6 L/min
D. Administer oxygen via non-rebreathing mask

30. A patient with COPD and a history of hypercapnia is receiving oxygen via simple mask in the recovery room following admission for pneumonia. Upon transfer to the medical floor, he is noted to be increasingly drowsy and difficult to arouse. The nurse requests that you give him a breathing treatment with a bronchodilator. The most appropriate action would be to
A. Administer the breathing treatment as requested
B. Obtain an arterial blood gas sample
C. Change the oxygen to 2 L/min via nasal cannula
D. Change the oxygen to 40% via venturi mask

There are many variations of this type of question regarding chronic hypercapnia and oxygen administration on both the Entry-Level and Registry examinations! You may also expect:

31. A patient is being mechanically ventilated following craniotomy. During a suctioning procedure, the intracranial pressure monitor shows a sudden increase in ICP. The patient becomes restless and agitated. What is the most appropriate immediate action for the RCP in this situation?
A. Increase the FIO_2 on the ventilator to deliver 100% oxygen
B. Recommend administration of a sedative
C. Increase rate and volume of ventilation with a resuscitation bag
D. Ask the RN to page the physician "STAT"

Experiment

This exercise will seem simple, but it will help you understand control of breathing. It's even better if you have a pulse oximeter, some oxygen, and a non-rebreathing mask. *Remember to be safe—sit down when you do this, and have a partner!* Put the oximeter probe on your finger. Breathe normally. Now inhale deeply and hold your breath. Time how long you can hold your breath. Next, inhale and exhale deeply several times. Fill your lungs and time how long you can hold your breath.

32. How long could you hold your breath the first time? What about the second try?

33. What were the pulse oximetry readings before, during, and at the end of breath holding?

34. Compare the results and explain the differences in the breath-holding time and why you had to breathe. What is the meaning of the pulse oximeter readings?

Now, breathe 100% oxygen for several minutes. At the end of the time, hyperventilate while breathing the oxygen. Now hold your breath.

35. What happened to the time of breath-hold?

36. Given a vital capacity of 5 L and an oxygen consumption of 250 ml/min, what is the theoretical maximum breath-holding time of a normal adult?

If you really want to try this experiment at its best, see your instructor about breathing from a high-flow CPAP system at 100% oxygen, or use a ventilator!

Food for Thought

The reflexes and receptors that control breathing are important. So is the input of conscious thought. The higher brain centers have a definite effect on how we breathe.

37. Why do we take the patient's respiratory rate without telling them we are doing it?

38. Name as many factors as you can that involve the higher brain centers increasing the rate of ventilation. (Hint: How do you breathe when a police officer pulls up behind you and turns on the flashing lights?)

Bedside Assessment

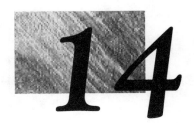

Patient assessment is the compass by which we steer in the clinical setting. Chapter 14 will help you learn the basics, but only practice will give you mastery. Your ability to evaluate using your senses will make all the difference in your career. This material is so important that I've packed this chapter full of questions, cases, and more questions!

Word Power

Chapter 14 starts off with a list of nearly 40 new words for you to learn. Power up your medical terminology by reading the chapter and solving the crossword puzzle on p. 90.

Start at the Very Beginning . . .

Successful assessors have developed a systematic way of evaluating patients. Except in life-threatening emergencies, most practitioners begin by interviewing the patient. The interview may be short or long, depending on the situation. The increasing use of protocols requires us to conduct more in-depth interviews. Let's review the essentials of interviewing and history-taking.

1. What information would you gather prior to entering the patient's room?

2. Describe how to *start* the ideal interview. Be sure to discuss space, privacy, and introductions.

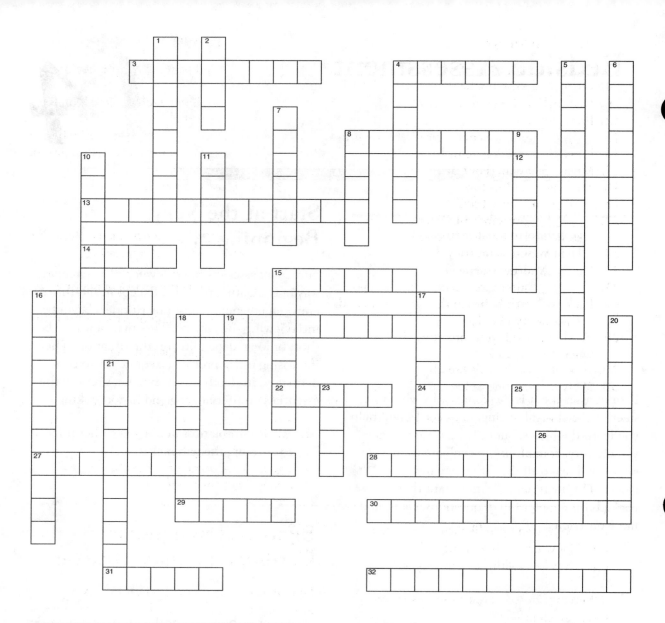

3. Circle the *best approach* from each set of choices in the following list:
   A1. "Hi Bob, good morning."
   A2. "Good morning Mr. Johnson."
   B1. Stand at the foot of the bed
   B2. Sit in a chair at the bedside
   C1. Make room for your notes on the bed-side table
   C2. Keep your clipboard on your lap
   D1. "Do you need anything right now?"
   D2. "I'll tell your nurse to check on you."
   E1. "I'll be back to see you in 1 hour."
   E2. "I'll return in a while to check on you."

Are You Asking the Questions Right?

The way you ask questions will determine your relationship with the patient and the amount and quality of the information you gather.

4. Circle the *best approach* from each set of choices in following list:
   A1. "What are you coughing up?"
   A2. "You didn't cough up blood, did you?"
   B1. "I understand you don't like your breathing treatments."

ACROSS	DOWN

ACROSS

1. Bluish discoloration of the skin
4. Mucus from the tracheobronchial tree
8. Discontinuous abnormal breath sounds
12. Prefix for fast
13. _____emphysema is air under the skin
14. Look for distended veins here
15. Mucus that comes out the mouth
16. Medical term for slow
18. Extra, or abnormal sounds
22. _____pressure, the difference between systolic and diastolic blood pressure
24. Level of consciousness
25. Designed to expel mucus
27. _____alternans occurs when you go back and forth between the diaphragm and the accessory muscles!
28. You have this if your breathing is labored when you lie down
29. Auscultation reveals breath_____
30. Body temperature below 32° Celsius
31. Stay at least 2-4 feet away to give the patient a personal_____space during the interview
32. Sweaty stuff

DOWN

1. _____pressure, when the heart contracts
2. Dys, ortho, hypo, tachy—are all prefixes that go with this one
4. Abdominal _____, occurs when th[e] diaphragm is tired and the belly sinks in with each breath
5. Abnormal voice sounds heard over consolidation
6. Slow respiratory rate
7. _____ of monkeys (also a chest shap[e] associated with air trapping)
8. Treasure, pigeon, or barrel
9. High-pitched continuous upper airway sound
10. Patient's perception of difficult breathing
11. Foul smelling
15. Another name for fainting
16. Heart rate below 60
17. Got pus?
18. Pattern of end-stage muscle fatigue
19. _____signs
20. Rapid breathing pattern
21. Coughing up blood
23. Primary organ of gas exchange
26. I've got the fever

B2. "Why don't you like these treatments?"
C1. "How is your breathing today?"
C2. "Is your breathing better today?"

5. When are 'closed' questions most useful? Give an example.

Signs and Symptoms of Cardiopulmonary Disease

Five things come to mind when I think of common symptoms of heart and lung disease. I am sure there are more, but if you can remember these, you can use them to your benefit as part of the interviewing process.

 "I feel short of breath. . ."

6. Describe the dyspnea (Borg) scale. Why would this be useful?

7. How else can you identify the degree of dyspnea a patient feels?

8. What are the possible causes of these common types of cough?

Cough	Cause(s)
A. Dry cough	_____
B. Loose, productive	_____
C. Acute, self-limiting	_____
D. Chronic	_____

9. What is the difference between mucus and sputum?

10. What are the three characteristics of sputum that should be documented and reported to the physician?
    A. _____
    B. _____
    C. _____

"Cough it up, honey!"

11. Define *nonmassive* hemoptysis and give three common causes.
    A. _____
    B. _____
    C. _____

12. Define *massive* hemoptysis and give three possible causes.
    A. _____
    B. _____
    C. _____

"It hurts when I take a deep breath!"

13. What is the most serious kind of nonpleuritic chest pain?

14. How does pleuritic chest pain differ from nonpleuritic pain?

"Hot stuff!"

15. Significant elevation of temperature will have what result on metabolic rate, oxygen consumption, CO_2 production, and breathing pattern?

16. Along with fever, what are two signs that are highly suggestive of respiratory infection?

A. _____

B. _____

Medical History

Whether you personally take medical histories or not, you will need to be familiar with the standard format used in this process that is *always* conducted at some point (usually early on) during a patient's admission to the formal healthcare setting.

17. What do the initials "CC" and "HPI" stand for? List at least five important areas described in the HPI.

18. What do the initials "PMH" stand for? List at least five important areas described in the PMH.

General appearance is assessed during the first few seconds of *every* encounter with a patient. During your first encounter, you might look at their body as a whole, facial expression, anxiety level, positioning, and personal hygiene.

19. Describe the significance of the findings for each of the areas of general appearance listed below.

Finding	Significance
A. Weak, emaciated and diaphoretic	_____
	_____
	_____
B. Appears anxious	_____
	_____
C. Sitting up, leaning with arms on table	_____
	_____

Is Anyone Home?

What's the difference between stuporous and lethargic? Obtunded and comatose? Alert and confused? These aren't completely subjective terms and you will see them used frequently in the medical record. After taking a look at the overall appearance, you need to determine the level of consciousness. For starters, the patient is either obviously conscious or not when you look at them. If they are conscious, you have to find out the level of alertness. If they don't seem to be obviously conscious, you need to find out how depressed their sensorium is, and describe this with commonly accepted terms.

20. What does the phrase "oriented × 3" mean?

21. Compare and contrast the terms *lethargic* and *obtunded*.

22. What is the difference between a "stuporous" patient and a "comatose" patient?

There are special rating systems like the Glasgow Coma Scale to help further identify the degree of coma. You also need to keep in mind that there are special circumstances (such as deafness) that may make assessment more difficult.

Vital Information

23. What is the first thing an RCP should evaluate in cases of a depressed level of consciousness?

Temperature, pulse, respiratory rate, and blood pressure are the traditional vital signs. Cheap, useful, and easy to obtain. (People are starting to call pulse oximetry the "fifth vital sign" because it is taken so often.) Vital signs offer great clues about response to therapeutic interventions, but they're not as simple as you might think, considering how often they are measured. Let's start with the basics.

24. Fill in the correct normal adult values (or terms) in the chart below.

Sign	Avg. Normal	Low	High
Temperature			Hyperthermia
	72/minute		
Respiratory rate		12/minute	
Systolic BP		90 mm Hg	
			90 mm Hg

25. Name the four common sites for temperature measurement. Give a *disadvantage* of each site.

Site	Disadvantage
A. _____	_____
B. _____	_____
C. _____	_____
D. _____	_____

26. Match these pulsating terms to their throbbing definitions!

Term
_____ A. Tachycardia
_____ B. Bruits
_____ C. Amplitude
_____ D. Paradoxical pulse
_____ E. Pulsus alternans
_____ F. Bradycardia

Definition

1. Palpable vibrations in the pulse
2. Strength of the pulse
3. Pulse rate below 60
4. Drop in amplitude with inspiration
5. Pulse rate above 100
6. Alternating strong and weak pulses

27. Match these flowing respiratory patterns to their whooshing definitions! (Hint: I cheated! Try the glossary!)

Terms

_____ A. Tachypnea
_____ B. Eupnea
_____ C. Orthopnea
_____ D. Trepopnea
_____ E. Hyperpnea
_____ F. Bradypnea

Definitions

1. Difficulty breathing in a supine position
2. Abnormally low respiratory rate
3. Deep breathing
4. Normal breathing pattern
5. Abnormally high respiratory rate
6. Labored breathing in an upright position

28. How can you prevent the patient from becoming aware (and thus consciously altering) that you are taking their respiratory rate?

29. What condition may result in syncope in the hypovolemic patient? How can you prevent this from happening? How is it treated medically?

30. What does it mean when patients show larger (>6-8 mm Hg) than normal drop in systolic pressure during inspiration?

Examining the Chest and Lungs: The Big Four

This is like learning the 10 Commandments, only there are four:

Thou shalt inspect the chest!
Thou shalt palpate the chest!
Thou shalt percuss the chest!
Thou shalt auscultate the chest!

It sounds so easy when you put it that way, doesn't it? Before you start to assess, make sure you have enough *light*, enough *privacy*, enough *time*, and enough *quiet*. *Of course, you can't always get what you want!* Chapter 14 describes the *ideal* evaluation of a patient. You will have to modify to meet the circumstances every time!

See Me

There's a lot you can see when you take a quick look at the patient. Practice looking. Let's find out if you know what to look for in a patient with respiratory problems.

31. Write a description for the following six abnormal chest shapes.
    A. Barrel

    B. Kyphosis

    C. Kyphoscoliosis

    D. Pectus carinatum

E. Pectus excavatum

F. Scoliosis

32. Breathing patterns are important, too. Describe the pattern that goes with these six conditions.
    A. Asthma

    B. Atelectasis

    C. Chest trauma

D. Epiglottitis

E. Increased ICP

F. Metabolic acidosis

Experiment

To get good at this, you might try going to the mall. Yes, the mall. If you sit with a nice cup of espresso and watch passersby, you can see chest shape, breathing pattern, and all the rest. Compare adult patterns with those of children. Compare the chest shape of an elderly person with that of a young adult. After you try this exercise, answer the following questions.

33. Did you observe anyone breathing with their diaphragm? How could you tell?

34. Did you observe the use of accessory muscles? How could you tell?

35. How does the chest shape of a young adult differ from that of a senior?

36. What unusual chest shapes did you observe? Anyone on portable oxygen?

Feel Me

Palpation is the art of touching the chest wall. Palpation is an art (and a useful one) because it's so subjective. You have to get a feel for it (sorry). Don't practice this at the mall, please!

37. Explain the difference between vocal, tactile, and rhonchial fremitus.

38. Describe the difference in fremitus between emphysema and pneumonia.

39. How does subcutaneous emphysema form? What is the feeling of air under the skin called?

Experiment

You should learn palpation in the laboratory setting of your program. Since disrobing is necessary, gowns and privacy will be needed. (As well as professionalism.) Assess tactile fremitus by asking your classmate to repeat the word "ninety-nine" while you palpate under the clavicles, between the shoulder blades, along the sides, and over the lower lobes. Measure chest expansion as demonstrated in Figure 14-4 in your text. Now answer these questions.

40. Describe the temperature of your partner's skin.

41. Were there any areas of abnormal fremitus? Why (why not?)?

42. Estimate the amount of chest expansion in centimeters. What is normal adult expansion?

Touch Me

Or tap me. Diagnostic percussion of the chest is another art form that is rarely practiced these days. Still, it can be useful in detecting some important abnormalities, and your board examinations expect you to be able to interpret the results of percussion findings!

43. Identify the percussion notes for these conditions.
    A. Emphysema

    B. Atelectasis

C. Pleural effusion

D. Pneumothorax

E. Pneumonia

44. What are the limitations of percussion?
     What can't you feel?

Experiment

You should do this in the lab while you are performing the palpation and auscultation exercises. Place your left middle finger on the intercostal space on the side of the chest. Rapidly strike it with your index finger or middle finger of your

right hand. Do this on both sides of the chest. Repeat over the lower lobes in the back. Have your partner take a really deep breath and hold it while you tap. Have them exhale fully, then tap. Try tapping over something solid like the scapula. Try tapping over the abdomen. Tap on your own head. Is it hollow? It takes practice to get good at percussion. *Don't include this procedure in a routine examination of a patient unless other observations suggest an appropriate problem. Have an expert present when you try this in the clinical setting!*

45. What happened to the resonance when your partner inhaled deeply? On exhalation?

Hear Me

This is it. This is the big one. Auscultation seems so easy, and identifying breath sounds so difficult.

Follow these 10 Commandments to improve your technique.

I.   Sit the patient up whenever you can.
II.   Turn off the TV, radio, or other external sources of noise.
III. Ask the patient to breathe slowly and deeply through his or her mouth.
IV.   Listen to skin whenever you can.
V.   Listen to the lower lobes first.
VI.   Listen to one full inspiration and exhalation in each spot.
VII. Listen to both sides in each spot.
VIII. Auscultate lower, middle, and upper portions of the lung.
IX.   Listen to front and back of the chest.
X.   Compare right and left lungs; compare upper and lower lobes.

Simple, right? Now you try it.

Experiment

You should try this in the laboratory before going to the bedside. You can listen at home too. The more normal sounds you auscultate, the better you will be at recognizing abnormal sounds. All you need is your stethoscope, a partner (you can even start on yourself), and a quiet place to listen. Adjust the earpieces so they are pointing slightly forward, not straight into your ears. Check to make sure the diaphragm is "on" (not the bell). Now, listen.

1. Place your partner in a sitting position (or high Fowler's).

2. Ask your partner to breathe in and out slowly through the mouth.

3. Listen on skin over the posterior lower lobes (below the shoulder blade).

4. In and out, right side and left side!

5. Listen on the side of the chest (still lower lobes).

6. Listen between the shoulder blades (not over the spine!).

7. Listen on the front to the middle lobe and lingula (anterior, below nipple).

8. Listen on the front below the collar bone (above nipples).

9. Listen over the trachea.

Look at Fig. 14-6 on page 311 in Egan. You can auscultate 20 or more places on the chest, but we don't usually do this much auscultation in the clinical setting. It takes too long for a routine evaluation. Always listen to upper, middle, lower, front, and back. When you hear abnormal sounds, or have a critically ill patient, you should expand your assessment.

Now that you've read the chapter and practiced, try answering these questions.

46. Fill in the chart below with descriptions of your favorite breath sounds.

Breath Sound	Pitch	Intensity	Where is it Heard?
A. Vesicular			
B. Bronchial			
C. Broncho-vesicular			

47. Compare the mechanisms and causes of coarse, low-pitched crackles and fine end-inspiratory crackles.

48. Contrast monophonic and polyphonic wheezes in terms of mechanisms, phase of ventilation, and conditions that produce these different musical sounds.

49. How do rhonchi differ from crackles?

Extremity Exam

You will almost always want to take a look at the patient's fingers. For one thing, it goes hand in hand with pulse oximetry. Cardiopulmonary disease may alter the fingers and other extremities.

50. How do you test for capillary refill? (Test your own while you're at it.) What is a normal capillary refill time?

51. Where should you check for edema caused by right heart failure? Why?

52. Compare and contrast the significance of peripheral cyanosis and central cyanosis.

Case Studies

Case 1

George Brush is an alert 67-year-old politician who is admitted for dyspnea and hemoptysis. While interviewing the patient you discover that he is coughing up small amounts of thick, blood- streaked mucus several times per day for the last few days. Mr. Brush has a history of 100 pack years of cigarette smoking. Physical examination reveals a barrel chest, use of accessory muscles, and digital clubbing.

53. Mr. B's history and chest configuration suggest what primary pulmonary disorder?

54. Along with enlargement of the ends of the fingers, what sign helps you recognize clubbing?

55. What does the presence of clubbing suggest in this case?

Case 2

Marla Stewart is a 47-year-old homemaker admitted for a systemic infection 3 days after cutting herself in the kitchen while preparing some chicken. She complains of dyspnea and has a fever. Her vital signs are: pulse 110; respiratory rate 28; and blood pressure 76/58 mm Hg. The nurse's notes reveal that Ms. Stewart was alert on admission, but she is now confused and anxious. Her extremities are warm and capillary refill is normal.

56. Why do you think Ms. Stewart's mental status has deteriorated?

57. What other "vital sign" should be evaluated?

58. Which abnormal vital sign has the most clinical significance in this case?

Case 3

You are called to the medical ward to evaluate John Hopkins, a 29-year-old medical student who was admitted for shortness of breath and is now complaining of chest pain. Mr. Hopkins tells you that the pain came on suddenly and is worse when he inhales. Your interview reveals that this pain is on the right side and feels like a sharp, stabbing sensation. Temperature is normal, but blood pressure, heart rate, and respiratory rate are elevated. Palpation reveals crepitus over the right lateral chest wall.

59. What other physical assessments would be useful in determining the nature of the problem?

60. What immediate treatment should you initiate in this situation?

61. What diagnostic test would be helpful in determining the cause of the pain?

62. What does the finding of crepitus on palpation indicate?

Case 4

Harry Garcia, a 59-year-old rock star, is recovering from open-heart surgery performed 2 days ago. Mr. Garcia is alert and oriented × 3. He complains of dyspnea (a lot of people seem to complain about that) and a dry cough. Vital signs reveal a pulse of 104 and a respiratory rate of 32 with a shallow pattern. Mr. Garcia tells you that the difficulty breathing started yesterday and has been gradually getting worse. Auscultation reveals decreased breath sounds in both bases with end-inspiratory crackles.

63. What is the most likely cause of the dyspnea?

64. What diagnostic test is indicated to confirm the diagnosis?

65. What respiratory care intervention(s) are indicated?

What About those Board Exams?

Whole sections of each test are devoted to this subject. The NBRC exam matrix is filled with "assess by inspection," "assess by palpation," "assess by auscultation," and "interview the patient," Even the most conservative estimate would project 12 questions on this subject alone! When you combine this portion of the test with other questions that require you to use assessment information to make decisions, you can expect a minimum of 10% of the Entry-Level Examination to be on the material in Chapter 14! I know you will be looking at this subject more closely later on as you prepare for your boards. For now, let me give you some sample questions.

66. During a chest examination of an intubated patient, the RCP palpates vibrations on exhalation over the upper chest. What action should be taken at this time?
    A. The patient should be given a bronchodilator
    B. The patient should be suctioned
    C. The patient should be given supplemental oxygen
    D. The patient should be placed on mechanical ventilation

67. A patient's medical record indicates that he has orthopnea. Which of the following best describes this condition?
    A. Difficulty breathing at night
    B. Difficulty breathing when upright
    C. Difficulty breathing on exertion
    D. Difficulty breathing when lying down

68. A child is brought to the emergency department for severe respiratory distress. Upon entering the room, the respiratory care practitioner hears a high-pitched sound when the child inhales. This is most likely:
   A. Wheezing
   B. Stridor
   C. Rhonchi
   D. Crackles

69. A respiratory care practitioner is asked to evaluate a patient for oxygen therapy. The RCP notices that the patient is sleepy, but arouses when questioned. This level of consciousness is best described as:
   A. Confused
   B. Obtunded
   C. Stuporous
   D. Lethargic

70. Which of the following breath sounds is most likely to be heard during acute exacerbation of asthma?
   A. Wheezes
   B. Crackles
   C. Stridor
   D. Rhonchi

71. All of the following physical findings are consistent with pneumonia except:
   A. Dull percussion note
   B. Presence of inspiratory crackles
   C. Bronchial breath sounds over the affected area
   D. Bradypnea

72. Which of the following findings suggest that a patient is oriented?
   I. Awareness of the correct date
   II. Ability to correctly state his own name
   III. Awake when you enter the room
   A. I only
   B. I and II only
   C. I and III only
   D. I, II, III

73. During an interview, the patient states he has been coughing up thick, foul-smelling sputum. This finding is most consistent with:
   A. A bacterial infection of the lung
   B. A diagnosis of lung cancer
   C. Obstructive lung disease
   D. Pulmonary tuberculosis

74. An RCP is inspecting the chest of a child with respiratory distress. The practitioner notes that the child has a large, concave depression of the sternum. This finding should be documented as:
   A. Barrel chest
   B. Pectus carinatum
   C. Pectus excavatum
   D. Kyphoscoliosis

75. All of the following physical findings are consistent with complete upper airway obstruction *except*:
   A. Inability to speak
   B. Stridor
   C. Supraclavicular retractions
   D. Flaring of the nostrils

76. While assessing a patient who is dyspneic and tachypneic, an RCP notices a bluish discoloration of the lips and oral mucosa. The practitioner should document which of the following in the medical record?
   A. Presence of cyanosis
   B. Presence of hypoxemia
   C. Presence of increased work of breathing
   D. Presence of orthopnea

Food for Thought

My brain is full, how about yours?

Electrocardiogram and Laboratory Assessment

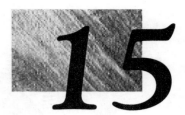

15

In the clinical setting, laboratory assessment directly follows the interview and physical assessment. The NBRC's Clinical Simulation Examinations often follow a similar format. A lot of students struggle with this, but I know you'll be on top of it when you finish these exercises.

A Picture is Worth . . .

I don't see any really new words we haven't already covered, so let's go right to the picture. Label all these heart parts and conduction clues on p. 106.

Heart Parts

1. _____

2. _____

3. _____

4. _____

5. _____

6. _____

7. _____

8. _____

9. _____

Conduction Clues

10. The natural "pacemaker" of the heart is the _____.

11. The _____ conducts impulses through the atria.

12. The _____ carries impulses across the right atrium.

13. _____ is the "backup pacemaker."

14. _____, why not "hers?"

15. _____ carries impulses to the left ventricle.

16. _____ carries impulses to the right ventricle.

17. _____ fingerlike projections penetrate the ventricles.

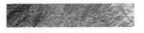

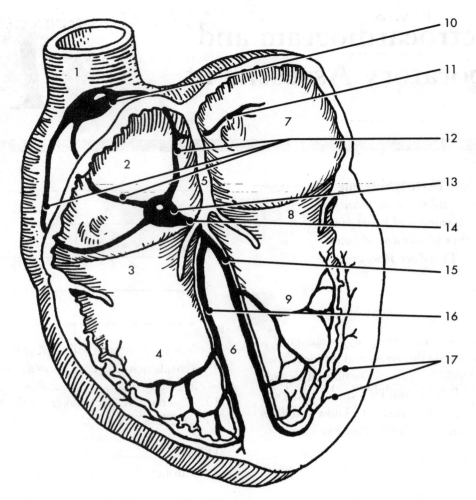

Anatomy of the electrical conduction system of the human heart.

More Pictures?

Let's get the basic identification perfect. Label these four common waves and indicate the event they represent. Space for your answer is provided on the next page.

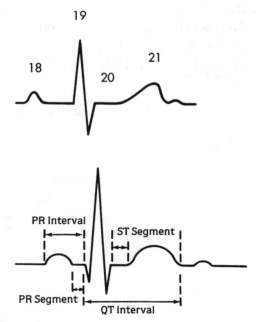

Normal configuration of ECG waves. (From Wilkins RL, Krider SJ, Sheldon, RL: *Clinical assessment in respiratory care*, ed 3, St Louis, 1995, Mosby.)

Wave	Represents
18. _____	_____
19. _____	_____
20. _____	_____
21. _____	_____

22. Where is atrial repolarization?

23. What is the maximum duration of the P-R Interval?

24. What pathological abnormality results in a depressed or elevated S-T segment?

Making Measurements

The ECG paper is made up of tiny boxes or grids that allow you to measure time on the horizontal axis, and millimeters of deflection on the vertical axis. A darker line occurs every five boxes.

25. What is the normal paper speed for an ECG?

26. The time (horizontal) represented by one small box is _____ seconds, and by one large box is _____ seconds.

27. One millivolt of electrical energy will produce a deflection of _____ small boxes or _____ large boxes.

Start at the very beginning . . .

Since many respiratory care practitioners perform ECGs on patients, or take care of monitored patients, you will need to be able to evaluate the rhythms you see to maintain safe patient care. Successful assessors have developed a systematic way of evaluating the electrocardiograph.

 Step 1: Evaluate the rate

You can do this manually, or rely on the electronic data. There are time marks every 3 seconds. So, the number of QRS complexes in 6 seconds can be multiplied by 10. When the rate is regular, you can divide 300 by the number of large boxes between 2 QRS complexes.

Try It, You'll Like It!

Count the rate in the pattern below by both manual methods.

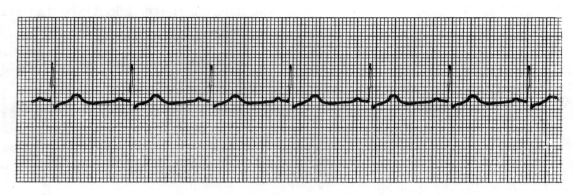

Pattern 1

28. The number of QRS complexes in this 6-second strip is _____. Multiply by 10 to get a rate of _____.

29. There are _____ heavy lines between complex A and complex B. 300 divided by this number is _____. That's the average rate!

Does every P wave have a QRS that follows it? That indicates a sinus rhythm!

30. If the rate is below 60 it is called sinus _____.

31. If the rate is above 100 it is called sinus _____.

 ## Step 2: Measure the PR Interval

Count the number of small boxes between the start of the P wave and the start of the QRS complex. Remember the normal value of less than 0.20 seconds (5 small boxes). A P wave, followed by a QRS but separated by a prolonged P-R Interval, represents a delay at the A-V node. This is called a first-degree heart block. No treatment is usually needed. We just monitor for a worsening block.

Try It, You'll Like It!

Measure the P-R interval in the sample below.

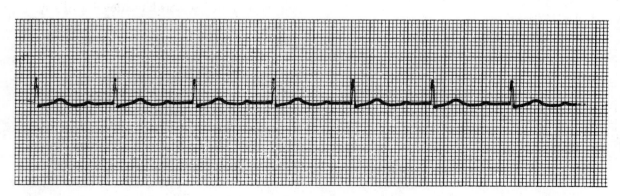

Pattern 2

32. The time from the P wave to the QRS complex is _____ seconds.

33. What arrhythmia does this represent?

Step 3: Evaluate the QRS Complex

The normal QRS is no more than 0.12 seconds (three small boxes) in width. Wide QRS complexes are abnormal and do not result in good ventricular contractions.

Try It, You'll Like It!
Measure the QRS complex in the sample below.

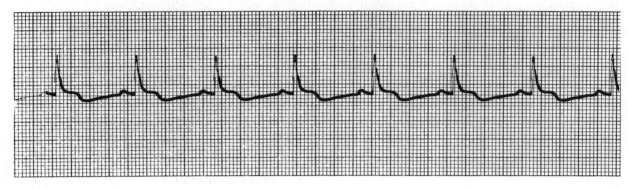

Pattern 3

34. The duration of the QRS complex is _____ seconds.

Step 4: Evaluate the T wave

Normal T waves are upright and rounded. Inverted T waves represent poor blood flow to the heart muscle. Strangely shaped T waves may be caused by hyperkalemia.

35. The T wave in *Pattern 1* is upright/inverted. (Circle one.)

Step 5: Evaluate the ST segment

A normal ST segment is basically flat, or Isoelectric. Elevated or depressed ST segments are bad! They represent oxygenation problems and are seen in conditions such as myocardial infarction (MI). (That's a heart attack.)

Try It, You'll Like It!
Evaluate the ST segment seen below.

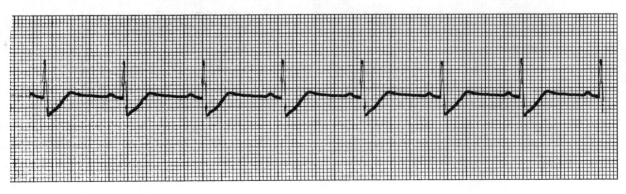

Pattern 4

36. The ST segment in this pattern is elevated/flat/depressed. (Circle one.)

 Step 6: Identify the R to R interval

You are looking for a regular relationship. If the R's are not the same distance apart, you have an irregular rhythm.

Try It, You'll Like It!

Evaluate the R-R interval seen below.

37. The R-R interval in this pattern is regular/irregular. (Circle one.)

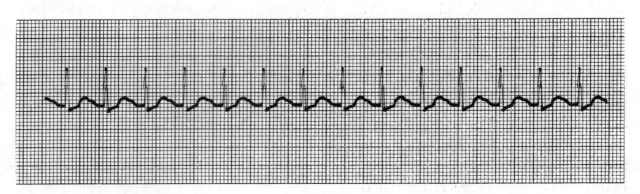

Pattern 5

Recognizing Arrhythmias

Now that you have the basic idea, let's take a look at the major arrhythmias that you will encounter. This is pattern recognition, so look for the "picture" each rhythm shows.

Normal sinus rhythm

Upright P wave. Normal PR interval. Each P is followed by a normal QRS. R-R intervals are regular and the rate is between 60-100 beats/min. No treatment is needed for this rhythm!

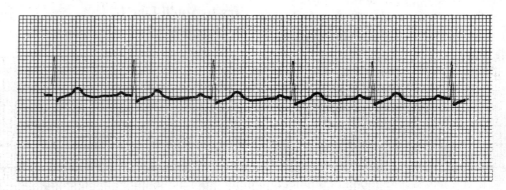

Pattern 6

Sinus bradycardia

Upright P wave. Normal PR interval. Each P is followed by a normal QRS. R-R intervals are regular, *but the rate is less than 60*. This is *absolute bradycardia*. It is only a problem if the blood pressure drops. You might see this rhythm during suctioning as a result of vagal stimulation. Stop suctioning! Intravenous atropine is a treatment for this arrhythmia.

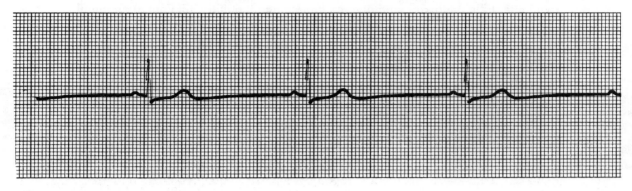

Pattern 7

Sinus tachycardia

Upright P wave. Short PR interval. Each P is followed by a normal QRS. R-R intervals are regular, *but the rate is over 100!* This is *sinus tachycardia*. Tachycardia is the first sign of hypoxemia in most patients. Consider whether you are doing something to cause it, such as suctioning. Look back at the pattern 5 to see an example of sinus tachycardia.

First-degree heart block

Upright P wave. *Prolonged* PR interval. Each P is followed by a normal QRS. R-R intervals are regular. Only a problem if signs and symptoms such as low BP, chest pain, and so on come with it. May be caused by drugs or MI. Look back at the pattern 2 to see an example of a first-degree block.

Second-degree heart block

Our block is moving lower down the conduction pathway. Not good! There are two types.

Second-degree Type I

This one is called Wenckeback or Mobitz Type I. The P waves have a progressively prolonged transmission (prolonged P-R interval) followed by a P with no QRS. There is usually a repeated pattern, for example, three P's and one lost QRS.

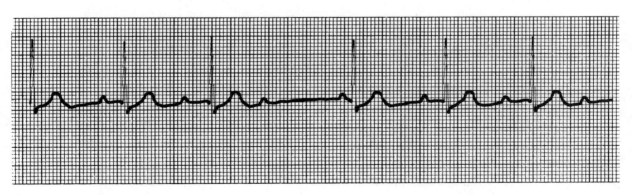

Pattern 8

Second-degree Type II

Mobitz Type II. Definitely not a good sign. This block is worse. You will see some P's conducted (followed by a QRS) and some P's with no QRS following.

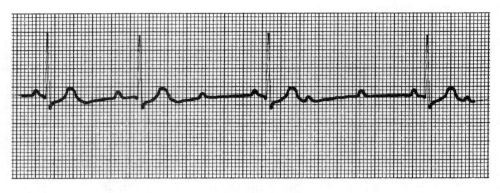

Pattern 9

Third-degree block

Also called complete heart block, this rhythm is definitely life-threatening. No impulses from the SA node are conducted. Since the ventricles have their own intrinsic rate, you will see the atria paced by the SA node (P waves) and the ventricles (QRS) pacing themselves. These QRS complexes are often wide. Blood pressure is poor, and an artificial pacemaker is needed.

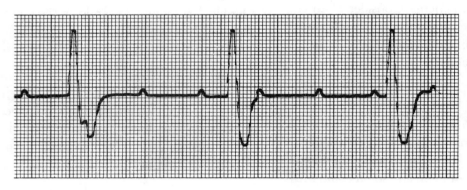

Pattern 10

A little story

An easy way to keep the blocks straight is a love story gone wrong.

A couple gets married. At first, you have a normal sinus rhythm. She (P) is at home, and he (QRS) comes home on time (Pattern 11, A). After a while, he is spending more time with his secretary after work. She (P) is at home, he is coming home late. A first-degree block (Pattern 11, B). Eventually, while she (P) is at home, he (QRS) comes home later, then later, and one night, he does not come home (missed QRS)! A second-degree type one block (Pattern 11, C). She (P) is rightfully furious, and tells him to mend his ways or else. He (QRS) starts coming home on time, but then goes back to his old ways and does not come home. A second-degree type two block (Pattern 11, D). After this final insult, she (P) is at home, and he (QRS) is at home, but they are sleeping in separate bedrooms and have nothing to do with each other. Third-degree block! (Pattern 11, E.) A pacemaker (or a divorce lawyer) is needed in this situation.

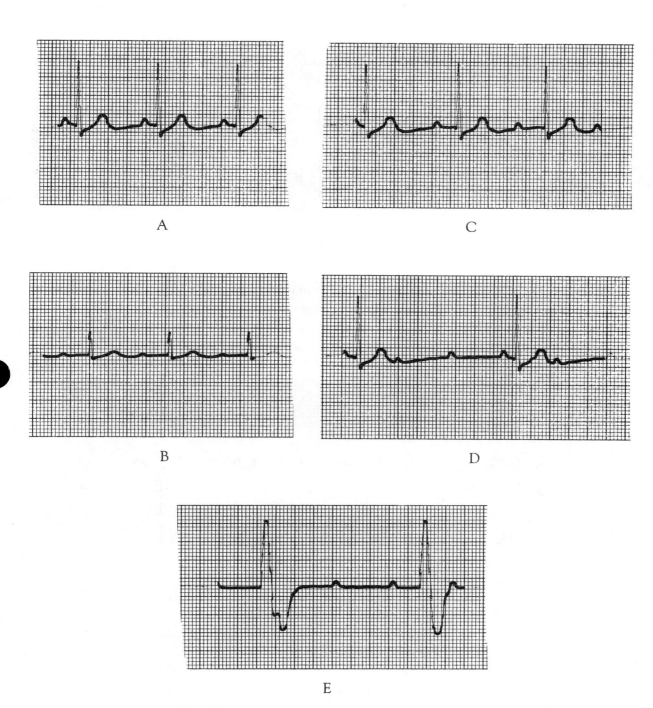

A

C

B

D

E

Pattern 11

Atrial arrhythmias

Atrial fibrillation is an erratic quivering of the atria that does not deliver a good preload to the ventricles. Clots may also form in the atria. Sometimes the ventricle responds to fibrillation with a rapid rate as well. No P wave is seen, but the QRS probably looks OK. Drugs (such as digitalis) or electrical treatments are used. (Notice the R-R intervals.)

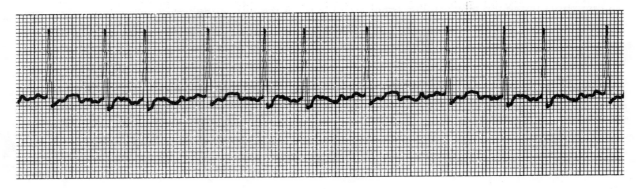

Pattern 12

Atrial flutter is a very rapid (250) atrial rate. You can spot it every time by noting the "sawtooth" or "picket fence" pattern of the atrial discharge. Drug or electrical treatments are used.

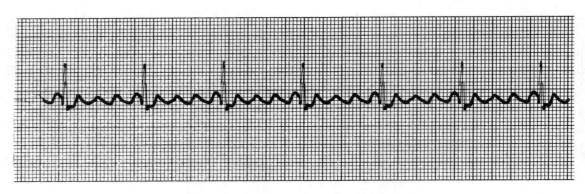

Pattern 13

Premature Ventricular Contractions

You will want to notice these abnormal QRS complexes, because they are often caused by hypoxemia. In other words, if you are suctioning and the patient experiences premature ventricular contractions (PVCs), STOP! Oxygenate the patient. There are other causes, such as stress, caffeine, and nicotine. Intravenous lidocaine is the therapy for too many PVCs (Usually more than 6 per minute).

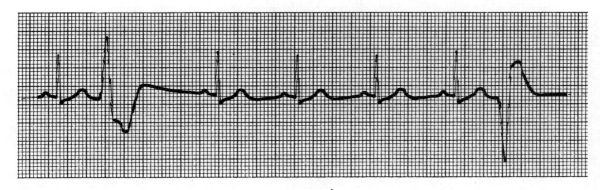

Pattern 14

Ventricular Tachycardia

Tachycardia, of course, is a rate above 100. But this rhythm shows no P waves, wide QRS, and does not usually have a pulse. *This is life threatening!* Stop, call for help, check for a pulse, and act appropriately. Lidocaine or defibrillation is needed.

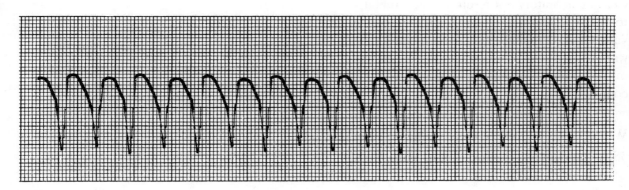

Pattern 15

Ventricular Fibrillation

The only rhythm worse than this is a flatline (asystole). There is no pulse, cardiac output, or blood pressure. Only defibrillation will really help, but you can do CPR and give oxygen and drugs as well.

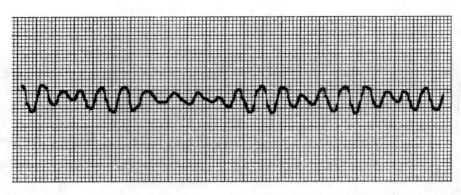

Pattern 16

Practice recognizing the important arrhythmias. After a while, these basic patterns will be easy to spot, just like a Van Gogh painting, and you won't have to think too hard!

Labba Dabba Doo!

Certain laboratory test results are very useful to the RCP. You will need to learn the normal values and what abnormal results mean if you want to pass your boards, or get the big picture in the hospital. Let's start with complete blood counts.

White

38. What does a large elevation in white blood count (WBC) suggest?

    A.

    B.

39. Name three common causes of low WBC.

    A. _____

    B. _____

    C. _____

40. What specific type of WBC is elevated in bacterial pneumonia? Viral?

Red

41. What term describes a low red blood count (RBC)? What is the treatment for this disorder?

42. What is a normal hemoglobin level and why are RCPs especially interested in hemoglobin levels?

43. What blood abnormality is caused by chronic hypoxemia?

44. Prior to performing an ABG you would be wise to check what two values?

    A. _____

    B. _____

Lytes, Camera, Action

RCPs are interested in electrolyte values because they affect acid-base balance and muscle function. We covered electrolytes in Chapter 11. See how much you remember.

45. What is the normal range for serum potassium?

46. Why is potassium of particular interest to patients being weaned from mechanical ventilation?

47. What value on the venous chemistry panel represents bicarbonate?

48. What other test is indicated when a chemistry panel shows abnormal anion gap?

49. What are the two tests that together indicate renal function?

A. _____

B. _____

Enzymes

Enzymes are present everywhere in the body. They make reactions happen. (remember carbonic anhydrase?). Specific enzymes are released when tissues are damaged. Myocardial infarction is a good example.

50. Name the two common liver enzymes that might be elevated in patients with hepatitis. Give the old names (what most people remember, like your old teachers!) and the new names.

	Old	New
A.	_____	_____
B.	_____	_____

51. What specific enzyme found only in the heart is suggestive of a myocardial infarction?

Sputum is our Bread and Butter!

You will probably be asked to obtain many sputum specimens during your career. Sputum samples are needed when lung infections are suspected. Gram stain, culture, and sensitivity are almost always performed, but only if you get the right stuff!

52. Why would the laboratory reject your sputum specimen?

53. What is the purpose of growing the bacteria on a culture plate?

Case Studies

Case 1

Joan, a student, is suctioning a patient orally with a tonsil suction. The monitor shows sinus bradycardia. Blood pressure is falling. Alarms are sounding.

54. What should Joan do?

55. What physiological mechanism was responsible for the drop in rate?

Case 2

Nate, a student, is suctioning a patient via the endotracheal tube. The monitor shows sinus tachycardia with frequent PVCs. Alarms are sounding. The patient is agitated.

56. What should Nate do?

57. What physiological mechanism was responsible for the increased rate and arrhythmias?

Case 3

While performing a ventilator check on a patient in the coronary care unit, Jeff, a student, observes that the rhythm on the monitor has changed from atrial fibrillation to ventricular fibrillation.

58. What should Jeff do first?

59. Name at least three responses indicated to treat this rhythm.
   A. _____
   B. _____
   C. _____

What About Those Board Exams?

Actual pictures of ECG rhythms usually appear in the Clinical Simulation Exam and occasionally on the other written exams. Cardioversion and defibrillation are on the Written Registry as well. You will need to supplement the text with more information to understand these subjects. The Advanced Cardiac Life Support material from the American Heart Association is a good resource. The Entry-Level Exam doesn't have too much on the heart, only the basics. Here are some sample questions from Chapter 15 that you might run into.

60. Sputum culture and sensitivity would be indicated for which of the following conditions?
   A. ST segment elevation
   B. Pleural effusion
   C. Pneumothorax
   D. Bronchitis

61. A patient presents in the emergency room with vomiting. Blood gas results reveal a metabolic alkalosis. Based on this information, you would also suggest
   A. A stat chest radiograph
   B. Electrolyte analysis
   C. Blood cultures
   D. Urinalysis

62. While receiving a nebulized bronchodilator treatment in the telemetry unit, a patient experiences an episode of pulseless ventricular tachycardia. The immediate treatment of this rhythm is
   A. Administration of oxygen
   B. Administration of intravenous epinephrine
   C. Defibrillation
   D. Placement of a chest tube

Food for Thought

You want more? Try this.

63. A young adult patient presents with symptoms of hypoxemia and signs of pneumonia. What are several possible reasons the white blood count is severely depressed?

64. What type of individual might have absolute bradycardia without symptoms and would not need any treatment?

Analysis and Monitoring of Gas Exchange

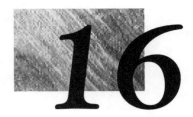

16

"Vision is the art of seeing the invisible."
Jonathan Swift

Analyzing and monitoring gas exchange is one of the most important areas of the respiratory care profession. In Chapter 12 we talked about interpreting the acid-base balance of arterial blood gases. Naturally, there's more to it than that. Chapter 16 will cover the equipment used to analyze blood and much more. For example, there are noninvasive methods to monitor gas exchange, such as capnometry and pulse oximetry. So, whether you're talking about clinical practice or thinking about credentialing examinations, you're going to need a firm grasp on this slippery subject.

Life's a Gas

You'll have to learn the specialized terminology of invasive and noninvasive monitoring if you want to get the most mileage out of this material. Solve the crossword puzzle on p. 122 to test your understanding of the key terms in Chapter 16.

First Things First . . .

First, you have to make a choice between analysis and monitoring. Analysis usually means obtaining a sample of body fluid and putting it in some type of lab analyzer to get results. Properly done, these measurements have a high degree of accuracy. Unfortunately, they are like a snapshot of a single event. Monitoring is usually done at the bedside and is a continuous process, much like watching a video. Next, you have a choice of invasive or noninvasive techniques. Invasive techniques are probably more accurate, but they also have a greater risk of harm to the patient. They are a good way to establish a baseline. Noninvasive methods are often used for monitoring, and are especially useful when used together with invasive techniques. Conclusion? No one method is best. Your role as a clinician is to get the right balance. My role is to help you figure out how to do that!

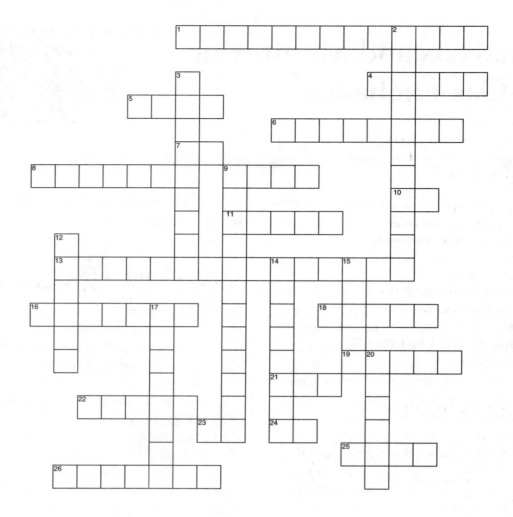

ACROSS

1. Oxygen analyzer that measures the flow of electrons between negative and positively charged poles.
4. _____ of care, testing blood at the bedside instead of in the lab.
5. Systematic errors in measurement.
6. Artery in the arm that's not your first choice.
7. _____ vivo, inside the body.
8. Big artery in the groin that is used for drawing blood when other choices fail.
9. Allen's, for example.
10. _____ vivo, outside the body.
11. Never do this with a used needle.
13. Pulse oximeters use this principle to detect arterial pulsation.

16. Device that provides ongoing information to clinicians.
18. Oxygen analyzing electrode.
19. Preanalytical ones, bubble in sample for example.
21. _____ invasive monitoring doesn't hurt!
22. Modify this test and perform before radial puncture.
23. Quality control.
24. Oximeter used to measure carbon monoxide in the blood.
25. Point-of-_____: method of testing blood at the bedside.
26. Measure blood values in the laboratory.

Continues.

DOWN

2. External quality control testing program.
3. Alternative to arterial sampling in infants.
9. Clot buster.
12. Sensor that works on optical detection instead of electrochemical properties.
14. Oxygen analyzer that doesn't use a battery.
15. Non-invasive oximeter commonly used to measure hemoglobin's saturation with oxygen.
17. Determine the saturation of hemoglobin with a photoelectric device.
20. Artery of choice for puncture or cannulation.

3. Explain the differences between the two types of analyzers in terms of principle of operation and response time.

4. Describe the two-step process for calibrating an oxygen analyzer.

Meet the Objectives

You've read the chapter, and now you're feeling a little overwhelmed. I don't blame you! Answer the following questions and you will get a grip on the good stuff.

1. In your own words, explain how an electro-chemical analyzer converts the number of oxygen molecules (PO_2) into a measurable reading.

5. What is the gold standard of gas exchange analysis? What does this mean?

6. List four reasons why the radial artery is the preferred site for ABG sampling.
   A. _____
   B. _____
   C. _____
   D. _____

2. There are two common types of electro-chemical analyzers. Name them.
   A. _____
   B. _____

7. Describe the modified Allen test and the definition of a positive result.

8. Name four other sites you can use if the radial artery is unavailable or has a poor pulse.
   A. _____
   B. _____
   C. _____
   D. _____

9. How long should you wait after changing the FIO_2 before performing an ABG on a patient with healthy lungs? What about a patient with COPD?

10. What technique can help prevent hyperventilation from pain or anxiety from altering the sample results?

11. The AARC's ABG sampling guidelines describe several medications that may result in prolonged bleeding. These are anticoagulants (clot preventors) and thrombolytics (clot busters). Give two examples of each of these classes of drugs.
    A. Anticoagulants
       1. _____
       2. _____
    B. Thrombolytics
       1. _____
       2. _____

12. Name the four things you can do to avoid most pre-analytical sampling errors.
    A. _____
    B. _____
    C. _____
    D. _____

13. What precaution should you take when handling any laboratory specimen?

14. What are the three primary parameters measured by a blood gas analyzer?
    A. _____
    B. _____
    C. _____

15. If you wanted to measure actual hemoglobin saturation, what type of analyzer would be needed?

16. What is the range of accuracy for most commercially available pulse oximeters?

      B. Control media

      C. Proficiency testing

17. Describe three noninvasive ways you can determine the reliability of a pulse oximeter at the bedside.
    A. _____
    B. _____
    C. _____

18. According to the AARC guidelines, what action should you take to verify the results when pulse oximetry is unreliable or does not confirm suspicions about the patient's clinical state?

20. In what patient population is capillary sampling appropriate?

21. What are the two most common errors committed during capillary sampling?
    A. _____
    B. _____

19. Describe the three main quality assurance procedures used to maintain consistently accurate blood gas results.
    A. Automated calibration

22. Explain what variables are reliable and unreliable in capillary sampling as compared with arterial sampling.

23. What are the primary advantages and disadvantages of transcutaneous gas monitoring over arterial sampling?
    A. Advantages

    B. Disadvantages

24. When would you choose a pulse oximeter over a transcutaneous monitor for monitoring an infant's oxygenation status?

25. When would the transcutaneous monitor be preferred over the pulse oximeter?

26. Describe proper placement of a capnometer sampling chamber or adaptor for a patient who is being mechanically ventilated.

27. What are the normal values for end-tidal CO_2 for healthy individuals and how do they compare to arterial CO_2?

28. An end-tidal CO_2 of zero may indicate a serious problem. Name two life-threatening causes of a zero value for end-tidal CO_2.
    A. _____
    B. _____

29. While performing end-tidal CO_2 measurements, you notice that the baseline does not return to zero on inspiration. Interpret this result.

30. While performing end-tidal CO_2 measurements, you notice that no real plateau is reached. Give two possible interpretations of this result.

A. _____

B. _____

Chapter Highlights

The questions you just answered covered many of the important points; however, this chapter was really crammed with details. Here are a few more questions that highlight some of the main points we haven't already covered.

31. What are the three most common causes of oxygen analyzer malfunctions?

A. _____

B. _____

C. _____

32. Blood gases provide more information than other methods of gas exchange analysis. What are the three general areas that a blood gas helps to assess?

A. _____

B. _____

C. _____

33. What is the maximum ideal time between ABG sampling and analysis?

34. What are the two primary benefits and hazards of indwelling peripheral arterial lines?

A. Benefits

1. _____

2. _____

B. Hazards

1. _____

2. _____

35. What is the point of care testing and what are the potential benefits of this method of testing blood samples?

36. What is the difference between capnography and capnometry?

Case Studies

Now that you have the information, let's see if you can apply it to the following scenarios.

Case 1

Biff Hoser, a 34-year-old firefighter, is brought to the emergency room for treatment of smoke inhalation while fighting a house fire. Heart rate is 126, respirations are 28 and labored. SpO_2 is 100% on 6 L by nasal cannula. Blood pressure is 145/90. Breath sounds are coarse with inspiratory crackles in both bases. Biff's face is smudged with soot and he is coughing up sputum with black specks in it.

37. What clinical signs of hypoxemia does Mr. Hoser display?

38. Explain why the pulse oximeter is reading 100% in spite of these signs.

39. What is the most probable cause of the hypoxemia?

40. What blood test would you recommend to confirm your suspicions?

Case 2

Little Maggie Simmons is a premature infant. She is wearing supplemental oxygen. Her doctor is concerned about the effects of hyperoxia on her lungs and eyes. Maggie is being monitored by a pulse oximeter, which shows a saturation of 100%.

41. What range of pO_2 is possible with an SpO_2 of 100%?

42. What type of noninvasive monitoring would you recommend in this situation?

Case 3

Grandpa Miller is an elderly patient admitted for acute exacerbation of his long-standing COPD. He is wearing a nasal cannula at 2 L/min.

43. What is the simplest way to quickly assess his oxygenation status?

44. Why would you recommend an ABG for this patient?

Case 4

Jimmy Dornor was riding his motorcycle without a helmet when he crashed. Now he has a head injury and is being mechanically ventilated. His doctor asks you to make recommendations regarding monitoring his gas exchange.

45. What are the advantages of using capnometry to monitor CO_2 in this situation?

46. Where would you place the capnometer probe in the ventilator circuit?

47. During monitoring, you notice that the capnograph does not return to "0" when Jimmy inhales. What does this indicate?

48. A few minutes later Jimmy's exhaled CO_2 levels begin to rise. So does his blood pressure. Jimmy becomes agitated. What action would you take?

49. Why do rising CO_2 levels cause increases in ICP?

In some centers patients are not hyperventilated because injured areas of the brain may already have advanced perfusion.

What About Those Board Exams?

The NBRC has a strong affinity for monitoring gas exchange. So should you! You will find pulse oximeters and oxygen analyzers on the Entry-Level Exam. Capnography and transcutaneous monitoring go into the Registry Exams. So do mixed venous sampling, co-oximetry, blood gas analyzers, and quality control. Here's a baker's dozen of what you can expect.

50. An RCP is preparing to perform pulse oximetry. Which of the following would be LEAST beneficial for assessing accuracy of the device?
   A. Checking the capillary refill time
   B. Assessing skin color and temperature
   C. Performing an Allen test on the patient
   D. Assessing pulse rate

51. Which of the following would you perform after obtaining an arterial blood gas sample?
    I. Remove air bubbles from the sample
    II. Mix the sample by rotating the syringe
    III. Maintain site pressure for at least one minute
    IV. Add heparin to the sample
    A. I only
    B. I, II only
    C. I, II, III only
    D. I, II, III, IV only

52. A pulse oximeter is being used to monitor a patient who was rescued from a fire. The SpO_2 is 90%; however, the patient is unconscious and shows signs of respiratory distress. What additional test should the RCP recommend?
    A. CT scan
    B. Electrolyte measurement
    C. Co-oximetry
    D. Hemoglobin and hematocrit levels

53. A polarographic oxygen analyzer fails to calibrate when exposed to 100% oxygen. The first action the RCP should take would be to:
    A. Replace the battery
    B. Replace the membrane
    C. Replace the fuel cell
    D. Try another oxygen source

54. An infant is placed on a transcutaneous oxygen monitor. The $tcPO_2$ is reading 40 mm Hg less than the PaO_2 obtained from an arterial sample. All of the following could cause this problem *except*:
    A. Improper calibration of the transcutaneous electrode
    B. Room air contamination of the transcutaneous electrode
    C. Inadequate heating of the skin at the electrode site
    D. Inadequate perfusion of the skin at the electrode site

55. Which of the following analyzers is calibrated to a value of zero when exposed to room air?
    A. Clark electrode
    B. Galvanic oxygen analyzer
    C. Capnometer
    D. Geisler-type nitrogen analyzer

56. Which of the following would be most useful in assessing proper tube placement following endotracheal intubation?
    A. Transcutaneous monitoring
    B. Arterial blood gas analysis
    C. Pulse oximetry
    D. End-tidal CO_2 monitoring

57. Complications of arterial puncture include all of the following *except*:
    A. Pulmonary embolus
    B. Hematoma
    C. Infection
    D. Nerve damage

58. A galvanic oxygen analyzer is placed in the ventilator system to continuously measure the delivered FIO_2. The set FIO_2 is 40%; however, the analyzer is reading 32%. Which of the following is the most likely cause of this discrepancy?
    A. The batteries in the analyzer need to be changed
    B. The electrode membrane has water condensation on its surface
    C. The analyzer needs to be calibrated
    D. The ventilator requires servicing

59. Which of the following will affect the accuracy of pulse oximeter measurements?
    I. Increased bilirubin levels
    II. Decreased hematocrit levels
    III. Dark skin pigmentation
    IV. Exposure to sunlight
    A. I, II only
    B. II, III only
    C. III, IV only
    D. II, III, IV only

60. An arterial blood gas is drawn from a patient who is breathing room air. Analysis reveals the following results: pH, 7.45; $PaCO_2$, 35 mm Hg; PaO_2, 155 mm Hg. Which of the following best explains these results?
   A. Too much heparin was added to the sample
   B. An air bubble has contaminated the sample
   C. Analysis of the sample was delayed for more than 60 minutes
   D. The patient was hyperventilating during the puncture

61. Which of the following sites would be the best for continuous monitoring of exhaled CO_2 during mechanical ventilation?
   A. Exhalation valve
   B. Inspiratory side of the ventilator circuit
   C. Expiratory side of the ventilator circuit
   D. Endotracheal tube connector

62. Which of the following is true concerning the use of a transcutaneous PO_2 monitor?
   A. $tcPO_2$ should be checked with arterial blood samples
   B. The skin temperature control should be maintained at 37° Celsius
   C. The site should be changed every 24 hours
   D. The low calibration point is determined using room air

Food for Thought

63. How would you modify your technique if you had to perform ABGs on a patient receiving anticoagulants?

64. What problems may occur as a result of icing ABG samples?

65. Switching probes from one brand of pulse oximeter to another is strongly discouraged. What could happen if you do this?

66. Why can you use a capnometer during CPR but not a pulse oximeter?

Pulmonary Function Testing

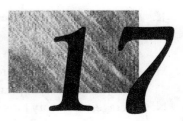

17

> "Most teachers would
> continue to lecture on
> navigation while the ship
> is going down."
> **James Boren**

Remember when you were a child, and blowing out those candles on your birthday cake was an exciting but difficult task? That was your first pulmonary function test. If you could blow out the candles, you passed and got your wish. I wish everybody liked PFTs as much as I do, but I admit it is a tough subject. In the last few years lung testing has taken on even greater importance. Multiskilling, assessment-based protocols, increasing asthma concerns, disability and legal issues, and a strong focus on the credentialing examinations are just a few reasons for the resurgence of interest in the science of diagnosing and quantifying pulmonary disorders.

Initially . . .

A quick glance at the Key Terms in Chapter 17 should leave you breathless with desire (or despair) to know what all those abbreviations mean. In fact, it would be pretty difficult to have a conversation with a pulmonary technologist without speaking in acronyms. Do not pass go until you can match the right definitions and terms or symbols.

_____ 1. DL
_____ 2. ERV
_____ 3. VT
_____ 4. IRV
_____ 5. RV
_____ 6. TLC
_____ 7. VC
_____ 8. IC
_____ 9. FRC
_____ 10. MVV
_____ 11. FVC
_____ 12. PEFR
_____ 13. $FEF_{200-1200}$
_____ 14. FEV_1
_____ 15. $FEF_{25\%-75\%}$
_____ 16. FEV_1/FVC

A. Volume inspired with a normal breath
B. Greatest amount of air you can breathe in 12 to 15 seconds
C. Largest amount of air the lungs can hold
D. Fastest flow rate generated at the very beginning of forced exhalation
E. Milliliters of gas the lung can transfer to the blood
F. Amount of air you can exhale after a maximum inspiration
G. Ratio of volume exhaled in 1 second to total volume exhaled
H. Average expiratory flow during the early part of forced exhalation
I. Amount of air you can inhale after a normal exhalation
J. Amount of air you can inhale after a normal inspiration

K. Air left in the lungs after a maximum exhalation

L. Air left in the lungs after a normal exhalation

M. Amount of air you can forcefully exhale after a maximum inspiration

N. Average expiratory flow during the middle part of forced exhalation

O. Volume of air you can forcefully exhale in 1 second

P. Amount of air you can exhale after a normal exhalation

First Things First . . .

As if learning all those acronyms wasn't enough, we can't really go on until you put the four lung volumes and four lung capacities into perspective with their normal values in a healthy adult. Use the box I've provided below. *Memorize this information! It will serve you well on your board exams!*

17. Fill in the names and normal values that go with each letter in the box.

Volume/Capacity	Value
A. _____	_____
B. _____	_____
C. _____	_____
D. _____	_____
E. _____	_____
F. _____	_____
G. _____	_____
H. _____	_____

Now see if you can draw the box and fill in the values on a separate sheet of paper without looking. Check your answers. Do this until you have it absolutely wired!

Meet the Objectives

Answer these questions to find out if you have grasped the important points for each area of lung testing.

Lung Volumes

Lung volume measurement is an important adjunct to spirometry and helps quantify and determine a diagnosis of restriction or obstruction. Specialized equipment is needed to perform these tests.

18. Which volumes cannot be measured with a spirometer?

19. Which capacities cannot be measured with a spirometer?

20. Name the three tests used to determine the volumes and capacities that can't be measured.
    A. _____
    B. _____
    C. _____

21. What is thoracic gas volume?

22. How will volumes or capacities for a patient with air trapping obtained by helium dilution or nitrogen washout differ from those obtained with a body plethysmograph?

23. What effect will an air leak have on the values obtained by helium dilution or nitrogen washout?

Spirometry

Spirometry is the most commonly performed pulmonary function test, and vital capacity (or Forced Vital Capacity [FVC]) is the most commonly obtained value. Many types of spirometers exist, but any one that meets the standards and is working properly can be used.

24. What four variables are used to calculate normal values for spirometry?
    A. _____
    B. _____
    C. _____
    D. _____

25. What is meant by an "acceptable" FVC and what is the minimum number of acceptable FVC maneuvers?
    A. Duration
    B. Variance of two best FVCs
    C. Satisfactory start
    D. Minimum number

26. Which FVC should you report? Which FEV$_1$?
    A. FVC

    B. FEV$_1$

27. Which flow rate is the greatest?

28. Which flow rate represents large airways?

29. Which flow rate represents the middle range?

30. A spirometer is considered accurate if the volume is verified to be within what percentage of a known value?

31. What device is used to verify the volume of a spirometer?

32. What is the normal value for MVV? How is this test performed?

Diffusion

Diffusing capacity represents the ability of the lung to transfer gas into the blood. This test requires breathing a special gas mixture.

33. What gas is usually used to measure the lung's ability to transfer gas to the blood?

34. What other special gas is used in this test? Why?

35. What blood test results are needed to ensure accuracy of diffusion studies?

Interpretation Fundamentals

In a minute, we'll go to our case studies and board exam questions to test your ability to put all the information together. First, see if you have the basic ideas straight.

36. What are the two major categories of pulmonary disease classification? Fill in the chart below to compare the effects of each category. (Hint: see Table 17-3!)
    A.
    1. Anatomy
       _____
       _____
    2. Phase
       _____
       _____
    3. Pathophysiology
       _____
       _____
    4. Measure
       _____
       _____

B.
    1. Anatomy
       _____
       _____
    2. Phase
       _____
       _____
    3. Pathophysiology
       _____
       _____
    4. Measure
       _____
       _____

37. Fill in the corresponding percent of predicted for the degrees of impairment.

Degree of Impairment	%Predicted
A. Normal	_____
B. Mild	_____
C. Moderate	_____
D. Severe	_____

38. The original normal values for pulmonary functions were probably based on a 6 ft, 20-year-old white male. How are normal values corrected for non-whites?

39. Compare the FEV_1/FVC ratios you would see in normal, obstructed, and restricted patients.
    A. Normal

    B. Obstructed

    C. Restricted

Case Studies

Now that you have the information, let's see if you can apply it to the following scenarios. Use the algorithm on page 398 (Fig. 17-17), until you have the basics down pat.

Case 1

Spirometry is performed on Wendy Wheezer, a 24-year-old who complains of a "tight chest" and cough. Simple spirometry shows:

Test	Actual	Predicted	%Predicted
FVC	3.2 L	4.0L	80%
FEV_1	1.6 L	3.2L	50%
FEV_1/FVC	50%	70%	

40. Interpretation?

41. What other test should be performed in light of the results and the clinical information?

Case 2

Jim is a 34-year-old RCP. His instructor requires him to undergo pulmonary function testing as part of a course. Here are the results.

Test	Actual	Predicted	%Predicted
FVC	3.9 L	4.8 L	81%
FEV_1	3.1 L	4.1 L	76%
FEV_1/FVC	79%	70%	

42. Interpretation?

43. What patient history would be helpful in interpreting these results?

Case 3

Mr. A.B. Stosis is a 60-year-old shipyard worker. He complains of dyspnea on exertion and dry cough. Here are his spirometry results:

Test	Actual	Predicted	%Predicted
FVC	2.0 L	4.0 L	50%
FEV_1	1.5 L	3.4 L	44%
FEV_1/FVC	75%	70%	

44. Interpretation?

45. What additional tests would be helpful?

46. What additional history would be helpful?

Case 4

Miss D. Zeeze presents in her doctor's office complaining of dyspnea on exertion. Spirometry and lung volume results show:

Test	Actual	Predicted	%Predicted
FVC	1.5 L	3.0 L	50%
FEV_1	.75 L	2.5 L	30%
FEV_1/FVC	50%	70%	
TLC	2.6 L	3.8 L	68%

47. Interpretation?

48. What additional history would be helpful?

Case 5

Paul Puffer is a 70-year-old male with a 100 pack-year smoking history. He complains of a dry cough and dyspnea on exertion. Results of lung tests:

Test	Actual	Predicted	%Predicted
FVC	2.9 L	4.4 L	65%
FEV_1	1.3 L	3.7 L	35%
FEV_1/FVC	59%	70%	
TLC	6.6 L	5.5	120%
FRC	4.5 L	2.2	
RV	3.7 L	1.1 L	
DLCO	16	25	64%

49. Interpretation (be complete!)

50. What disease state do the lung volumes and history suggest?

51. Why is the vital capacity lower than predicted?

There are lots more case studies in Chapter 17 in your textbook!

What About Those Board Exams?

I estimate that up to 10% of the Written Registry exam questions are on the subject of pulmonary function testing! That could be the difference between passing and. . .

The Entry-Level Examination matrix says: "Perform and interpret the results of spirometry before/and after bronchodilator." The matrix goes on to mention performing and/or interpreting FEV_1 and pulmonary function values. Try your hand at some questions in the NBRC style.

52. Which of the following tests would be helpful in assessing the effects on cigarette smoking on the smaller airways?
    A. FVC
    B. FEF_{25-75}
    C. FEV_1
    D. $FEF_{200-1200}$

53. A patient's physician asks you to recommend a pulmonary function test to help assess the effects of a possible tumor in the trachea. Which of the following would you recommend?
    A. Spirometry with volume-time curves
    B. Spirometry before and after bronchodilator
    C. Lung volume studies via nitrogen washout
    D. Spirometry with flow-volume loops

54. A pulmonary function technologist tests a spirometer by injecting 3.0 L of air from a large-volume syringe. The spirometer measures a result of 2.94 L. Which of the following is true regarding this situation?
    A. The results are within normal limits
    B. The spirometer has a leak
    C. The air was injected too slowly
    D. The BTPS corrections were not made properly

55. Which of the following values is incorrectly calculated?

Test	Actual	Predicted	%Predicted
FVC	4.4 L	4.8 L	92%
FEV_1	3.5 L	4.1 L	80%
FEV_1/FVC	80%	70%	
TLC	5.2 L	5.5	
FRC	2.0 L	2.4	
ERV	1.2 L	1.2 L	
RV	1.0 L	1.2 L	

    I. TLC   A. I, II
    II. FVC   B. I, IV
    III. FRC   C. II, III
    IV. RV   D. II, IV

56. Which of the following pulmonary measurements is usually the smallest?
    A. Inspiratory capacity
    B. Vital capacity
    C. Functional residual capacity
    D. Total lung capacity

57. The following results were obtained from spirometry of an adult female smoker with chronic bronchitis. What is the correct interpretation?

Test	Actual	Predicted	%Predicted
FVC	4.2 L	4.8 L	88%
FEV_1	2.9 L	4.1 L	71%
FEV_1/FVC	69%	70%	

    A. Results indicate a mild diffusion defect
    B. Results are within the normal range
    C. A mixed obstructive/restrictive defect is present
    D. Results show obstructive lung disease

58. What percent increase in forced spirometric volumes or flow rates after a bronchodilator is administered is the *minimum* indication that reversible airway obstruction is present?
    A. 5%
    B. 10%
    C. 15%
    D. 20%

59. Which of the following can be measured during spirometric testing?
    A. Residual volume
    B. Tidal volume
    C. Total lung capacity
    D. Functional residual capacity

60. An increased total lung capacity combined with a decreased diffusing capacity are strongly indicative of which of the following conditions?
    A. Emphysema
    B. Pneumonia
    C. Pulmonary fibrosis
    D. Pleural effusion

Food for Thought

Of course there is more! We have just scratched the surface of a complex area of testing. Entire textbooks are devoted to pulmonary function testing! Here are a few more questions to fill up the corners of your brain.

61. What effect does smoking have on the results of a diffusion test? Why?

62. What lung volume or capacity is useful in predicting normal values for incentive spirometry?

63. Calculate your normal values for FVC, FEV_1, and FEF_{25-75} using Fig. 17-13 in Egan. Do it using the nomogram and the regression equation.

	FVC	FEV_1	FEF_{25-75}
A. Nomogram	_____	_____	_____
B. Equation	_____	_____	_____

Show your work for the regression equation (be sure to *use* a calculator!)
Formula: _____
Calculation: _____

A Synopsis of Thoracic Imaging: Chest X-ray, CT, and MRI

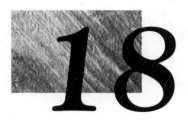

> "In the field of
> observation, chance
> favors the prepared mind."
> L. Pasteur

Thoracic imaging provides a window for the practitioner to view structures and events inside the chest that we normally cannot see. The chest radiograph is especially important to the respiratory care practitioner for the purpose of confirming placement of tubes, or diagnosis of certain conditions such as pneumothorax. You should also understand the usefulness other common imaging techniques you will encounter in clinical practice, such at computed tomography and magnetic resonance imaging.

Word Wizard

The chest _____ is more commonly called a chest film, or radiograph. It is one of the most common methods for evaluating the lungs and other structures in the thorax. Air-filled lung tissue appears mostly dark on the film because it is easily penetrated, or _____. The dense bone tissue of ribs appears white. Dense matter that is not easily penetrated is referred to as _____ Soft tissues such as blood vessels appear more grayish because they have an intermediate density. Abnormal conditions may be spotted through observation of certain densities in the wrong location. Accumulation of fluid in the pleural space, or _____, appears white and may obscure the angle where the ribs meet the diaphragm. Alveoli appear white when filled with pus or blood. On the chest film these areas are called pulmonary _____. Air in the pleural space, or _____, is another example of an abnormal density. This condition appears as a black area with none of the usual grayish markings of blood vessels in the lung tissue.

Step-by-Step

Every primer on chest radiograph interpretation recommends you develop a systematic method for approaching interpretation. The first step is to make sure you are looking at the right film (patient) with the time and date you need. If you are handling an actual film, as opposed to a digitized one, make sure it is placed on the viewer correctly. The "left" side of the film (usually where the heart is) should be facing your right hand side, as if the patient was standing facing you. A marker is normally placed on the film to indicate the left side.

1. What structures offer clues to help identify whether the patient is straight or rotated?

2. What appearance in the lung fields suggests overexposure of the chest film?

3. What appearance of the vertebral bodies suggests underexposure?

4. What effect does underexposure have on the appearance of lung tissue?

5. Systematic observation divides the chest anatomy into what three areas?

    A. _____

    B. _____

    C. _____

6. The pleura appear at the edge of chest wall. (Although the pleura themselves are usually difficult to see.) What are the two major pleural abnormalities detected on the chest film?

    A. _____

    B. _____

7. Following trauma, you should examine the ribs for what abnormality?

8. Why is lung tissue difficult to evaluate?

9. What is the maximum size of the heart shadow on a posterior-anterior (PA) projection?

10. What important muscle of ventilation should be evaluated in the chest film?

13. What view is most sensitive for detecting pleural fluid? How is the patient positioned to obtain this view?

Identifying Abnormalities

The second part of Chapter 18 covers evaluation of abnormalities seen in the three major anatomic portions seen in chest imaging. After you read the material, answer the following questions that highlight the important points.

14. When is sonography (ultrasound) indicated in the evaluation of pleural abnormalities?

Evaluation of the Pleura

11. What is the costophrenic angle?

15. What other imaging procedure may be helpful?

12. What sign will help you recognize the presence of fluid in the pleural space? Describe this sign.

16. Air in the pleural space is always abnormal. Name the three common causes of this condition.
    A. _____
    B. _____
    C. _____

17. What breathing maneuver will help identify a small pneumothorax on a chest film?

18. Tension pneumothorax is immediately life-threatening. Name at least two radiographic signs of tension pneumothorax.
    A. _____
    _____
    B. _____
    _____

19. What is the treatment for tension pneumothorax?

Evaluation of Lung Parenchyma

20. What are the two components of the lung parenchyma?
    A. _____
    B. _____

21. How will alveolar infiltrates appear on the chest film?

22. What is the difference between the radiographic appearance of pneumonia and pulmonary hemorrhage?

23. What causes airways to become visible, and what is this sign called?

24. Honeycombing, nodules, and volume loss are all x-ray hallmarks of what type of lung disorder?

25. Describe the silhouette sign. Discuss the difference between a right lower and right middle lobe infiltrate as seen on a chest film.

26. List three important indirect signs of volume loss, or atelectasis, seen on the chest radiograph.

    A. _____

    B. _____

    C. _____

27. You can count on your ribs to tell you about lung volumes. Fill in the chart below based on what anterior ribs you would see above the diaphragm depending on the degree of lung inflation.

Lung Volume	Anterior Ribs
A. Poor inspiration	_____
B. Good effort	_____
C. Hyperinflation	_____

28. Ribs aren't the only way to assess COPD with hyperinflation. List the two primary and three secondary radiographic signs seen with emphysema.

    A. Primary

        1. _____

        2. _____

    B. Secondary

        1. _____

        2. _____

        3. _____

29. Compare the sensitivity of the chest radiograph and computerized tomography for detection of obstructive airway disease?

Catheters, Lines, and Tubes

30. The endotracheal tube is made of soft plastic. Why is the chest film useful in deciding correct tube position after intubation?

31. Where is the distal tip of an ideally placed endotracheal tube in relationship to the carina?

32. Where will the endotracheal tube usually end up if it is placed too far into the trachea?

33. What pulmonary complication may be identified on a chest film when a CVP catheter is placed via the subclavian vein?

34. A pulmonary artery catheter (Swan-Ganz) that is seen to extend too far into the lung fields of a chest x-ray may have what unwanted results?

37. Based on your knowledge of the silhouette sign, in what lobe is the infiltrate located?

38. What diagnosis does the presence of air bronchograms suggest?

The Mediastinum

35. Where does the mediastinum lie within the chest?

39. What physical assessments could confirm the information in the chest film?

36. What imaging technique is most favored for assessing mediastinal masses?

Case Studies

Case 1

You are asked to perform postural drainage and clapping on Jane Dough, a patient with a large, right-sided pulmonary infiltrate. Evaluation of the chest radiograph shows a patchy white density with air bronchograms in the right lung. The right border of the heart is visible in the film.

Case 2

Grandpa Miller presents in the emergency room with acute exacerbation of his long-standing COPD. A decision is made to intubate him. It is difficult to auscultate breath sounds, and chest movement is minimal; however, your impression is that breath sounds are more diminished on the left. A chest radiograph is obtained, which shows the tip of the endotracheal tube 1cm above the carina. The left lung field is slightly smaller than the right. Both diaphragms appear flat, and you are able to count eight anterior ribs above the diaphragms.

40. Where should the tip of the tube be in relationship to the carina?

●

41. With regard to the endotracheal tube, what action should you take?

42. What is the significance of the flattened diaphragms and number of ribs seen above the diaphragm?

●

What About Those Board Exams?

I have carefully reviewed the NBRC's examination matrices and come to the conclusion that *no* one textbook contains all the x-ray information indicated to be part of the examinations! Chapter 18 covers some of this material, and you will find much of the rest in later chapters on lung diseases and pediatric/neonatal respiratory care.

I'll give you some sample questions based on the material covered in this chapter, but you will need to carefully review each examination matrix to identify all the areas you need to know. The Certification Examination requires you to "Inspect the chest x-ray to determine the position of endotracheal or tracheostomy tube." You must also know when to "recommend a chest x-ray", and when to "review existing data in the patient record" such as the "results of chest x-rays." The Registry Examinations agree, but take this a step further, asking you to "inspect the chest x-ray to determine":

1. Pneumothorax or subcutaneous air
2. Consolidation or atelectasis
3. Diaphragm position
4. Hyperinflation
5. Pleural fluid
6. Pulmonary infiltrates

There's more! How many questions will you see on this topic? A review of available practice exams suggests one to three on the Certification Exam and up to five on the Registry. Each examination can vary considerably, but you are *guaranteed* to be tested on this material in some fashion! Try these questions.

43. A patient has dyspnea and tachycardia following thoracentesis to treat a pleural effusion. Evaluation of this patient should include:
A. A CT scan
B. An MRI
C. A chest radiograph
D. A bronchoscopy

44. A pneumothorax would appear on a chest radiograph as:
A. A white area near the lung base
B. A white area that obscures the costophrenic angle
C. A dark area without lung marking
D. A dark area with honeycomb markings

●

45. The medical record of an intubated patient indicates that the morning chest film shows opacification of the lower right lung field with elevated right diaphragm and a shift of the trachea to the right. These findings suggest:
    A. Left-sided pneumothorax
    B. Right-sided pleural effusion
    C. Right mainstem intubation
    D. Right-sided atelectasis

46. On a chest radiograph, the tip of the endotracheal tube for an adult patient should be:
    A. 2 cm above the vocal cords
    B. 2 cm above the carina
    C. At the carina
    D. 2 cm below the carina

47. A patient is believed to have a pleural effusion. Which of the following radiographic techniques would be most useful in making a confirmation?
    A. Computed tomography
    B. Decubitus radiographic projection
    C. Magnetic resonance imaging
    D. A-P radiographic projection

Naturally, chest film interpretation will appear as part of the information in questions that are not specifically about radiographs (as with blood gases). Remember: Chest radiographs are diagnostic, not therapeutic. If a patient is circling the drain from a tension pneumothorax, the radiograph will not be life-saving—a chest tube will!

Food for Thought

48. The author states that head position is very important in assessing the tip of an endotracheal tube on a radiograph. What happens to the tube if the head moves up (extension) or the chin goes down (flexion)?

Pulmonary Infections

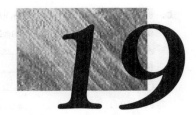

"Captain of the men
of death. . ."
Sir William Osler

A hundred years after these words were said,
pneumonia is still a leading cause of death. In
fact, it is the sixth leading cause of death in the
United States. There is a tremendous clinical
interest in ventilator-associated pneumonia
right now. Respiratory care practitioners play a
key role in the research and prevention of this
serious complication of life in the intensive care
unit. Pneumonia is simple to understand, right?
There are only two types: community and nosocomial. Or is it viral and bacterial? Or is it acute
and chronic? Typical and atypical? Or perhaps
aspiration and. . .read on, and you will meet
"the old man's friend" in its many forms.

Classification and Pathogenesis

1. What does the term *empirical therapy* mean?

2. Give the textbook definition of nosocomial
   pneumonia.

3. How common is hospital-acquired pneumonia?

4. List two patient populations that are at special risk for fatal forms of nosocomial pneumonia.
   A. _____
   B. _____

5. Name four diseases acquired via inhalation
   of infectious particles.
   A. _____
   B. _____
   C. _____
   D. _____

6. List four of the patient populations at risk for aspiration of large volumes of gastric fluids.
   A. _____
   B. _____
   C. _____
   D. _____

7. What group of respiratory patients is at special risk for aspiration of small amounts of colonized secretions?

8. Describe the role of suctioning in lower respiratory tract infection.

9. Give the prime example of reactivation of a latent infection.

Microbiology

10. Why is it so important to know what organisms are commonly associated with pneumonia?

11. What organism is most commonly identified as the cause of community-acquired pneumonia?

12. Name two atypical pathogens.
    A. _____
    B. _____

13. Why is no microbiological identification made in so many cases of pneumonia?

14. Name two viruses associated with pneumonia. When are they encountered?

Clinical Manifestations

15. Patients with community-acquired pneumonia typically have fever and what three respiratory symptoms?
    A. _____
    B. _____
    C. _____

16. What other two other common respiratory problems show the same symptoms?
    A. _____
    B. _____

17. What is the classic, typical presentation of community-acquired pneumonia?

18. In intubated patients, nosocomial pneumonia usually shows up as what three changes in the patient's condition?
    A. _____
    B. _____
    C. _____

19. Describe the common radiographic abnormalities associated with pneumonia.

20. Why is the chest film of limited use in diagnosing pneumonia in critically ill patients?

Risk Factors

21. Fill in the data for each of the following risk factors for mortality associated with community-acquired pneumonia.

Factor	Description
A. Age	_____
B. Gender	_____
C. Vital signs	_____
D. Arterial pH	_____
E. High-risk causes	_____
F. Comorbid illness	_____

22. A number of factors predispose the hospital patient to pneumonia, including poor host defenses such as underlying illness. Name five such conditions.
    A. _____
    B. _____
    C. _____
    D. _____
    E. _____

23. List four factors that expose the lung to large numbers of microorganisms.
    A. _____
    B. _____
    C. _____
    D. _____

Diagnostic Studies

24. Why is determining the predominant causative organism via sputum Gram stain, culture, and sensitivity so useful in treating pneumonia patients?

25. Describe the process for collecting a good specimen by expectoration.

26. Describe the satisfactory specimen.

27. Name the organism identified by each of the following specialized tests.

Test	Organism
A. Acid-fast stain	_____
B. Direct fluorescent stain	_____
C. Toluidine blue	_____
D. Potassium hydroxide	_____

28. When should HIV testing be recommended in cases of community-acquired pneumonia?

29. When should fiberoptic bronchoscopy be recommended in cases of community-acquired pneumonia?

30. Name four techniques useful in confirming the diagnosis nosocomial pneumonia.
    A. _____
    B. _____
    C. _____
    D. _____

Therapy

31. What is the primary medical treatment for pneumonia?

32. What is the agent of choice for treating the following organisms?

Organism	Agent of Choice
A. Pneumococcal infection	_____
B. *Mycoplasma*	_____
C. *P. carinii*	_____
D. *Legionella*	_____

33. How long is a typical course of treatment for pneumonia?

34. How long does it take for the radiograph to show resolution of pneumonia in young individuals? In older patients?

Prevention

35. Immunization is one of the primary strategies for preventing community-acquired pneumonia. Individuals are immunized against what two organisms?
   A. _____
   B. _____

36. Identify 3 groups that should be immunized.

37. Identify the three "probably effective" strategies for the prevention of nosocomial pneumonia.
   A. _____
   B. _____
   C. _____

38. What positioning technique is useful in preventing pneumonia in patients?

39. What is the current medication for GI bleeding prophylaxis that may be effective in preventing pneumonia?

Case Studies

Case 1
Abe Drinker is a 55-year-old male who shows up at the clinic complaining of chills, fever, and chest pain on inspiration. Abe is coughing up

rusty-colored sputum. He admits to a history of heavy smoking and regular use of alcoholic beverages. Physical examination reveals a HR of 125, RR of 30, and a temperature of 104° Fahrenheit. He has inspiratory crackles in the right lower lobe. Blood gases reveal a pH of 7.34, $PaCO_2$ of 50, and a PaO_2 of 58.

40. What is the most likely diagnosis? Support your answer based on the clinical signs and symptoms.

41. What immediate treatment should you initiate?

42. Give at least five reasons why Mr. Drinker is at risk of dying from his condition.
    A. _____
    B. _____
    C. _____
    D. _____
    E. _____

Case 2

Mickey Souris is intubated and on the ventilator following a head injury. On the third day following his craniotomy, Mr. Souris develops a fever. During routine suctioning you notice his secretions are thick and yellow. Breath sounds are decreased in the left lower lobe.

43. What is the role of the artificial airway in development of pneumonia?

44. What test would you recommend at this time to help confirm a diagnosis?

What Does the NBRC Say?

Interestingly enough, they don't say much about pneumonia. Certain lung infections may appear on the boards in the context of their treatment and recognition. For example, the use of Ribavirin to treat RSV. Or inhaled pentamidine in HIV patients with pneumonia. Isolation procedures for tuberculosis patients is a possible area of testing as well as general methods to prevent the spread of infection. You should certainly recognize when a patient has a lung infection and pay attention to basic microbiology.

Food for Thought

45. What is the role of the respiratory therapist in educating at-risk populations about methods to prevent pneumonia?

46. Have you had your flu shot?

Obstructive Lung Disease: COPD, Asthma, and Related Diseases

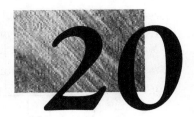

20

I first learned about obstructive lung disease by watching some of my family members develop it as a consequence of heavy smoking. As a child, I thought that coughing was normal! The conditions discussed in Chapter 20, chronic obstructive pulmonary disease (COPD) and asthma, are so common that you probably know someone who has them too. (Of course, lots of famous people had COPD as well. If "honest Abe" had Marfan's syndrome, he might have developed lung disease!) RCPs spend a lot of their time working with COPD patients, and I am sure you will pay special attention to the information in this chapter, as you get to know the "pink puffers" and "blue bloaters."

Sputum Power

Before we start on the long dark journey into the lungs, take a shot at the COPD crossword puzzle on p. 158.

Chronic Obstructive Pulmonary Disease

If you talk about each type of COPD as if it was "pure emphysema" you would be oversimplifying in many cases. The Venn diagram on page 442 in Egan demonstrates this nicely. Many patients show signs of having mixed disease states. Asthma is classified as separate from COPD, but those with long-standing, poorly controlled asthma will often present with signs of COPD later in life. So, while it is convenient to talk about emphysema, chronic bronchitis, or asthma, in the clinical setting, you will see patients who have varying degrees of pathology that represent each of these important components of the spectrum of COPD. Remember that most COPD patients have a smoking history, so you will want to explore this issue. (You can calculate pack-years by multiplying packs per day times years smoked.)

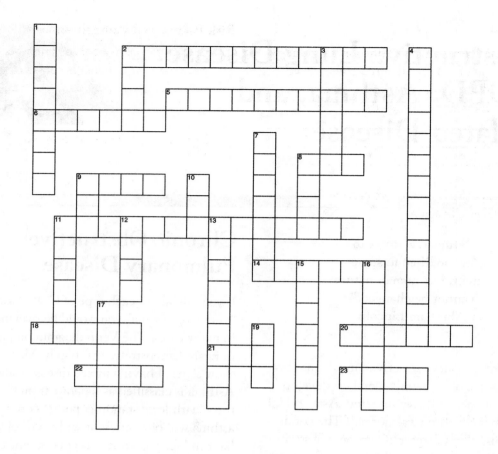

ACROSS

1. abdominal smooth muscle contraction in the airways.
5. chronic form shows productive cough for 3 months in 2 consecutive years.
6. the only thing that increases survival of end-stage COPD patients.
8. late asthma response.
9. another four letter word for COPD!
11. results in permanent dilation of the airways.
14. this fibrosis is the most frequently lethal genetic disease of white children.
18. _____ one antitrypsin deficiency, a genetic form of emphysema.
20. where COPD stands as a killer
21. asthma you get when you exercise
22. common bedside test used to manage asthma
23. these puffers really have emphysema

DOWN

1. cystic _____, known in Europe as mucoviscidosis.
2. bloater, or patient with chronic bronchitis.
3. complex lung disease associated with wheezing and airway inflammation
4. drug that opens the airways
7. passed on from parents to children via DNA.
8. abbreviation for surgery that removes part of the emphysematous lung.
9. _____pulmonale, the heart failure associated with hypoxemia.
10. most common way to deliver drugs to the airway
11. COPD chest shape
12. famous oxygen therapy study that proved increased survival with oxygen.
13. enlargement and destruction of the distal airways and alveoli
15. Stop it
16. the "C " in COPD
17. lung butter
19. early asthma response

Overview

1. Chronic bronchitis is defined as a productive cough for 3 months in 2 consecutive years. What three other causes of chronic cough have to be excluded?

   A. _____

   B. _____

   C. _____

2. Compare the incidence of chronic bronchitis with emphysema.

3. What is the difference between the death rates for heart attack and stroke compared with that of COPD?

4. What is the approximate cost of health care associated with COPD?

Risk Factors and Pathophysiology

5. Besides cigarette smoking (number 1), name two other possible causes of COPD.

   A. _____

   B. _____

6. Describe the "susceptible smoker."

7. Explain the protease-antiprotease hypothesis of emphysema (briefly, please!).

8. Describe the three mechanisms of airflow obstruction in COPD.

   A. _____

   B. _____

   C. _____

Clinical Signs

9. Name four common symptoms of COPD.

   A. _____

   B. _____

   C. _____

   D. _____

10. Compare the onset of dyspnea in typical cases of COPD with that of alpha$_1$-antitrypsin deficiency.

11. What physical change in the chest wall occurs as a result of prolonged hyperinflation?

12. Name three other late signs of COPD.
    A. _____
    B. _____
    C. _____

13. Compare chronic bronchitis, emphysema, and alpha$_1$-antitrypsin deficiency in terms of the following features.

Features	Chronic Bronchitis	Emphysema	Alpha$_1$
A. Age of onset	_____	_____	_____
B. Family History	_____	_____	_____
C. Smoker	_____	_____	_____
D. Lung volume	_____	_____	_____
E. DLCO	_____	_____	_____
F. FEV$_1$/FVC	_____	_____	_____
G. Radiograph	_____	_____	_____

Management

Your text lists five general goals of management for COPD. In addition, we need to think about how to avoid complications when the patient has an acute exacerbation of their condition.

14. Why would it be important to differentiate asthma from other forms of COPD?

15. What is the minimum spirometric standard for demonstrating significantly improved airflow following bronchodilator administration?

16. Why is bronchodilator therapy recommended for COPD? What types of drugs are used? What is the effect on decline of lung function and survival?
    A. Why

B. What drugs

C. Outcome

17. Discuss the role of inhaled steroids in COPD.

18. What is the primary effect of theophylline (methylxanthines) on patients with COPD? What serum blood levels are currently recommended to avoid side effects?

19. Name the four important elements of managing an acute exacerbation of COPD due to purulent bronchitis.
A. _____
B. _____
C. _____
D. _____

20. What is the primary goal of pulmonary rehabilitation?

21. What is the effect of pulmonary rehabilitation programs on survival and pulmonary function?

22. A comprehensive smoking cessation program usually includes what three elements?
A. _____
B. _____
C. _____

23. What is the only treatment for COPD that has been shown to prolong survival?

24. What is the relationship between bronchodilator therapy and home oxygen therapy?

25. What two vaccines are recommended for patients with COPD? Which one is given annually?

A. _____

B. _____

26. Describe the two surgical options for end-stage COPD. Discuss the outcomes of each of these options.

A.

B.

Asthma

——— "All that wheezes is not asthma." Anonymous RCPs ———

Asthma is on the rise, and all of our drugs and technology have not been able to solve the problem. A number of interesting theories exist to explain why industrialized countries are experiencing worse problems than underdeveloped nations. For RCPs, however, the situation is a wonderful opportunity to apply our special expertise to help educate the public and our clients regarding prevention, treatment, and control.

Overview

27. What is the difference between older definitions and the more current view of asthma?

28. What percentage of people living in the United States are believed to have asthma?

29. What is the difference between the death rate for asthma and that of other common, treatable conditions?

Etiology and Pathogenesis

30. What are the two primary effects of asthma that result in airflow obstruction?

A. _____

B. _____

31. What happens when a patient with asthma inhales an allergen to which he is sensitized?

32. Describe the early and late asthmatic reactions.

    A. Early

    B. Late

Clinical Signs

33. What factor plays a key role in suggesting and establishing a diagnosis of asthma?

34. What are the four classic symptoms of asthma?

    A. _____

    B. _____

    C. _____

    D. _____

35. List five conditions that can mimic the wheezing of asthma.

    A. _____

    B. _____

    C. _____

    D. _____

    E. _____

36. How is reversibility of airflow obstruction demonstrated?

37. Bronchial provocation is the specialized test regimen used to demonstrate obstruction in suspected asthmatics who are symptom free at the time of testing. Name the drug used for this test and what response indicates hyperresponsiveness.

    A. Drug

B. Response

38. Describe the role of arterial blood gases in the diagnosis of asthma.

Management

The goal of asthma management is to maintain a high quality of life without symptoms or limitations. The patient should be relatively free of side effects from treatment. To achieve this, a four-step approach has been recommended by the National Institutes of Health.

39. Complete the chart below to show your understanding of the stepwise approach.

Severity	Symptoms	Long-term meds
A. 1-intermittent	_____	_____
B. 2-mild persistent	_____	_____
C. 3-moderate persistent	_____	_____
D. 4-severe persistent	_____	_____

40. Explain control of asthma in terms of the following criteria:
A. Symptoms

B. Beta$_2$ agonists

C. Exercise

D. PEFR

41. Give the criteria and actions for green, yellow, and red peak flow zones.

Zone	PEFR % predicted	Treatment/Action
A. Green	_____	_____
B. Yellow	_____	_____
C. Red	_____	_____

42. Compare the use of inhaled corticosteroids and bronchodilators in asthma.

43. Name the two common side effects of inhaled steroids and two ways to control them.
    A. _____
    B. _____
    C. _____

44. Discuss the use of cromolyn sodium in asthma treatment.
    A. Indications—Adults

    B. Indications—Children

C. Acute attacks

45. When is use of nedocromil indicated?

46. What type of drugs are the first-line treatment for all types of acute bronchospasm?

47. What is the primary indication for salmeterol?

48. Describe the use of methylxanthines such as theophylline in the treatment of asthma.

C. Symptoms

D. Discharge medications

49. What is the benefit of using ipratroprium in the day-to-day management of asthma?

52. How can you prevent allergic reactions in asthmatic patients?

50. Name three factors you should monitor in a patient hospitalized with acute asthma.
   A. _____
   B. _____
   C. _____

51. Give the criteria for hospital discharge for each of the following.
   A. PaO_2

53. Name three common outdoor and indoor allergens.
   A. Outdoor
      1. _____
      2. _____
      3. _____
   B. Indoor
      1. _____
      2. _____
      3. _____

   B. PEFR

54. What is EIA? List three prophylactic drug treatments.
   A. _____
   B. _____
      1. _____
      2. _____
      3. _____

55. Define occupational asthma. What is the most common cause?

56. What is the only way to eliminate occupational asthma once an individual is sensitized?

57. What drug is particularly helpful in the treatment of cough-variant asthma?

58. List three medications that may be helpful in treating nocturnal asthma.
   A. _____
   B. _____
   C. _____

59. What recommendations would you make to a patient who has aspirin sensitivity?

60. What is the effect of pregnancy on asthmatics?

61. Discuss the use of asthma medications during pregnancy.

Bronchiectasis

Bronchiectasis is a condition in which airways are deformed and destroyed by chronic inflammation.

62. What is the clinical hallmark of bronchiectasis?

63. What test is now considered definitive for diagnosing bronchiectasis?

64. List the causes of local and diffuse bronchiectasis.
    A. Local
       1. _____
       2. _____

    B. Diffuse
       1. _____
       2. _____
       3. _____

65. Name the two primary treatments for bronchiectasis.
    A. _____
    B. _____

66. What treatment is indicated in severe cases of bronchiectasis associated with massive hemoptysis?

Cystic Fibrosis

65 Roses . . . that's what young children are taught to call their illness when they can't pronounce the medical name. This colorful term has become a part of the national campaign against CF, which is the most common lethal genetic disease in the United States.

67. What is the "triad" of cystic fibrosis?
    A. _____
    B. _____
    C. _____

68. What is the hallmark of CF?

69. Discuss the changes in lifespan of CF patients that have occurred over the last 30 years.

70. How is a diagnosis of CF confirmed?

71. List four classic respiratory treatments for CF.
   A. _____
   B. _____
   C. _____
   D. _____

72. What two organisms are frequently responsible for lung infections associated with this disorder?
   A. _____
   B. _____

73. What is the most likely diagnosis?

74. Calculate Mr. Henry's "pack-years."

75. What factor should you focus on to help Mr. Henry control his condition?

Case Studies

Case 1

Forest Henry is a 70-year-old male whose chief complaint is dyspnea on exertion. He has a smoking history of 2 packs per day for the last 50 years. Mr. Henry has a barrel-shaped chest and very decreased breath sounds. His chest radiograph shows hyperinflation, especially in the apices, flattened diaphragms, and a small heart. He admits to a morning cough but denies significant sputum production.

Case 2

Billy-Bob Thorn is a 60-year-old man who has smoked a pack of cigarettes per day since he was a teenager. He complains of a chronic productive cough that is producing thick yellow sputum. He is admitted to the medical floor with a fever and shortness of breath. Blood gases reveal pH 7.35, $PaCO_2$ 50 mm Hg, PaO_2 57 mm Hg. Physical exam shows pedal edema, distended neck veins, and use of accessory muscles of ventilation. He has scattered wheezing and rhonchi on auscultation.

76. What type of COPD is most likely in Mr. Thorn's case?

77. What should you do with his sputum the next time he coughs productively?

78. What is the immediate respiratory treatment in this case?

79. What other respiratory medications would you recommend?

Case 3

Aaron Defaut is a 44-year-old man who complains of dyspnea on exertion. He is a nonsmoker, but drinks wine with his meals. Mr. Defaut has a barrel-shaped chest and very decreased breath sounds. His chest radiograph shows hyperinflation, especially in the bases. History reveals that his father and uncle both died of "lung problems."

80. What is the most likely cause of Mr. Defaut's COPD symptoms? Justify your answer based on the information presented.

81. What treatments are available for this condition?

Case 4

Pierre Poussif is a 15-year-old male who complains that he cannot catch his breath when he exercises. He states that he coughs a lot, especially in winter. Pierre's breath sounds are clear, and his physical examination is unremarkable.

82. What do you suspect is the problem?

83. How could a definitive diagnosis be made?

85. The arterial blood gas results indicate the presence of
    A. Acute respiratory alkalosis
    B. Acute metabolic alkalosis
    C. Chronic respiratory acidosis
    D. Acute respiratory acidosis

86. You are asked to initiate oxygen therapy. What would you recommend?
    A. Simple mask at 10 L/min
    B. Non-rebreathing mask at 15 L/min
    C. Nasal cannula at 2 L/min
    D. Air entrainment mask at 50% FIO_2

87. What therapy would you recommend after the oxygen is in place?
    A. 2 puffs Atrovent (ipratropium) via MDI
    B. 0.5 ml Proventil (albuterol) via SVN
    C. Intravenous aminophylline (theophylline) administration
    D. Intravenous antibiotics

What Does the NBRC Say?

It will come as no surprise that the board exams place a special emphasis on COPD and asthma. The Clinical Simulation Examination Matrix states that you will see at least "two problems involving adult patients with COPD." You may also see a pediatric patient with asthma or cystic fibrosis. *All* aspects of managing these patients may be included from pulmonary function testing to rehabilitation. Multiple-choice exams, such as the Written Registry and Entry-Level Examinations, do not specifically mention COPD or asthma in the matrices, however, diagnosis and management of these patients is heavily tested. Here are some sample questions.

A 20-year-old woman who has a history of asthma is brought to the emergency department in respiratory distress. Your assessment of the patient reveals: pH, 7.47; $PaCO_2$, 33 mm Hg; PaO_2, 72 mm Hg; HCO_3, 23 mEq/L; RR, 28; HR, 115; PEFR, 200 L/min.

84. Which of the following breath sounds would you expect to hear in this patient?
    A. Inspiratory crackles
    B. Expiratory wheezing
    C. Inspiratory stridor
    D. Expiratory rhonchi

88. Blood gases are repeated 30 minutes after the oxygen therapy is initiated. They indicate: pH, 7.42; $PaCO_2$, 38 mm Hg; PaO_2, 86 mm Hg; HCO_3, 23 mEq/L; RR, 24; HR, 88; PEFR, 210 L/min. Which of the following has shown significant improvement based on this information?
    A. Compliance
    B. Resistance
    C. Oxygenation
    D. Ventilation

89. Intravenous steroids and repeated bronchodilators have been given. The patient is now receiving 40% oxygen. Blood gas values are as follows: pH, 7.34; $PaCO_2$, 53 mm Hg; PaO_2, 74 mm Hg; HCO_3, 26 mEq/L; RR, 18; HR, 125; PEFR, 110 L/min. What would you suggest at this point?
    A. Increase the FIO_2 to 50%
    B. Continuous nebulization of bronchodilators
    C. Administration of intravenous bicarbonate
    D. Intubation and mechanical ventilation

90. An RCP is asked to administer a mucolytic agent to a patient with cystic fibrosis. The physician asks for your recommendations. Which of the following are appropriate?
    I. Hypertonic saline
    II. Mucomyst
    III. Pulmozyme
    IV. Decadron
    A. I, II
    B. II only
    C. II, III
    D. II, III, IV

91. A patient with COPD and CO_2 retention is admitted for an acute exacerbation of her disease. The physician requests your suggestion for initiating oxygen therapy. Which of the following would you recommend?
    A. Nasal cannula at 6 L/min
    B. Air-entrainment mask at 28%
    C. Simple mask at 2 L/min
    D. Partial rebreathing mask at 8 L/min

92. A PFT on a 65-year-old female indicates airflow obstruction with mild air-trapping. The patient is coughing up thick sputum. Which of the following diagnoses is most likely?
    A. Cystic fibrosis
    B. Pneumonia
    C. Pulmonary fibrosis
    D. Bronchiectasis

93. A PFT on a 56-year-old male with a history of smoking shows increased TLC and RV. The DLCO is reduced. What diagnosis is suggested by these findings?
    A. Emphysema
    B. Pneumonia
    C. Sarcoidosis
    D. Pneumoconiosis

94. Spirometry is performed before and after bronchodilator administration. Which of the following indicates a therapeutic response?
    I. FEV_1 increased by 10%
    II. FVC increased by 300 ml
    III. PEFR increased by 50 L/min

A. I only
B. II only
C. I, II only
D. III only

Food for Thought

95. Since only 15% of smokers actually show big declines in airflow, why should we encourage all patients to quit smoking?

96. Patients with alpha$_1$-antitrypsin deficiency may be eligible for intravenous augmentation therapy. Discuss the pros and cons of this treatment.

97. Leukotriene inhibitors are now being considered as potential tools for controlling asthma. How do they work?

Interstitial Lung Disease

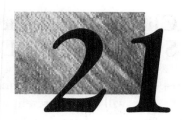

"I do the very best I know
how—the very best I can;
and I mean to keep on
doing so until the end."
Abraham Lincoln

There are an unbelievable number of interstitial lung diseases (ILD). Individually, they are not very common, but as a group, they represent a significant set of lung disorders.

Sooner or later you will encounter some of the members of this broad category of restrictive conditions. Fortunately, there are many common elements in the clinical signs, PFT abnormalities, and treatment of ILD.

Game, Set, and Match!

Since there are so many new terms related to ILD in Chapter 21, a quick review will probably help you keep them straight.

_____ 1. Asbestosis
_____ 2. Corticosteroids
_____ 3. Cytotoxic agents
_____ 4. Eosinophilic granuloma

_____ 5. Hypersensitivity pneumonitis
_____ 6. Idiopathic pulmonary fibrosis (IPF)
_____ 7. Interstitial lung disease
_____ 8. Lupus erythematosus (systemic)
_____ 9. Occupational lung disease
_____ 10. Pneumoconiosis
_____ 11. Rheumatoid arthritis
_____ 12. Sarcoidosis
_____ 13. Silicosis

A. Formation of scar tissue in the lung without known cause
B. Respiratory disorder characterized by fibrotic infiltrates in the lower lobes
C. Inflammatory reaction provoked by inhalation of organic dusts
D. Chemical that is lethal to living cells
E. Interstitial lung disease associated with inhalation of small inorganic particles
F. Restrictive disorder associated with pleural abnormalities and lung tumors
G. Disorder of unknown origin that results in formation of epithelioid tubercles
H. Hormones associated with control of body processes
I. Bone growth associated with numerous histiocytes and specific WBCs
J. Serious pulmonary form of the inflammatory skin disease
K. Occupational disease most commonly seen in coal workers
L. Disorder caused by long-term exposure to sand and stone dust
M. Connective tissue disease associated with inflammation of the joints

Clinical Signs and Symptoms of ILD

14. Patients with ILD of many different etiologies will usually present with what two common complaints?

    A. _____

    B. _____

15. Describe the breath sounds usually heard in interstitial lung disease.

16. What two explanations does Egan give for wheezing heard in patients with ILD?

    A.

    B.

17. Name at least two of the late signs of ILD.

    A. _____

    B. _____

18. Physical signs of underlying connective tissue disease include what four features?

    A. _____

    B. _____

    C. _____

    D. _____

19. Describe the classic radiographic findings in idiopathic pulmonary fibrosis. What are the late-stage findings?

20. Discuss the effects of ILD on the following pulmonary function variables.

Variable	Effect of ILD
A. FEV_1	_____
B. FVC	_____
C. FEV_1/FVC	_____
D. DLCO	_____
E. Lung volumes	_____
F. Pao_2	_____
G. Compliance	_____

Specific Types of ILD

Since there are so many causes of ILD, it will help you to look at the primary groupings and some representative examples of each category.

21. What are the three most common types of occupational ILD?

    A. _____

    B. _____

    C. _____

22. What do these examples have in common?

26. What is the name for chronic exposure to inhaled organic material that may result in progressive scarring of the lung?

23. Give at least one specific example for each of the following general categories of drugs that are associated with the development of ILD.

	Category	Example
A.	Antibiotic	_____
B.	Antiinflammatory	_____
C.	Cardiovascular	_____
D.	Chemotherapeutic	_____
E.	Illegal drugs	_____
F.	Miscellaneous agents	_____

27. What is the key to identifying the cause of this condition?

28. What is meant by the term *idiopathic*?

24. Why is pulmonary involvement in connective tissue disorders often undetected until late in the course of the disease?

29. Let's compare the two ILDs discussed in Egan.

	IPF	Sarcoidosis
A. Age	_____	_____
	_____	_____
B. Symptoms	_____	_____
	_____	_____
C. Treatament	_____	_____
	_____	_____
D. Prognosis	_____	_____
	_____	_____

25. Name three common connective disorders associated with lung disease.
   A. _____
   B. _____
   C. _____

Treatment

30. Discuss the treatment for hypersensitivity pneumonitis and occupational lung disease.

31. What is the traditional primary medical therapy for ILD?

32. When the traditional medicine isn't enough, what type of drugs are used?

33. What condition is colchicine being used to treat?

34. What is the treatment of last resort for end-stage ILD?

Case Studies

Case 1

Herb Foin is a 48-year-old man admitted for dyspnea on exertion and a dry cough of unknown origin. The chest radiograph shows bilateral reticulonodular infiltrates. Pulse oximetry indicates mild hypoxemia on room air. History reveals that Mr. Foin is a hay farmer.

35. What is the most likely diagnosis?

36. What is the most likely cause of the lung disease? What are some other possible causes?

Case 2

Vincent Kealoha is a retired Pearl Harbor ship-yard worker. He states that he has had a cough for some time, but recently began expectorating some blood. He has bibasilar inspiratory crackles, with otherwise clear breath sounds. A chest radiograph shows reticulonodular infiltrates in both lower lobes. The radiologist also notes the presence of a small right-sided pleural effusion and the presence of pleural plaques and pleural fibrosis. PFTs reveal a normal FEV_1%, decreased TLC and RV, and a decreased DLCO.

37. What is most likely the pulmonary diagnosis?

38. What other information would be helpful in making a determination?

39. What type of disorder is suggested by the PFT results?

What About Those Board Exams?

The NBRC thinks you should know your pulmonary function testing and physical examination findings pretty well! Interstitial lung disease doesn't have a particular category on the boards, but it may be included as a side issue to material such as interpreting PFT results.

Food for Thought

40. What is the general term for all lung diseases that cause a reduction in lung volumes without a reduction in flow rates?

41. The text listed only three occupations that might cause ILD. Can you think of at least three other possibilities?
    A. _____
    B. _____
    C. _____

Pleural Diseases

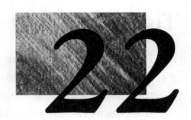

22

"Some men dream of
doing great things.
Others stay awake
and accomplish them."

Imagine a piece of cake enclosed in Saran Wrap.
Or, if you prefer collapsed lungs, a sandwich
covered in that thin, tough clear stuff we use
to store food. Thinking about pleura always
makes me think of plastic wrap. Like that clingy
food protector, a breach in the pleura has important consequences. I hope you get a chance to
play with some lungs while you're in training,
but if you don't, you can always head for the
kitchen!

Hey Buddy, Got a Match?

Chapter 22 introduces lots of important new
terms. Match these pleural puzzlers to their definitions. You're going to need the glossary, but it will
be worth it. Many of these words are commonly
seen on board exams or in clinical practice.

_____ 1. Bronchopleural fistula
_____ 2. Chylothorax
_____ 3. Empyema
_____ 4. Exudative effusion
_____ 5. Hemothorax
_____ 6. Parietal pleura
_____ 7. Pleural effusion
_____ 8. Pleurisy
_____ 9. Pleurodesis
_____ 10. Pneumothorax

_____ 11. Primary spontaneous
             pneumothorax
_____ 12. Re-expansion pulmonary edema
_____ 13. Secondary spontaneous
             pneumothorax
_____ 14. Tension pneumothorax
_____ 15. Thoracentesis
_____ 16. Transudative pleural effusion
_____ 17. Visceral pleura

A. Pleural effusion high in protein
B. Air leak from the lung to the pleural space
C. Membrane covering the surface of the chest
   wall
D. Pleural fluid rich with triglycerides from a
   ruptured thoracic duct
E. Pleural pain
F. Pus-filled pleural effusion
G. Blood in the pleural space
H. Abnormal collection of fluid in the pleural
   space
I. Pneumothorax without underlying lung disease
J. Air under pressure in the pleural space
K. Procedure that fuses the pleura to prevent
   pneumothorax
L. Air in the pleural space
M. Occurs when the lung is rapidly inflated after
   compression by pleural fluid
N. Pneumothorax that occurs with underlying
   lung disease
O. Low-protein effusion caused by CHF or cir-
   rhosis
P. Chest wall puncture for diagnostic or thera-
   peutic purposes
Q. Membrane that lines the lung surface

The Pleural Space

18. How do the pleura of the American buffalo and humans differ? What is the clinical significance for the buffalo and when are humans in the same situation?

19. Describe the so-called "pleural space."

20. What is normal intrapleural pressure and what effect does this have on fluid movement?

21. Explain why pleural pressures are different at the apex and lung bases.

Pleural Effusions

22. Give a brief explanation of how each of the following conditions can cause transudative pleural effusions.

Condition	Mechanism
A. CHF	_____
B. Hypoalbuminemia	_____
C. Liver disease	_____
D. Lymph obstruction	_____
E. CVP line	_____

23. What is the most common cause of clinical pleural effusions?

24. What is the general cause of exudative pleural effusions?

25. Give a brief explanation of the cause of these exudative pleural effusions.

Effusion	Cause
A. Parapneumonic	_____
B. Malignant	_____
C. Chylothorax	_____
D. Hemothorax	_____

26. What change in pulmonary function is associated with pleural effusion?

27. In what specific portion of the upright chest film is pleural effusion visualized?

28. Describe the specific type of chest film used to improve visualization of pleural effusions.

29. What type of imaging is the most sensitive test for identification of pleural effusions?

30. What are the three major risks of thoracentesis?
    A. _____
    B. _____
    C. _____

31. Identify the purpose of each of the chambers in the three-bottle chest tube drainage system shown below.
    A. _____
    B. _____
    C. _____

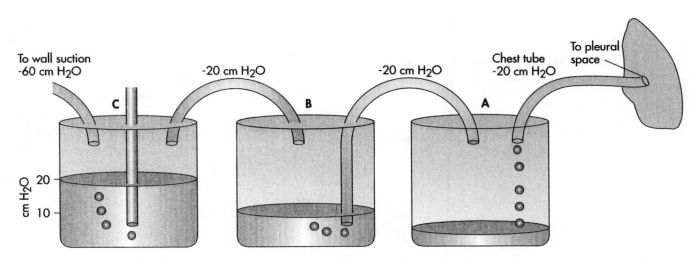

The standard three-bottle system is the basis for all commercial chest tube drainage systems.

Pneumothorax

32. What two symptoms are common to almost all cases of pneumothorax?

    A. _____

    B. _____

33. What is the most common type of traumatic pneumothorax and how is it treated? Give three specific examples.

34. Compare blunt and penetrating chest trauma as causes of pneumothorax. How does treatment differ in these two situations?

35. What special technique may be helpful to visualize pneumothorax in a newborn?

36. Compare the two major types of spontaneous pneumothorax.

37. Tension pneumothorax can be a life-threatening medical emergency.

    A. Definition

    B. Radiographic finding

    C. Clinical signs

    D. Treatment

38. Compare the outcomes of early clinical diagnosis and treatment of tension pneumothorax with delayed diagnosis.

39. How does oxygen administration assist in resolution of a pneumothorax?

40. What is BPF? How does mechanical ventilation perpetuate this problem? What special modes of ventilation may be indicated?

41. What do you think is wrong with Dink's right lung? Support your conclusion with at least five pieces of information from the case.
   A. "I think Mrs. Dink has
      1.

      2.

      3.

      4.

      5.

Case Studies

Case 1

Mrs. Ima Dink, a mathematics instructor with a history of CHF, is admitted with a complaint of pain on inspiration. Her respirations are rapid and shallow. Heart rate is 104. The pulse oximeter shows a saturation of 93% on room air. Breath sounds are very decreased on the right side, crackles in the left base. Chest wall movement is markedly less on the right. The chest radiograph shows calcification of the right lung, with shift of mediastinal structures to the left. Diagnostic percussion reveals a dull note on the right side.

42. What would you recommend as the first respiratory intervention?

43. How could this disorder be resolved?

Case 2

Steve Fink, a tall, thin, young male RCP, is admitted with a complaint of pain on inspiration. His respirations are rapid and shallow. Heart rate is 104. The pulse oximeter shows a saturation of 93% on room air. Breath sounds are very decreased on the right side, clear in the left base. Chest wall movement is markedly less on the right. The chest radiograph shows a dark area without lung markings on the right side, with shift of mediastinal structures to the left. Diagnostic percussion reveals increased resonance on the right side.

44. What do you think is wrong with Fink's right lung? Support your conclusion with at least five pieces of information from the case.
A. "I think Mr. Fink has
   1.

   2.

   3.

   4.

   5.

45. What would you recommend as the first respiratory intervention?

46. How could this disorder be resolved?

What Does the NBRC Say?

Since pneumothorax can be caused iatrogenically, and in mechanically ventilated patients may be life-threatening, you will be expected to know how to recognize and treat this problem. While there is no special category called "pneumothorax," you can expect at least three questions related to this topic. In addition, you are expected to understand the causes of pleural effusions, and how effusions are diagnosed and treated.

47. Immediately after insertion of a central line via the subclavian vein an intubated patient becomes dyspneic. The RCP should recommend which of the following diagnostic tests?
    A. 12-lead ECG
    B. Chest radiograph
    C. ABG
    D. Bedside spirometry

48. The middle bottle of a three-bottle chest drainage system is used as
    A. A water seal
    B. A fluid collection
    C. A means of applying vacuum to the chest
    D. A measurement of improvement of the pneumothorax

49. A chest tube is placed anteriorly between the second and third ribs. The tube is probably intended to treat a
    A. Chylothorax
    B. Hemothorax
    C. Transudative pleural effusion
    D. Pneumothorax

50. A patient is suspected of having a pleural effusion. Which radiographic position is most appropriate to confirm this diagnosis?
    A. A-P chest film
    B. Lateral decubitus chest film
    C. Apical lordotic chest film
    D. P-A chest film

51. Thoracentesis is performed and 1500 ml of fluid is removed from the right chest. Which of the following is likely to occur as a result?
    A. Pulmonary edema in the right lung
    B. Stridor and respiratory distress
    C. Pneumothorax in the right lung
    D. Atelectasis in the right lung

52. All of the following would be useful in differentiating right mainstem intubation from left-sided pneumothorax *except:*
    A. Chest radiograph
    B. Diagnostic percussion
    C. Auscultation
    D. Lung compliance measurement

53. Following an IPPB treatment a COPD patient complains of sudden severe chest pain. What is the RCP's first priority in this situation?
    A. Notify the physician of the problem
    B. Initiate oxygen therapy
    C. Recommend a chest radiograph
    D. Perform an arterial blood gas

54. A patient develops subcutaneous emphysema following a motor vehicle accident involving multiple rib fractures. What action should the RCP take in this situation?
    A. Perform bedside spirometry
    B. Initiate oxygen therapy
    C. Recommend a chest radiograph
    D. Perform an arterial blood gas

Believe me, there are *endless* variations on these themes. The subject material in Chapter 22 is limited, and probably seems pretty straightforward. Be prepared to encounter this topic many times in both the clinical and board examination settings.

Food for Thought

55. What is meant by the term *ascites*? Besides causing effusions, how could this affect respiratory function?

56. How is thoracentesis modified to prevent re-expansion pulmonary edema?

57. What is subcutaneous emphysema and what relationship does it have to pneumothorax?

Pulmonary Vascular Disease

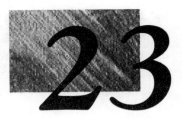

23

The invisible miles of delicate vessels in the lung remain hidden and ignored as they play their vital role in gas exchange and pressure regulation. Then a clot breaks loose and lodges in the pulmonary vascular highway, an accident that frequently has fatal consequences. Rarely recognized, pulmonary embolism results in thousands of deaths each year in the United States. Chapter 23 reviews the incidence, pathophysiology, and treatment of pulmonary embolus and pulmonary hypertension, two conditions the RCP will encounter many times in the hospital setting.

Word Power

When the pressure inside the lung vessels is elevated, a condition called pulmonary _____ exists. This could be caused by a blood clot that travels to the lung, or pulmonary _____. Other less common causes include bits of fat or air. If this process results in death of the lung tissue, it is called a pulmonary _____. Chronic elevation of pulmonary blood pressure will eventually cause a form of right heart failure known as cor _____.

Meet the Objectives

1. How many patients are admitted to the hospital each year in the United States for venous thromboembolism?

2. What is the yearly incidence of mortality related to thromboembolism?

3. Where do most pulmonary emboli originate?

4. Blood clots to the brain or heart often cause death of the tissue. Why is this uncommon in the lung?

5. Explain how pulmonary embolism (PE) increases alveolar dead space?

6. Why does hypoxemia develop in some cases of PE?

7. What is the primary hemodynamic consequence of pulmonary embolism?

8. The combination of what two symptoms should raise the suspicion of PE?
   A. _____
   B. _____

9. What are the three most frequent physical findings associated with PE?
   A. _____
   B. _____
   C. _____

10. What is the incidence of hemoptysis associated with PE?

11. What percent of patients with PE have a normal ECG?

12. Name the two most common ECG abnormalities associated with PE.
    A. _____
    B. _____

13. How is the chest radiograph helpful in diagnosing pulmonary embolism?

14. How helpful are ABGs in ruling out PE? What benefit does an ABG provide in these cases?

15. What are the three modalities most widely used for diagnosing DVT?
    A. _____
    B. _____
    C. _____

16. Which test is considered the "gold stan-dard" for the diagnosis of DVT?

17. What is the test of choice for diagnosis of symptomatic proximal DVT?

18. Because of the high mortality rate, it is important to make a definitive diagnosis of pulmonary embolus. What two invasive tests are reasonably sensitive and reliable in confirming this diagnosis?
    A. _____
    B. _____

19. What is the relationship of the ventilation (V) and perfusion (Q) portions of scans in making a high probability diagnosis of PE?

20. Name two relatively new, noninvasive imaging techniques that show promise in the detection of pulmonary embolism.
    A. _____
    B. _____

21. Prophylaxis for DVT is either pharmacolog-ical or mechanical. Give three examples of each.
    A. Pharmacological prophylaxis
       1. _____
       2. _____
       3. _____
    B. Mechanical prophylaxis
       1. _____
       2. _____
       3. _____

22. What is the standard pharmacological ther-apy for existing thrombosis or embolism? What is the mechanism of action? What are the risks?
    A. Drug

    B. Action

    C. Risks

23. How are thrombolytics different than anti-coagulants? Can they be given together?

24. Give three examples of thrombolytic drugs.
    A. _____
    B. _____
    C. _____

25. List the mechanical options available for treatment of massive PE.

26. When are vena cava filters indicated?

27. Define PPH.

28. Describe the epidemiology of PPH in terms of age, gender, symptoms, mortality, and genetic factors.
    A. Age: _____
    B. Gender: _____
    C. Genetics: _____
    D. Symptoms: _____
    E. Mortality: _____

29. How is this condition diagnosed?

30. Give three medical treatments for PPH
    A. _____
    B. _____
    C. _____

31. What is the only real cure for PPH?

32. Pulmonary hypertension is a frequent complication of COPD. What percentage of elderly patients with COPD will develop significant pulmonary hypertension?

33. Explain the role of alveolar hypoxia in the development of pulmonary hypertension.

34. What other factors seen in COPD contribute to this condition?

35. What is the only treatment that improves the survival rate in patients with COPD and pulmonary hypertension?

Chapter Highlights

36. Venous _____ is an important cause of morbidity and _____ in hospitalized patients.

37. One third of all deaths caused by pulmonary _____ occur within _____ hour(s) of the symptoms.

38. The point of origin of pulmonary embolism is a deep venous thrombosis of the _____ extremities or _____ in _____% of the cases.

39. The clinical presentation of PE and DVT is _____-_____.

40. _____ therapy reduces the risk of venous thromboembolism.

41. Treatment of venous thromboembolism includes anticoagulants such as _____ or _____.

42. Primary pulmonary hypertension is a rare disease that affects _____ patients.

43. Drug treatment of PPH includes _____ and vasodilators such as _____ channel blockers.

Case Studies

Case 1
Mortimer Kent is a 60-year-old who underwent total knee replacement. Two days after surgery he complains of dyspnea and anxiety. Physical examination reveals a heart rate of 110, respiratory rate of 28, blood pressure 115/80, and SpO_2 of 93% on room air. Breath sounds are clear except for faint inspiratory crackles in both bases.

44. Why is this patient at risk for pulmonary embolism?

45. What additional diagnostic tests would be helpful in ruling out other potential pulmonary problems?

46. What treatment would you provide as an RCP?

47. What medical treatment should be initiated if a diagnosis of PE is confirmed?

What Does the NBRC Say?

Pulmonary embolism is so nonspecific in its clinical presentation that it does not have any separate category in the registry examination matrices. On the other hand, dead space-to-tidal volume ratios (VD/VT) are definitely included. Evaluation of dyspnea, pulmonary hypertension, hypoxemia, and ventilation/perfusion scans are all mentioned. Cor pulmonale associated with COPD is a possible inclusion on the exam as well. Recommending anticoagulants is included in the pharmacology section. You are expected to be able to make a differential diagnosis between heart attack, pneumothorax, and PE when a patient complains of sudden chest pain. I don't see any of this included at the entry level.

48. A patient who is being mechanically ventilated shows an increased VD/VT ratio. Which of the following disorders could be responsible?
    A. Atelectasis
    B. Pneumonia
    C. Pulmonary embolism
    D. Pleural effusion

49. Which of the following is the most appropriate test to confirm the presence of a suspected pulmonary embolism?
    A. Chest radiograph
    B. Pulmonary angiography
    C. Bronchogram
    D. Arterial blood gas

50. A ventilation/perfusion scan reveals a defect in perfusion in the right lower lobe without a corresponding decrease in ventilation. Which of the following is the most probable diagnosis?
    A. Right lower lobe atelectasis
    B. Acute pulmonary embolus
    C. Pneumothorax
    D. Pneumonia

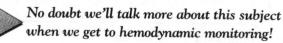 *No doubt we'll talk more about this subject when we get to hemodynamic monitoring!*

Food for Thought

51. What is the most common cause of pulmonary hypertension worldwide?

52. Discuss the pros and cons of moving a critically ill ventilator patient to Imaging for a V/Q scan to confirm a suspected diagnosis of PE.

Acute Lung Injury, Pulmonary Edema, and Multiple System Organ Failure

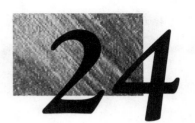

1. ALI

Pulmonary edema is a difficult clinical problem that you will encounter frequently in the emergency room and intensive care units. Although the symptoms and initial goals may be similar, cardiogenic (hydrostatic) and non-cardiogenic (non-hydrostatic) pulmonary edema have very different etiologies and treatments. These are complex syndromes that will challenge you to use every skill and apply all you've learned. In spite of all we have learned over the years, a fairly high mortality rate still exists, especially for ARDS.

2. APRV

3. ARDS

Acronym Soup

My favorite acronym is "snafu": Situation Normal, All Fouled Up. Unfortunately most medical acronyms aren't all that much fun, but you still need to learn them. Write out the definitions of Chapter 24's alphabet soup.

4. CHF

5. ECMO

6. ECCO2R

7. GIT

8. HFV

9. MODS

10. PMNs

11. PEEP

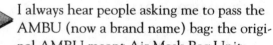 I always hear people asking me to pass the AMBU (now a brand name) bag: the original AMBU meant Air Mask Bag Unit.

Meet the Objectives

General Considerations
Let's talk about how to distinguish these two conditions and what causes them.

12. Name two common conditions leading to hydrostatic pulmonary edema for each of the following general categories:

     Conditions
     A. Cardiac
         1. _____
         2. _____
     B. Vascular
         1. _____
         2. _____
     C. Volume overload
         1. _____
         2. _____

13. List four primary and secondary risk factors for ALI/ARDS.
     A. Primary
         1. _____
         2. _____
         3. _____
         4. _____
     B. Secondary
         1. _____
         2. _____
         3. _____
         4. _____

14. Compare CHF and ARDS in terms of the following criteria for diagnosis.

                       CHF   ARDS
     A. Chest x-ray
         1. Heart _____
         2. Effusions _____
         3. Infiltrates _____
     B. PCWP _____
     C. BALF _____

15. Briefly describe the pathophysiology of hydrostatic pulmonary edema.

16. Briefly describe the pathophysiology of non-hydrostatic pulmonary edema.

17. What five areas must be addressed to avoid secondary lung injury in ARDS?
     A. _____
     B. _____
     C. _____
     D. _____
     E. _____

18. What two general approaches are used to maintain adequate tissue oxygen delivery in ARDS?
     A.

     B.

Ventilator Strategies

Most patients with ARDS will require artificial ventilatory support. The following questions address the currently accepted methods for providing mechanical ventilation.

19. How does optimal PEEP differ from PEEP that delivers the best PaO_2?

20. In general, what level of PEEP is considered optimal?

21. What is the overall goal of PEEP therapy in terms of oxygen toxicity?

22. PEEP should be adjusted to maintain what FiO_2 and PaO_2?

23. Compare tidal volumes delivered in conventional mechanical ventilation versus volumes delivered to ARDS patients.

24. What is meant by "permissive hypercapnia?" What is the goal of this ventilator strategy?

25. In what two conditions is permissive hypercapnia contraindicated? Why?
   A.

   B.

Innovative Strategies

When the techniques described above are not successful, we will have to try something different. Each of these methods has had some limited success. None are foolproof for every patient.

26. Describe high-frequency ventilation.

27. How does IRV differ from conventional ventilator modes?

28. What is the effect of IRV on survival of ARDS patients?

29. What pharmacological interventions are needed with IRV?
    A. _____
    B. _____

30. What are the two ways APRV optimizes ventilation in ARDS patients?
    A.

    B.

31. How does APRV compare to IRV?

32. How can patient positioning be radically altered to improve gas exchange?

33. Both ECMO and ECCO$_2$R facilitate gas exchange via what type of device?

34. What is the recommendation regarding ECMO and ECCO$_2$R in routine management of ARDS?

35. How is liquid ventilation accomplished?

36. What quality of perfluorocarbon compounds makes them attractive for use in ARDS?

Pharmacologic Treatments

A variety of drugs have been used to try to turn the tide in ARDS. A few have had some limited success.

37. What type of surfactant is being administered in ARDS clinical trials? How is it being delivered?

38. What is the potential role of nitric oxide (NO) in treating ARDS?

39. What type of patients would benefit most from NO?

40. What type of abnormal hemoglobinemia is associated with administration of NO?

41. What is the consequence of sudden discontinuation of inhaled NO?

42. What specific role do corticosteroids play in the treatment of ARDS?

Chapter Highlights

43. CHF and ARDS are common causes of acute _____ failure that have similar initial _____ presentations.

44. CHF associated pulmonary edema is due to elevated _____ pressures in the pulmonary _____.

45. ARDS associated pulmonary edema results from _____ injury to the lungs.

46. It may be necessary to perform _____ or _____ in order to distinguish CHF from ARDS.

47. Recommendations regarding the treatment of ARDS have focused on supporting _____ and systemic _____ function until the patient recovers from the underlying illness.

48. Ventilator strategies for patients with ARDS are designed to minimize ventilator _____ lung _____ by using _____, low _____ volumes, and nontoxic levels of inspired _____.

Case Studies

Case 1

Allen is a 5'6" tall, 143 lb (65 kg) teenager who wouldn't listen when his mom told him not to pop his pimples. Now he is in the ICU with: fever of 103 degrees Fahrenheit, blood pressure of 80/50, heart rate 120, and an SpO_2 of 88% on 100% oxygen. His pulmonary capillary wedge pressure is 14 mm Hg and cardiac output is 8L/min. Breath sounds reveal coarse crackles throughout the lungs. Allen is intubated and currently being ventilated with a tidal volume of 800 ml, rate of 14, and PEEP of 0.

49. What is the most likely diagnosis? Why?

50. With regard to the oxygenation status, what changes would you recommend?

51. With regard to the volume, what changes would you recommend?

52. What is the maximum recommended peak pressure that should be delivered to this patient to prevent alveolar damage?

Case 2

Mabel Frother is a 65-year-old, 143 lb (65 kg) woman who was intubated after presenting in the emergency department with pulmonary edema and severe respiratory distress. Now she is in the ICU with: temperature of 97 degrees Fahrenheit, blood pressure of 80/50, heart rate 120, and an SpO_2 of 90% on 60% oxygen. Her pulmonary capillary wedge pressure is 24 mm Hg and cardiac output is 3 L/min. Breath sounds reveal coarse crackles throughout the lungs. Mabel is intubated and currently being ventilated with a tidal volume of 800 ml, rate of 14, and PEEP of 10.

53. What is most likely the diagnosis? Why?

54. With regard to the oxygenation status, what changes would you recommend?

What Does the NBRC Say?

Just like it says in Chapter 24. You need to be able to differentiate CHF and ARDS based on clinical presentation and diagnostic information. You should be able to maintain oxygenation and determine optimal PEEP. Interpretation of wedge pressure, shunt, and pulmonary edema on the radiograph are in the Written Registry Matrix. So are IRV, HFV, and APRV. The Clinical Simulation Examination Matrix specifically mentions CHF as a possible cause. ARDS is not specifically mentioned, but it is implied as a possible cause.

55. Which of the following would be useful in treating an elevated shunt in a patient with ARDS who is being mechanically ventilated?
    A. Initiating SIMV mode
    B. Initiating PEEP
    C. Increasing the FIO_2
    D. Adding expiratory retard

56. Which of the following indicates the optimal PEEP setting?

PEEP	PaO_2	Cardiac Output
A. 5 cm H_2O	53 mm Hg	4.5 L/min
B. 10 cm H_2O	60 mm Hg	4.3 L/min
C. 15 cm H_2O	74 mm Hg	4.0 L/min
D. 20 cm H_2O	88 mm Hg	3.4 L/min

57. A patient is admitted to the ICU with a diagnosis of pulmonary edema. Which of the following breath sounds is consistent with this diagnosis?
    A. Inspiratory stridor
    B. Inspiratory crackles
    C. Expiratory rhonchi
    D. Pleural friction rub

58. A patient with ARDS being ventilated with the following settings

Mode	Assist Control
FIO_2	.80
Rate	10
PEEP	15 cm H_2O
VT	600 ml
SpO_2	82%

    Which of the following would you recommend?
    A. Increase the tidal volume
    B. Decrease the PEEP
    C. Change to inverse ratio ventilation
    D. Increase the rate

59. Which of the following would provide necessary information regarding fluid management in a critically ill patient with pulmonary edema?
    A. Bedside pulmonary function testing
    B. Intake and output measurements
    C. Daily weights
    D. Pulmonary artery catheter

60. Chest radiograph changes associated with non-cardiogenic pulmonary edema include
    I. Pleural effusion
    II. Bilateral infiltrates
    III. Enlarged left ventricle
    A. I, II only
    B. II only
    C. II, III only
    D. I, II, III only

61. Which of the following ventilator techniques have been suggested as useful in treating ARDS that does not respond to conventional therapy?
   I. High-frequency ventilation
   II. Airway pressure release ventilation
   III. Inverse ratio ventilation
   IV. Pressure support ventilation
   A. I, II only
   B. I, III only
   C. I, II, III only
   D. I, II, III, IV

 We'll come back to this subject again when we get to the chapter on hemodynamic monitoring!

Food for Thought

Shock lung, Da Nang lung, Adult Respiratory Distress Syndrome, wet lung, liver lung, and non-cardiogenic pulmonary edema are all names for ARDS. This syndrome has been recognized ever since we began to save trauma victims during modern warfare.

62. What is the recommendation regarding IRV in routine management of ARDS?

63. Is ARDS a homogenous or heterogenous lung condition? Explain.

Lung Neoplasms

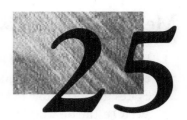

Respiratory cancer is a popular disease of the rich and famous. John Wayne, Humphrey Bog-art, Sigmund Freud; the list goes on and on. Yet there is hardly a more dreaded word in our society than cancer. Lung cancer is the most frequently diagnosed cancer in the world. Yet it is relatively easy to avoid . . .

New Words

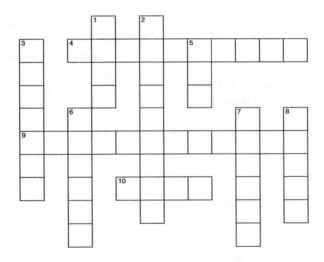

ACROSS

4. process by which tumor cells spread to distant parts of the body
9. Drug treatment to cure cancer
10. the "N" in the TNM staging system

DOWN

1. small _____ cancer, also called oat _____ cancer
2. treatment of neoplastic growth using gamma rays
3. _____ genic carcinoma—cancer originating in the airway
5. staging system
6. opposite of malignant
7. malignant tissue growth
8. type of nodes where cancer spreads

Meet the Objectives

1. How many new cases of bronchogenic carcinoma were newly diagnosed in the United States in 1997? How many cases does the WHO estimate worldwide?
   A. _____
   B. _____

2. What percent of cancer deaths are caused by bronchogenic cancer? Total deaths?
   A. _____
   B. _____

3. Compare the incidence of bronchogenic carcinoma in men and women.

4. What is the likelihood that a smoker will get lung cancer compared with that of a non-smoker?

5. What five smoking factors are related to the risk of developing cancer?
   A. _____
   B. _____
   C. _____
   D. _____
   E. _____

6. How many smokers are there in the United States? What percentage of the total population smokes? How many are men? How many are women?
   A. U.S. smokers: _____
   B. Percentage of population: _____
   C. Men: _____
   D. Women: _____

7. What is another name for passive exposure to smoke?

8. Describe the health risks of passive exposure to smoke.

9. Besides smoking, name the four other major influences linked to an increase in lung cancer.
   A. _____
   B. _____
   C. _____
   D. _____

10. What is meant by a "synergistic" relationship between smoking and the other factors? Give an example.

11. List the four major histopathological types of bronchogenic carcinoma along with the percentage of cases they represent and a brief description of the cells.

    Type of Cancer   *Percent*   *Description*
    A.

    B.

    C.

    D.

12. What are the two most common sites of metastasis of cancer originating in the lungs?
   A. _____
   B. _____

13. What percentage of patients with lung cancer are asymptomatic?

14. Local tumor growth in the central airways may cause many symptoms. Name five that a respiratory care practitioner could easily recognize.
   A. _____
   B. _____
   C. _____
   D. _____
   E. _____

15. Patients with pleural or chest wall involvement will typically have what three symptoms?
   A. _____
   B. _____
   C. _____

16. Bronchorrhea may be present with lung cancer. What is bronchorrhea, and what is the presence of this symptom likely to indicate?
   A. _____
   B. _____

17. Explain what is meant by the term *paraneoplastic syndrome.*

18. Give three examples of paraneoplastic syndromes commonly associated with bronchogenic carcinomas.
   A. _____
   B. _____
   C. _____

19. Name the four common methods for obtaining tissue for lung cancer diagnosis.
   A. _____
   B. _____
   C. _____
   D. _____

20. Why is tumor staging so important?

21. Explain the meaning of the TNM staging system.
   A. T

   B. N

   C. M

22. How is small cell cancer staged?

23. Why is surgical resection the treatment of choice for all non-small cell lung cancer?

24. What patients are not candidates for surgery in terms of staging?

25. How are RCPs involved in determining candidates for surgery?

26. What test values suggest a patient may safely undergo lobectomy or pneumonectomy?

27. Name two palliative therapy modalities.
    A. _____
    B. _____

28. What is the choice of therapy for small cell cancer?

29. What is the long-term disease-free survival rate in patients with extensive small cell disease?

Chapter Highlights

30. _____carcinoma is the leading cause of cancer deaths in the United States.

31. Approximately _____% of all lung cancer is linked to smoking.

32. _____ represents 30% to 35% of all lung cancer and currently is the most common type.

33. The _____ classification groups patients in stages or categories that correlate with _____.

34. Patients with _____ cancer are classified in two stages: limited or extensive.

35. The most commonly used modalities of treatment for patients with non-small cell lung cancer are surgical resection, _____, and _____.

36. The most effective way to prevent lung cancer is to prevent _____.

Case Studies

Chapter 25 has five excellent case studies in the form of Mini-Clini's, so I'm not going to reinvent the wheel. Four of these cases are particularly useful to the respiratory care practitioner.

37. Will you be caring for patients with weakness and drooping eyelids? How is this different in cancer than in neuromuscular disease?

38. Confusion and generalized weakness is often a sign of what type of serious neurological vascular accident?

39. What therapy modalities might improve lung function before surgery for lung resection?

40. What methods of diagnosis might be useful for the patient with copious amounts of clear, frothy sputum?

What Does the NBRC Say?

For once, the NBRC is relatively silent on this subject. Obviously you need to recognize that hemoptysis is an important sign of dysfunction that may relate to cancer or tuberculosis, among others.

Food for Thought

41. Besides lung cancer, what are the other significant health risks of smoking?

42. With the high incidence and known risk factors for lung cancer you would expect to see screening techniques. Discuss this issue.

43. What is brachytherapy?

Neuromuscular and Other Diseases of the Chest Wall

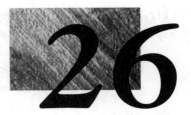

Even if your lungs are normal, diseases that affect the brain, nerves, muscles, or bony thorax can lead to respiratory failure or hypoxemia. There are so many unusual conditions that produce muscular weakness that it can be difficult to keep them all straight. You will do fine if you focus on the general principles that apply to assessment and maintenance of the airway in these complex and often sad cases.

Power Words

I've always wondered if neuromuscular really meant you had a strong mind. Let's find out when you try matching these diseases to their definitions.

_____ 1. Ankylosing spondylitis
_____ 2. Amyotrophic lateral sclerosis
_____ 3. Flail chest
___G___ 4. Guillain-Barre syndrome
_____ 5. Lambert-Eaton syndrome
_____ 6. Myasthenia gravis
_____ 7. Myotonic dystrophy
_____ 8. Polymyositis
_____ 9. Scoliosis

A. Neuromuscular conduction disorder that particularly affects the face, throat and respiratory muscles.
B. Chronic inflammatory disease that fuses the spine and affected joints.
C. Muscle-wasting disease characterized by delayed relaxation of contracted groups.
D. Degenerative disease of motor neurons characterized by progressive atrophy.
E. Inflammation of muscles caused by a rheumatological disorder.
F. Unstable chest due to rib fractures exhibiting paradoxical movement on inspiration.
G. Idiopathic polyneuritis characterized by ascending weakness.
H. Abnormal lateral curvature of the spine that may compromise ventilation.
I. Neuromuscular conduction disorder associated with underlying malignancy.

Meet the Objectives

General Principles

10. The brainstem centers receive numerous inputs as they control what three general sets of muscles in the respiratory system?
    A. _____
    B. _____
    C. _____

11. The three best recognized pulmonary dys-
functions of respiratory muscle weakness are:
A. _atelectasis_
B. _Hypoxemia_
C. _Ventilatory insufficiency_

12. What are the three common complaints of
patients with respiratory muscle weakness
due to neuromuscular disease?
A. _exertional dyspnea_
B. _Fatigue_
C. _orthopnea_

13. Give two representative diseases that affect
each of the following locations in the respiratory system.

Location	Diseases
A. Cortex, upper motor	Stroke
	trauma
B. Spinal cord	trauma
	ms
C. Lower motor neurons	ALS,
	muscular dystroph
D. Peripheral nerves	Guillain-Barré
	Lyme
E. Neuromuscular junction	Myastenia gravis
	botulism
F. Muscle tissue	MD (Duchennes)
	polymyositis
G. Interstitial lung tissue	Polymyositis
	Neurofibromatosis

14. Pulmonary function testing of patients with
neuromuscular disease and otherwise normal lung tissue will demonstrate what type
of ventilatory defect? _Restrictive_

15. What three specific tests are most useful in
monitoring ventilatory function in patients
with neuromuscular weakness?
A. _VC_
B. _IP_
C. _ABGS_

16. How well does pulmonary function testing
assess ability to protect the airway?

_It does not, Respiratory
muscle weakness is not uniform_

17. What signs and symptoms suggest performing
nocturnal oximetry or formal sleep testing?

_Cor palmonale, daytime
Somnulence, sleep
disturbances_

Specific Neuromuscular Diseases

18. What is myopathic disease? Give two exam-
ples.
A. _____
B. _____
C. _____

19. Discuss the role of nocturnal ventilation in
patients with myopathic diseases.

20. Most cases of myasthenia gravis arise from what abnormality at the cellular level?

21. What general category of drugs is used to treat myasthenia gravis?

22. What surgical treatment may be effective in some cases of myasthenia gravis?

23. List four predisposing factors to Guillain-Barre syndrome (GBS).
    A. viral infections
    B. pregnancy
    C. Hodgkins lymphoma
    D. general surgery

24. What percentage of patients with GBS will have respiratory muscle compromise?

one third

25. Bilateral interruption of the phrenic nerves that results in diaphragmatic paralysis is seen in what type of injury?

High servical cord inj.

26. Reversible unilateral diaphragmatic paralysis occurs frequently following what commonly performed surgery?

cardiac

27. Describe the chest radiographic presentation of unilateral diaphragmatic paralysis.

diaphram is still curved but displaced upward

28. How is the paralyzed diaphragm visualized during flouroscopy?

32. What is the hallmark sign of significant diaphragmatic weakness?

abdominal paradox

29. What is the percentage of new spinal cord injuries in the United States each year, and what percentage of these cases results in quadriplegia?

    A. _____

    B. _____

33. What percentage of patients with C3-C5 injury will ultimately become liberated from mechanical ventilation?

80%

30. Define the high and middle/low classification of cervical cord lesions.

    A. High

    B. Middle/Low

34. Both stroke and traumatic brain injuries lead to disordered breathing. What is a stroke?

31. Describe the muscle groups affected by each of the following spine injuries.

Level	Muscle Groups
A. C1-C2	_____
B. C3-C5	_____
C. C4-C8	_____
D. T1-T12	_____
E. T7-L1	_____

35. What are the two basic types of stroke?

    A. _____

    B. _____

36. Give examples of the effect on the respiratory system of strokes in the following locations in the brain.

Location	Effect on Respiration
A. Cerebral cortex	_____
	_____
B. Bilateral hemispheric infarct	_____
	_____
C. Lateral medulla	_____
	_____
D. Mid pons	_____
	_____

37. Aside from problems similar to stroke, brain trauma can cause what respiratory "fluid" problems?
   A. _____
   B. _____

Disorders of the Thoracic Cage

38. Describe these two chest wall deformations that often occur together.
   A. Kyphosis

   B. Scoliosis

39. Describe the ventilatory defects and pulmonary function changes associated with severe kyphoscoliosis.
   A. Ventilation

   B. Pulmonary function

40. How is kyphoscoliosis treated in younger patients?

41. Describe the role of nocturnal ventilation in treating patients with kyphoscoliosis.

42. Describe the paradoxical chest motion that is the hallmark of flail chest.

43. Name three other pulmonary injuries frequently associated with flail chest.
    A. _____
    B. _____
    C. _____

44. Regardless of the physiological mechanisms behind respiratory dysfunction, what are the mainstays of treatment for flail chest?
    A. _____
    B. _____
    C. _____

Chapter Highlights

45. The key components of the respiratory neuromuscular system are the *Brain*, the nerves, the *neuromuscular* junction, and the *muscles* of inspiration.

46. Weakness or *ventilatory* failure are the most important respiratory dysfunctions in many neuromuscular diseases.

47. Neuromuscular diseases can also cause *hyperventilation* or hypoventilation, sleep *apnea*, aspiration, *atelectasis*, and pulmonary hypertension.

48. Signs and symptoms of muscle weakness include exertional *Dyspnea, cough* orthopnea, soft vocalizations, and a weak *Cough*.

49. PFTs typically show a decreased *total* lung capacity, decreased *vital* capacity, and decreased *maximal* inspiratory pressures.

Case Studies

Case 1

Martha Greene is a 27-year-old woman who was admitted from her doctor's office following complaints of fatigue. Upon interview, Ms. Greene reports that she becomes weak after any exertion, especially in her arms. She also complains of difficulty swallowing. She denies any recent illness. Vital signs show a normal temperature, and slightly increased heart rate and respiration. Inspection reveals that she has drooping eyelids and appears to have little tone in her facial muscles.

50. Based on this information, what is the most likely diagnosis?

51. What drug therapy might help to confirm this diagnosis?

52. What test is the most sensitive indication of respiratory muscle strength?

55. What two treatment strategies have improved outcome in this syndrome?
A. IV Immuloglobulin infusin
B. plasmapheresis

What Does the NBRC Say?

One or two cases on the Clinical Simulation Examination will be devoted to adult patients with neuromuscular or neurological conditions. Myasthenia gravis, Guillain-Barre, tetanus, muscular dystrophy, and drug overdose are listed as examples in the matrix. You should be able to recommend or interpret the results of bedside tests such as vital capacity and maximum inspiratory pressure. So while there won't be too many multiple-choice questions on neuromuscular diseases, this is a very important part of the testing process. Chest and spinal trauma are also included on your boards. In particular, you should pay attention to the subject of flail chest.

Case 2

Gregory Brown is a 52-year-old male who was admitted from his doctor's office following complaints of fatigue. Upon interview, Mr. Brown reports that his feet felt numb yesterday, and his legs were weak when he got up this morning. He went to the doctor because he thought he might be having a stroke. He states that he had the flu about 2 weeks ago. Vital signs show a normal temperature and slightly increased heart rate and respiration.

53. Based on this information, what neuromuscular condition is likely?

54. How would analysis of CSF be useful in making a diagnosis? (Hint: you won't find this in the text in Chapter 26!)

56. A 23-year-old patient with flail chest is transferred to the ICU for observation following a motor vehicle accident. After 2 hours, the patient complains of increasing dyspnea, and arterial blood gas analysis is performed.

pH	7.33
$PaCO_2$	50 mm Hg
PaO_2	61 mm Hg

What action should the RCP recommend at this time?
A. Place the patient on oxygen therapy
B. Initiate mask CPAP
C. Administer a bronchodilator drug
D. Initiate mechanical ventilation

57. A patient with Guillain-Barre syndrome has had serial vital capacity measurements.

0900	3.1 L
1100	2.6 L
1300	2.1 L
1500	1.6 L

In regard to this data, what should the RCP recommend?
   A. Increase the monitoring to q1 hour
   B. Administration of Tensilon
   C. Intubation and mechanical ventilation
   D. Continue to monitor the patient q2 hours

58. A vital capacity below what value indicates the need for intubation and ventilation in a patient with acute neuromuscular disease?
   A. 30 ml/kg
   B. 20 ml/kg
   C. 15 ml/kg
   D. 10 ml/kg

59. A patient with myasthenia gravis presents in the emergency department with profound muscle weakness. Administration of which of the following will improve ventilation?
   A. Pancuronium
   B. Neostigmine
   C. Epinephrine
   D. Atropine

60. The presence of paradoxical chest motion on inspiration following a motor vehicle accident most likely indicates
   A. Flail chest
   B. Pulmonary contusion
   C. Pneumothorax
   D. Hypoxemia

Food for Thought

61. What is the long-term prognosis for the following conditions?
   A. Myasthenia gravis

   B. Guillain-Barre Syndrome

   C. Duchennne's muscular dystrophy

Disorders of Sleep

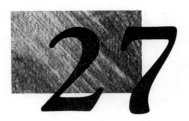

"Most people spend their lives going to bed when they're not sleepy and getting up when they are."
Cindy Adams

1. BiPAP

Introduction

Does someone you love snore excessively? Whenever I ask that question, hands go up in the audience. Does that mean the snorer has sleep apnea? Have you ever wondered just exactly what you do while you're sleeping? The polysomnography lab is just the place to find out. Many RCPs have found rewarding careers in the sleep or neurodiagnostic lab setting. Another reason RCPs are interested in disorders of sleep, are the cardiopulmonary consequences of sleep apnea. Finally, even in the acute care setting, you will be called on to deal with patients who utilize CPAP or bilevel airway pressure devices to control their apnea. Once again, you will find yourself in the position of being the expert on the assessment and equipment involved in treating this not-so-unusual condition.

2. CSA

3. CPAP

Acronym-o-philia

Give the full name of the following acronyms from Chapter 27 (Some of them should be old friends by now!).

4. EDS

5. EEG

6. EPAP

7. IPAP

8. OSA

9. PSG

10. UVPPP

11. UARS

Meet the Objectives

12. What is the definition of sleep apnea?

13. How does OSA differ from CSA?

14. What is the estimated incidence of OSA in the adult population?

15. Why does airway closure occur during sleep?

16. Name five cardiopulmonary consequences of untreated OSA.
    A. _____
    B. _____
    C. _____
    D. _____
    E. _____

17. Name four neurobehavioral consequences of untreated OSA.
    A. _____
    B. _____
    C. _____
    D. _____

18. List four factors that predispose a patient to OSA.
    A. _____
    B. _____
    C. _____
    D. _____

19. Describe the five common clinical features seen in many cases of OSA.
    A. _____
    B. _____
    C. _____
    D. _____
    E. _____

20. What is the current gold standard for making a diagnosis of OSA?

21. An apnea-hypopnea index of what value is consistent with moderate to severe sleep apnea? What is considered normal?

22. What are the three goals of treatment for OSA?
    A. _____
    B. _____
    C. _____

23. Discuss the behavioral options that should be pursued in all patients with sleep-disordered breathing.

24. Why do you think nocturnal CPAP has become the first-line medical therapy for OSA?

25. How does CPAP work to relieve OSA?

26. Discuss the issue of patient compliance with nasal CPAP therapy.

27. Explain how the titration of bilevel positive airway pressure therapy differs from that of CPAP.

28. Describe five of the common minor side effects of positive pressure therapy and what you can do to help the patient solve these annoying problems.

A. _____
_____

B. _____
_____

C. _____
_____

D. _____
_____

E. _____
_____

29. What is the role of tracheostomy in treating sleep apnea?

30. What is UPPP's success rate and what is the current recommendation regarding this procedure as a treatment for OSA?

Chapter Highlights

31. The three types of sleep apnea are obstructive, _____, and _____.

32. The predominant risk factor for airway narrowing or closure during sleep is a _____ or _____ upper airway.

33. The long-term adverse consequences of OSA include poor _____ functioning as well as increased risk of _____ morbidity and mortality.

34. Risk factors for OSA include _____ gender, age greater than _____ years, upper body _____, and habitual _____.

35. The first-line medical therapy for OSA is _____.

36. _____ positive airway pressure therapy may be useful in salvaging patients who have difficulty with standard positive pressure treatments.

37. _____ therapy may be an option for a select group of patients who have undergone extensive upper airway analysis and do comply with medical therapy.

Case Studies

KISS is another one of my favorite acronyms. Keep it simple . . . and this is simple. There is no way that I can improve on the four excellent cases in your textbook.

What Does the NBRC Say?

The NBRC usually considers CPAP to be a ventilator or freestanding strategy to improve oxygenation, but that is changing. Nasal CPAP and BiPAP (which, by the way, is a trademark registered by Respironics) are included on the Written Registry Examination. Remember that these techniques for raising airway pressure are also used to help prevent intubation and mechanical ventilation in the acute care setting. The Clinical Simulation Matrix does mention obesity-hypoventilation as a potential case. So, while this is a relatively new and not a large area of the boards, some of the information from Chapter 27 will be included.

38. An RCP notes in the medical record that a patient is receiving BiPAP therapy with a machine she brought from home. Which of the following is the most likely diagnosis for the patient?
    A. Pulmonary emphysema
    B. Congestive heart failure
    C. Obstructive sleep apnea
    D. Atrial fibrillation

39. A sleep study shows simultaneous cessation of airflow and respiratory muscle effort. These findings are consistent with
    A. Pulmonary hypertension
    B. Obstructive sleep apnea
    C. Congestive heart failure
    D. Central sleep apnea

40. Which of the following is true regarding BiPAP therapy?
    I. Expiratory pressure is always set above inspiratory pressure
    II. BiPAP units are pneumatically powered
    III. IPAP should be increased until snoring ceases
    A. I, III
    B. II only
    C. II, III
    D. III only

Food for Thought

41. What do tennis balls have to do with
obstructive sleep apnea?

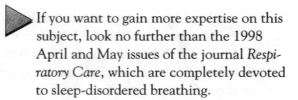 If you want to gain more expertise on this
subject, look no further than the 1998
April and May issues of the journal *Respiratory Care*, which are completely devoted
to sleep-disordered breathing.

Airway Pharmacology

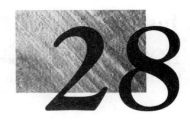

"All things are poison and poison is in all things. Whether it is a medication or . . . depends on the dose."
Paracelsus

When the first edition of Egan came out in 1969, only a limited number of drugs were available by inhalation. Most of those medications are no longer used, due to the advent of newer, more-specific agents with longer action and fewer side effects. New categories of inhaled medicines require the respiratory practitioner to have a strong grasp of pharmacological principles and the specific indications and actions for these newer tools for managing the airway. You will need to be able to advise physicians, nurses, and patients on methods and options for producing bronchodilation, reducing the inflammatory response, clearing secretions, and treating infection.

Better Living Through Chemistry

Try this matching exercise to test your ability to understand the new terms found in Chapter 28. (You may really have to dig for some of these—use the chapter, the glossary, and a medical dictionary if necessary!)

_____ 1. Indication
_____ 2. Tolerance
_____ 3. Adrenergic
_____ 4. Vasopressor
_____ 5. Pharmaceutical
_____ 6. Muscarinic
_____ 7. Pharmacodynamic

_____ 8. Side effect
_____ 9. Absolute contraindication
_____ 10. Leukotriene
_____ 11. Mydriasis
_____ 12. Agonist
_____ 13. Pharmacokinetic
_____ 14. Cholinergic
_____ 15. Antagonist
_____ 16. Tachyphylaxis
_____ 17. Onset
_____ 18. Peak effect
_____ 19. Duration
_____ 20. Half-life

A. How long to metabolize half of drug dosage
B. Drug may not be given for any reason
C. Effect of acetylcholine on smooth muscle
D. Reason for giving a drug to a patient
E. Undesired effect of a drug
F. Drugs that mimic the effect of epinephrine
G. Has receptor affinity and exerts an effect
H. Mimics the effect of acetylcholine
I. Drug that exerts a constricting effect on blood vessels
J. Phase related to route of administration
K. Dilation of the pupil of the eye
L. Phase related to mechanism of action
M. Maximum effect from a drug dosage
N. How long it takes a drug to start working
O. How long the drug's effect lasts
P. Increasing dose needed for effect
Q. Has receptor affinity but produces no effect
R. Rapidly developing tolerance
S. Compounds that produce allergic or inflammatory responses
T. Phase related to metabolism of a drug

Just Say Yes

21. What is the most common route of administration that is utilized by RCPs?

22. Name four advantages of this route.
    A. _____
    B. _____
    C. _____
    D. _____

23. Name two disadvantages.
    A. _____
    B. _____

24. How do medications delivered by this route usually end up in the systemic circulation?

25. Describe the two primary divisions of the autonomic nervous system in terms of name, neurotransmitter, and effect on bronchial smooth muscle.

A. Sympathetic
    1. Other name _____
    2. Transmitter _____
    3. Airwary muscle effect _____

B. Parasympathetic
    1. Other name _____
    2. Transmitter _____
    3. Airway muscle effect _____

Adrenergic Bronchodilators

26. State the three receptors of the sympathetic nervous system and their basic effects.

Receptor	Primary effect
A. Alpha	_____
	_____
B. Beta$_1$	_____
	_____
C. Beta$_2$	_____
	_____

27. Give the generic name, brand name, strength and dose for the following commonly used beta-adrenergic bronchodilators.

*Brand
Name*

A. Racemic epinephrine _____
   Strength/dose: _____
B. Metaproterenol _____
   Strength/dose: _____
C. Terbutaline
   (svn) _____
   Strength/dose: _____
   (MDI) _____
   Strength/dose: _____
D. Albuterol
   (svn) _____
   Strength/dose: _____
   (MDI) _____
   Strength/dose: _____
E. Bitolterol
   (svn) _____
   Strength/dose: _____
   (MDI) _____
   Strength/dose: _____
F. Pirbuterol
   (MDI) _____
   Strength/dose: _____
G. Salmeterol
   (MDI) _____
   Strength/dose: _____
H. Epinepherine
   (MDI) _____
   Strength/dose: _____

28. Epinephrine and racemic epinephrine are bronchodilators, but these drugs are usually administered to achieve what effects? Give examples of clinical conditions.

	Effect	Clinical uses
A.	_____	_____
B.	_____	_____

29. Discuss the use of Serevent in treating asthma. When should it be used? When should it be avoided? What patient teaching would be important with this drug?

30. It is especially important that you know how long it takes for a drug to start working, reach its maximum effect and how long the drug will last. Fill in the information for the drugs listed below.

Drug	Onset	Peak effect	Duration
A. Alupent	_____	_____	_____
B. Brethine	_____	_____	_____
C. Ventolin	_____	_____	_____
D. Serevent	_____	_____	_____

31. List the most common side effects of bronchodilator drugs.
    A. _____
    B. _____
    C. _____
    D. _____

32. Adverse reactions are more serious, but less frequently seen. List six potential adverse effects you must watch for in patients receiving adrenergic bronchodilators.
    A. _____
    B. _____
    C. _____
    D. _____
    E. _____
    F. _____

33. What should you monitor when administering any drugs via the aerosol route?

34. What specific tests or data can be obtained to monitor the effects of bronchodilator therapy?

Anticholinergic Bronchodilators

35. Generally, ipratropium is indicated for use in what types of patients?

36. Fill in the blanks to complete your knowledge of ipratropium.

Name	Brand Name	Strength	Dose
Ipratropium bromide			
MDI	_____	_____	_____
SVN	_____	_____	_____

37. Now try this one.

Drug	Onset	Peak effect	Duration
Ipratropium	_____	_____	_____

38. What medication is available by MDI with both ipratropium and albuterol? What are the possible advantages and disadvantages of this medication?

39. Describe the side effects and adverse reactions to watch for when administering this medication.

40. Why does Egan recommend that atropine no longer be used by inhalation?

Mucus-Controlling Agents

41. Describe the two drugs approved for inhalational treatment of secretion problems in the United States.

A. Generic name
    1. Brand name _____
    2. Dose _____
    3. Strength _____
    4. Indication _____
B. Generic name
    1. Brand name _____
    2. Dose _____
    3. Strength _____
    4. Indication _____

42. Bronchospasm is a common side effect of the administration of mucolytic agents. How would you recommend modifying the therapy to prevent or treat this problem?

43. What types of short- and long-term assessments should you make to monitor the effectiveness of these drugs?

Inhaled Corticosteroids

Like bronchodilators, there are a lot of inhaled steroids on the market. You can expect many of your patients to be receiving these medications. Physicians, patients, and family members have many misconceptions about steroids, including steroid phobia. Again, it's up to you to be the expert and be able to clearly explain the use of these very important tools in the fight against asthma.

44. How long will it take for inhaled steroids to have a noticeable effect on the symptoms of asthma?

45. What significance does this have in terms of patient education?

46. The most common side effects of inhaled steroids are local ones (as opposed to systemic). Name the four most common problems.
   A. _____
   B. _____
   C. _____
   D. _____

47. Why should reservoir devices always be used with the administration of aerosolized steroids via metered dose inhaler?

48. Describe the short- and long-term methods used to assess the effectiveness of inhaled steroids.

The National Institutes of Health 1997 Asthma Education and Prevention Program guidelines contain definitive information on the use of drug therapy for the treatment of asthma. You can get a copy of these guidelines from the American Lung Association or your instructors, or by downloading the information from the NIH web sites.

Mediator Antagonists

Drugs that prevent the release of histamine of block the release or effects of other mediators of inflammation are hot items right now. (New leukotriene receptor antagonists have just come into the marketplace.) These drugs, whether oral or inhaled, hold tremendous promise for treating asthma and preventing the long-term pulmonary consequences of this increasingly serious condition.

49. What is believed to be the mode of action of cromolyn sodium?

50. Which two mediator antagonists are recommended for use in children?

51. Which of these mediator antagonists is available by inhalation?

52. List the number one side effect for each of the following:

A. Cromolyn sodium (Intal)

B. Nedocromil (Tilade)

C. Zafirlukast

D. Zileuton

Treating Infection by the Aerosol Route

It should make sense to you that lung infections can be treated by aerosolizing medications. This technique for delivery is limited to very specific situations.

54. What agent may be nebulized to treat PCP seen in severely immunocompromised patients?

55. Discuss how to determine whether to give this drug via the oral, inhalational, or IV route.

56. What special precautions must be taken when administering this medication via aerosol?

57. What are the common undesired respiratory side effects of administration? What modification of therapy would you recommend if they occur?

58. While PCP is not a hazard to healthy people, patients with AIDS often have what other disease that is transmitted via the airborne route?

59. Describe the use of Ribavirin in terms of indication, patient population, and special equipment needed for administration.
   A.

   B.

   C.

   D.

60. What other anti-infective agents are aerosolized? What type of infection are they used against?

Case Studies

Case 1

Wendy Wheezer has asthma. She is admitted to the hospital for the second time in 2 months. She has not been able to get relief and is using her albuterol inhaler frequently.

61. In addition to inhaled beta-agonists, steroids are commonly administered to *reduce* inflammation associated with asthma. Name one inhaled steroid and recommend a dose.

62. What device is important to use along with MDIs to prevent deposition of these drugs in the mouth?

63. Why should Wendy rinse her mouth after using her inhaled steroid?

64. Recommend another drug that can be delivered by MDI as a long-term controller to prevent *release* of inflammatory mediators.

65. What long-acting bronchodilator may help Wendy sleep through the night without being awakened by dyspnea and wheezing?

Case 2

Cystic fibrosis is diagnosed in a 7-year-old white male. This patient has extremely thick mucus. Auscultation reveals scattered wheezing and rhonchi.

66. What drug would you recommend aerosolizing for treatment of the thick mucus?

67. What other drug should be given to treat the wheezing?

Case 3

Bob Bloater is a 67-year-old male with long-standing COPD characterized by chronic bronchitis. He is coughing up copious amounts of very thick white sputum. Bob complains that his chest feels tight and that he cannot catch his breath. His albuterol inhaler is not providing relief.

68. What bronchodilator is appropriate to add to the therapeutic regimen?

69. What mucolytic may be considered if other means of sputum clearance are ineffective? Why might this drug be counterproductive?

What About Those Board Exams?

Sure enough, those scholastic scoundrels at the NBRC have scattered a number of drug questions strategically throughout the tests. In fact, pharmacology appears in at least six different parts of the matrix!

70. A patient with *Pneumocystis carinii* pneumonia is unable to tolerate oral antibiotics due to gastrointestinal side effects. Which of the following would you recommend?
   A. Aerosolized acetylcysteine (Mucomyst)
   B. Aerosolized albuterol (Proventil)
   C. Aerosolized Dornase alfa (Pulmozyme)
   D. Aerosolized pentamidine iethionate (NebuPent)

71. An asthmatic patient presents in the emergency room with dyspnea, hypoxemia, and wheezing. All of the following are appropriate at this time *except*
   A. Administration of oxygen
   B. Nebulized cromolyn sodium (Intal)
   C. Nebulized albuterol (Ventolin)
   D. Measurement of peak expiratory flow rates

72. Following extubation, a patient has mild stridor. Which of the following would you recommend at this time?
   A. Administration of oxygen
   B. Aerosolized albuterol (Proventil)
   C. Aerosolized virazole (Ribavirin)
   D. Aerosolized racemic epinephrine (Vaponefrin)

73. After administering a corticosteroid via MDI, the respiratory care practitioner should ask the patient to perform which of the following actions?
   A. Rinse and gargle with water
   B. Breathe deeply and cough
   C. Inhale an adrenergic bronchodilator
   D. Inhale via a spacer device

74. The heart rate of a patient receiving an adrenergic bronchodilator rises from 80 to 94 beats per minute during the treatment. Which of the following actions is most appropriate?
    A. The RCP should discontinue the therapy
    B. Let the patient rest for 5 minutes and continue the therapy
    C. Continue the treatment
    D. Reduce the dosage of the bronchodilator in future treatments

75. A physician calls in an order for bronchodilator therapy for a patient with COPD. The order states ".05 ml of albuterol in 3 ml of normal saline via SVN four times per day." The respiratory care practitioner should
    A. Deliver the treatment as ordered
    B. Recommend substituting Atrovent
    C. Carefully monitor heart rate during the treatment
    D. Call the doctor to verify the order

76. Besides treatment of excessively thick mucus, what can Mucomyst be used for?

77. Primatene Mist is a commonly used asthma inhaler that is available without a prescription. What drug is found in this MDI? What are potential problems with patients taking this drug?

Food for Thought

You might be wondering how you can retain all this drug information. It's not easy! Especially when you might now use many of these medications on a regular basis. One suggestion I have for you is a time honored technique. Make drug cards. All you need are some 3 x 5 or 4 x 6 index cards. Write out the following on each card (or type on the computer and glue or tape to the card):
- Generic and brand names of the drug
- Routes (like MDI, oral, SVN)
- Dose
- Strength
- Adverse reactions and side effects
- Contraindications
- Patient teaching points

Airway Management

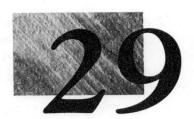

"When you can't breathe,
nothing else matters."
American Lung Association
motto

Airway management is one of my favorite subjects. It is very satisfying to help patients breathe better in such a dramatic fashion. While there is no substitute for experience, Chapter 29 (and 30) will help you learn how to use equipment, tubes and techniques to deal with airway emergencies. You will want to become an expert in every aspect of this subject so that you can become a skilled, knowledgeable provider and a resource for other health care professionals. Start off by learning the parts of the two most important artificial airways used to maintain adequate ventilation.

Tube Terms

_____ tubes are long, semirigid tubes, usually made of _____ chloride or some other type of plastic. A typical ET tube has nine basic parts. The proximal end (sticking out of the mouth) has a standard _____ mm adaptor. The body of the tube has _____ markings in centimeters. The tube ends in a _____ tip. There is a port, or slot, cut in the side of the tip called a _____ eye. This slot helps ensure gas flow if the tip is obstructed. Just above the tip, a _____ is bonded to the tube, which can be inflated to seal the airway to prevent aspiration or provide for _____ pressure venti-

lation. A small filling tube leads to a _____ balloon. This small balloon has a spring-loaded _____ with a connector where a syringe can be attached to allow inflation or deflation. A _____ indicator is embedded in the wall of the tube body to make it easier to see the tube position on a chest x-ray. Another commonly used tube, inserted through a surgical opening in the trachea, is called a _____ tube. These tubes are also made of plastic, or occasionally metal such as _____. The _____ cannula forms the primary structural unit of the tube. Like the ET tube, a _____ may be attached near the end to seal the airway. A _____ is attached to the proximal end to prevent slippage and provide a means to secure the tube to the neck. Many tubes have a removable _____ cannula with a standard _____ mm adaptor. This cannula can be removed for cleaning. A special device called an _____, has a rounded blunt end and is used to facilitate insertion.

Intubation Procedures

1. What is the preferred route for establishing an emergency tracheal airway?

2. Name the four practitioners who most commonly perform endotracheal intubation.
   A. _____
   B. _____
   C. _____
   D. _____

3. Why is suction equipment needed for intubation?

4. Describe two common troubleshooting procedures utilized when the laryngoscope doesn't light up properly.

5. How can you select the proper-sized ET tube for a patient?

6. Prior to insertion, how should the RCP test the tube?

7. How is the head positioned to align the mouth, pharynx, and larynx?

8. What other actions must be taken before making any attempt to intubate?

9. How long may you attempt intubation? Why?

10. Name at least two anatomic landmarks to be visualized prior to intubation.

11. Compare the use of the Miller and Macintosh laryngoscope blades during the intubation procedure.

12. Your textbook describes seven methods for clinically assessing correct tube position. While none of these methods absolutely confirms position, they are essential assessments to make right after the tube is placed. Name at least four of these methods.

A.

B.

C.

D.

13. What is the disadvantage of using capnographic or colorimetric analysis of carbon dioxide to assess intubation of a cardiac arrest victim?

14. What are the two methods used to absolutely confirm tube placement?

A.

B.

15. Give two examples of clinical situations in which nasotracheal intubation might be preferred over oral intubation.

A. _____

B. _____

16. Describe the two techniques used for nasal intubation.

    A.

    B.

17. Let's compare oral and nasal intubation. Each has advantages and disadvantages. Place a letter 'O' by items that match oral intubation, and a letter 'N' by items that go with nasal intubation.

    A. Avoids epistaxis and sinusitis   _____
    B. Greater comfort for long-term use _____
    C. Easier to suction   _____
    D. Larger tube   _____
    E. Greater risk of extubation   _____
    F. Improved oral hygiene   _____
    G. Bronchoscopy more difficult   _____
    H. Increased salivation   _____
    I. Reduced risk of kinking   _____
    J. Decreased laryngeal ulceration   _____
    K. Increased risk of sinusitis   _____

Tracheotomy

18. What is the primary indication for performing a tracheotomy?

19. When is tracheotomy the preferred route of airway management?

20. Describe the sequence for removing an endotracheal tube during the tracheotomy procedure.

21. Compare the location of placement in percutaneous and traditional surgical tracheostomy.

22. Name at least three advantages of the per-cutaneous technique compared with traditional surgical tracheotomy.

A.

B.

C.

Airway Trauma

23. Compare the following laryngeal injuries associated with intubation in terms of symptoms and treatment.

    A. Glottic edema
      1. Symptoms _____
      2. Treatment _____
    B. Vocal cord inflammation
      1. Symptoms _____
      2. Treatments _____
    C. Laryngeal ulceration
      1. Symptoms _____
      2. Treatments _____
    D. Polyp/granuloma
      1. Symptoms _____
      2. Treatments _____
    E. Vocal cord paralysis
      1. Symptoms _____
      2. Treatments _____
    F. Laryngeal stenosis
      1. Symptoms _____
      2. Treatments _____

24. Name the three most common tracheal lesions.
    A. _____
    B. _____
    C. _____

25. Compare tracheal malacia and tracheal stenosis in terms of cause, pathology, and treatment.

    A. Malacia
      1. Cause _____
      2. Pathology _____
      3. Treatment _____
    B. Stenosis
      1. Cause _____
      2. Pathology _____
      3. Treatment _____

26. Describe the T-E fistula in terms of cause, complications, and treatment.

27. Tracheoinnominate fistula is a rare but serious complication. What are the clues and what are the immediate and corrective actions taken? What is the survival rate?

Care and Feeding of Your New Airway

Once placement of an artificial airway is successfully completed the real fun begins. As an RCP, you will be expected to secure the airway, maintain adequate humidification, manage secretions, care for the cuff, and troubleshoot problems that arise–some of which are life-threatening.

28. What is the most common material used to secure endotracheal tubes? Tracheostomy tubes?

29. How do flexion and extension of the neck affect tube motion? What is the average distance the tube will move (in centimeters)?

30. What is the worst problem that results from inadequate humidification of the artificial airway?

31. What temperature range must be maintained in a heated humidification system to provide adequate inspired moisture?

32. What device can be used as an alternative to heated humidifiers for short-term humidification of the intubated patient?

33. State at least four reasons why tracheal airways always increase the risk of infection.
    A. _____
    B. _____
    C. _____
    D. _____

34. Describe three techniques that can be utilized to decrease the risk of infection.
    A.

    B.

    C.

35. What is the most common cause of airway obstruction in the critically ill patient?

36. Describe the shape of a modern tube cuff.

37. What is the recommended safe cuff pressure? What is the consequence of elevated cuff pressures?

38. Describe the two alternative cuff inflation techniques.
    A.

    B.

39. How is the methylene blue test performed?

40. State the three airway emergencies.
    A. _____
    B. _____
    C. _____

41. Give three reasons why a tube may become obstructed.
    A.

    B.

    C.

42. What simple technique is used to assess tube obstructions that are not relieved by repositioning the head?

43. If you cannot clear the obstruction, what action should you be prepared to take?

44. What additional troubleshooting step can often be performed on patients with tracheostomies?

45. What effects will occur with a cuff leak when a patient is being mechanically ventilated?

46. What action should you be prepared to take if the cuff is blown?

Extubation

Extubation is a procedure commonly performed by the RCP. You will need to be familiar with the indications for extubation and techniques used to minimize risk during this procedure.

47. Describe two methods for performing a "cuff-leak test."
   A.

   B.

48. List five types of equipment you will want to assemble *prior* to extubation.
   A. _____
   B. _____
   C. _____
   D. _____
   E. _____

49. You will need to suction what two places before extubating? Name them and describe the correct sequencing for this important step.

50. Describe the two different strategies for removing the tube itself.
    A.

    B.

51. What therapeutic modality is usually applied immediately after extubation?

52. The worst complication of extubation is laryngospasm. What can you do if this persists more than a few seconds?

53. A common complication of extubation is glottic edema. How will you recognize *and* treat this problem?

54. Oral feeding should be withheld for how long following extubation? Why?

55. State the three methods for weaning from a tracheostomy tube. Give one advantage and one disadvantage for each technique.

    A. Technique _____
       1. Advantage _____
       2. Disadvantage _____
    B. Technique _____
       1. Advantage _____
       2. Disadvantage _____
    C. Technique _____
       1. Advantage _____
       2. Disadvantage _____

Ten Commandments for Endotracheal Suctioning

I. Thou shall assess thy patient.

II. Thou shall use the correct vacuum setting.

III. Thou shall use the right-sized catheter.

IV. Thou shall preoxygenate and hyperinflate thy patient.

V. Thou shall withdraw 1 to 2 cm prior to suctioning.

VI. Thou shall suction on withdrawal only.

VII. Thou shall limit the duration to 10 to 15 seconds.

VIII. Thou shall reoxygenate and hyperinflate after each attempt.

IX. Thou shall only irrigate when indicated.

X. Thou shall monitor thy patient.

56. Discuss the advantages and disadvantages of closed-system multi-use catheters.

57. What special catheter is used to facilitate entry into the left mainstem bronchus?

58. Describe the cause and how to prevent each of the following complications.

    A. Hypoxemia
      1. Cause _____
      2. Prevention _____

    B. Cardiac arrhythmia
      1. Cause _____
      2. Prevention _____

    C. Hypotension
      1. Cause _____
      2. Prevention _____

    D. Atelectasis
      1. Cause _____
      2. Prevention _____

    E. Mucosal trauma
      1. Cause _____
      2. Prevention _____

    F. Increased ICP
      1. Cause _____
      2. Prevention _____

59. How should you position a patient for naso-tracheal suctioning?

60. What additional supplies will be needed to prevent trauma during this procedure?

61. What specialized airway is used to facilitate repeated nasal suctioning?

Bronchoscopy

62. State one advantage and three disadvantages of the rigid bronchoscope.

63. Give an example of a specific drug and the general goal for each of the following classes of premedication used in bronchoscopy.

   A. Tranquilizer
      1. Example _____
      2. Goal _____
   B. Drying agent
      1. Example _____
      2. Goal _____
   C. Narcotic-analgesic
      1. Example _____
      2. Goal _____
   D. Anesthetic
      1. Example _____
      2. Goal _____
   E. Vasoconstrictor
      1. Example _____
      2. Goal _____

64. What three types of cardiopulmonary monitoring devices are considered essential for this procedure?
   A. _____
   B. _____
   C. _____

Case Studies

Case 1

During your first day of clinical training in the ICU a patient suffers a cardiac arrest. Your clinical instructor asks you to assist in preparing the equipment needed for endotracheal intubation. The patient is a small 56-year-old female.

65. What size of endotracheal tube should you select?

66. How should you test the tube prior to insertion?

67. How will you test the laryngoscope and blade for proper function?

68. Once the tube is inserted, how can you quickly assess placement?

69. A colorimetric CO_2 detector is attached to the endotracheal tube. The end-tidal CO_2 is 2% on exhalation, and 0% on inhalation as the chest rises with bagging. What does this suggest regarding the effectiveness of the chest compressions?

Case 2

After your heart-pounding initiation into resuscitation, it is time to check the other ventilator patients on the unit. Mrs. Barbara Doll, a 19-year-old with a head injury, is receiving mechanical ventilation via a cuffed no. 8 tracheostomy tube with an inner cannula. As you enter the room, the high-pressure alarm is sounding.

70. How will you determine the need for suctioning in this situation?

71. What vacuum pressure should be set prior to suctioning?

72. What size suction catheter is suggested using the rule of thumb found in Egan?

73. How long, and with what FIO_2, should you preoxygenate this patient?

74. After suctioning, you will need to check the cuff pressure. What is a safe cuff pressure?

What About Those Board Exams?

Chapter 29 is the longest one we've had so far! That must mean this is extremely important material. The NBRC agrees! The Entry-Level Examination Matrix says you must perform procedures to achieve maintenance of the airway, including artificial airway care, adequate humidification, cuff monitoring, positioning, and removal of secretions. They go on to include modification of the management of artificial airways, including changing the type of humidification, inflating or deflating the cuff, and initiating suctioning. Finally, you should be able to assemble and check the function of the airways and the intubation equipment. The Registry Examination adds more complex questions in all these areas and concludes with assisting the physician in performing bronchoscopy, tracheostomy, and of course, intubation. The actual number of airway questions varies from exam to exam, but you should be prepared for at least 8 to 10 questions on any given test.

75. Which of the following will decrease the risk of damage to the trachea from the endotracheal tube cuff?
   I. Minimal leak technique
   II. Maintaining cuff pressures of 25 to 35 cm H_2O
   III. Minimum occluding volume technique
   A. I only
   B. I, II only
   C. I, III only
   D. I, II, III

76. The diameter of the suction catheter should be no larger than
   A. One-tenth the inner diameter of the endotracheal tube
   B. One-third the inner diameter of the endotracheal tube
   C. One-half the inner diameter of the endotracheal tube
   D. Three-fourths the inner diameter of the endotracheal tube

77. A patient with a tracheostomy tube no longer requires mechanical ventilation. All of the following would facilitate weaning from the tracheostomy except
   A. A fenestrated tracheostomy tube
   B. A cuffed tracheostomy tube
   C. A tracheostomy button
   D. An uncuffed tracheostomy tube

78. Extubation is performed on a patient with an endotracheal tube. Presence of which of the following suggests the presence of upper airway edema?
   A. Rhonchi
   B. Crackles
   C. Wheezes
   D. Stridor

79. All of the following are useful in nasotracheal intubation except
   A. Laryngoscope blade
   B. Stylette
   C. Miller blade
   D. Magill forceps

80. While performing endotracheal suctioning, a respiratory care practitioner notes that flow through the catheter is minimal and secretion clearance is sluggish. Which of the following are possible causes of this problem.
   I. The vacuum setting is greater than 120 mm Hg
   II. The suction canister is full of secretions
   III. There is a leak in the system
   A. I only
   B. I, II only
   C. II only
   D. II, III only

81. Rapid, initial determination of endotracheal tube placement can be achieved by
   I. Auscultation
   II. Arterial blood gas analysis
   III. Measurement of end-tidal CO_2
   IV. Measurement of SpO_2
   A. I, II only
   B. I, III only
   C. II, III, IV
   D. I, III, IV

82. A patient with a tracheostomy tube shows signs of severe airway obstruction. A suction catheter will only pass a short distance into the tube. The RCP should
   A. Remove the tracheostomy tube
   B. Deflate the cuff of the tube
   C. Ventilate the tube with positive pressure
   D. Remove the inner cannula

83. Which of the following can be used to measure the adequacy of pulmonary circulation during closed-chest cardiac compressions?
    A. Capnometry
    B. Arterial blood gas analysis
    C. Pulse oximetry
    D. Blood pressure monitoring

84. Prior to performing bronchoscopy, an RCP is asked to administer a nebulized anesthetic to a patient. What medication is most appropriate to place in the nebulizer?
    A. Versed
    B. Atropine
    C. Morphine
    D. Lidocaine

Food for Thought

85. What are the advantages and disadvantages of commercial tube holders or harnesses compared with tape or cloth ties for securing endotracheal or tracheostomy tubes?

Emergency Life Support

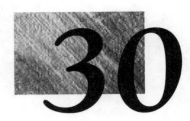

30

"We're in the resuscitation business, not the resurrection business."
Anonymous RCP

1. ABC

Nothing is more satisfying than being a part of the team that helps save someone's life! A successful resuscitation is an exciting event that you will remember forever. Of course, a poorly managed effort is completely frustrating, and attempting to save someone who should never have CPR in the first place is about as depressing as it gets. Since RCPs play an integral role in hospital resuscitations, you will want to know both the basic and advanced life support techniques. *There is no substitute for formal training and certification in basic and advanced life support!* Chapter 30 summarizes the important concepts of these two activities, and will provide you will knowledge skills you will be expected to demonstrate on your boards.

2. ACLS

3. AED

Acres of Acronyms

You must have noticed by now that medicine loves acronyms. I found 17 in Chapter 30 that will enable you to talk the talk. (Walking the walk is another story altogether!) Write out the full definition of each acronym below.

4. AHA

8. CDC

5. ARC

9. CNS

6. BLS

10. CPR

7. BVM

11. DNR

12. EMS

13. OSHA

14. PALS

15. PVC

16. RCP

17. SVT

Causes and Prevention of Sudden Death

18. What is the primary cause of sudden death in the United States?

19. Give an estimate for how many lives could be saved each year by a comprehensive community-wide system of life support implemented throughout the country.

20. Identify five types of accidental death in people under the age of 40 in the United States.
    A. _____
    B. _____
    C. _____
    D. _____
    E. _____

21. Discuss death by foreign body obstruction of the airway in children.

Basic Life Support

22. Use Box 30-1 on page 631 of Egan to help you describe the following steps of adult basic life support.

        Action   *Description*

A. Responsiveness

B. Activate EMS

C. Airway

D. Breathing

E. Circulation

23. Compare adult, child, and infant resuscitation for the following categories.
Adult
A. Obstructed
    1. Conscious _____
    2. Unconscious _____
B. Breathing _____
C. Compress
    1. _____
    2. _____
    3. _____
    4. _____
    5. _____
Child
A. Obstructed
    1. Conscious _____
    2. Unconscious _____
B. Breathing _____
C. Compress
    1. Hands _____
    2. Ratio _____
    3. Cycles _____
    4. Depth _____
    5. Rate _____

24. When is the jaw-thrust maneuver indicated?

25. How can you determine if a victim is breathing?

26. Describe the technique for mouth-to-mouth breaths for adults and children. What is the hazard to the victim in this procedure?
A. Adults

B. Children

C. Infants

D. Hazard

27. When is mouth-to-nose resuscitation indicated in adults?

30. How is hand positioning for chest compression different in adults, children, and infants?

A. Adult

28. Mouth-to-tube or stoma? You might be able to bring yourself to do this on a loved one, but in the hospital, you will want to modify this technique. What would you do?

B. Children

C. Infant

29. How is assessment of pulselessness different in adults and infants?

31. Describe the modifications to CPR that you need to consider under these special circumstances:
    A. Near drowning

    B. Electrocution

    C. Pacemaker

    D. Artificial heart valve

32. Once CPR is begun, it is normally stopped only for what three reasons?
    A. _____
    B. _____
    C. _____

33. A person with sudden cardiac arrest is probably in what rhythm?

34. What is the treatment for this rhythm?

35. The AHA has recommended the addition of the letter "D" to the ABCs. Explain what this means.

36. How can you easily and quickly determine the effectiveness of ventilations and compressions delivered during CPR?
    A. Ventilation

    B. Compression

37. State the three major common complications of CPR.

A. _____

B. _____

C. _____

38. CPR is contraindicated under what two circumstances?

A. _____

B. _____

39. What is the universal distress signal for foreign body obstruction of the airway?

40. When should back blows be used on an adult victim?

41. Give another name for the abdominal thrust maneuver. When should you avoid this maneuver in an adult?

A. _____

B. _____

42. Describe four ways you can tell that you have effectively removed a foreign body from the airway.

A. _____

B. _____

C. _____

D. _____

Advanced Cardiac Life Support

RCPs are often called on to perform oxygenation, assessment, and airway management techniques during resuscitation. In addition, I recommend that you take the American Heart Association course in Advanced Cardiac Life Support.

43. What concentration of oxygen should be administered during a life-threatening emergency?

44. Rank the following ventilation techniques in order with "1" representing the technique that delivers the largest volume.

A. _____ Bag-valve-mask

B. _____ Mouth-to-mouth

C. _____ Mouth-to-mask

45. List five characteristics of the ideal mask.

A. _____

B. _____

C. _____

D. _____

E. _____

46. What is the technique to select the best-sized oropharyngeal airway (OPA)?

47. Name and describe the two basic types of oral airways.

A.

B.

48. What could go wrong if you insert an oral airway in a conscious victim?

49. What airway would you choose for the patient who cannot tolerate an oral airway?

50. Describe two ways to insert an oral airway without pushing the tongue back.

A.

B.

51. How would you lubricate the following airways prior to insertion?

A. Oral

B. Nasal

52. Why is an endotracheal tube the preferred method for securing the airway during CPR?

53. What is the recommended maximum duration of an intubation attempt?

54. Describe the four ways to achieve a high FiO$_2$ with a self-inflating resuscitation bag.

A.

B.

C.

D.

55. When should the endotracheal route of drug administration be used?

56. What is the primary treatment for pulseless ventricular tachycardia and ventricular fibrillation?

57. Give three examples of drugs that can be delivered via the ET route.

A. _____

B. _____

C. _____

58. What modification to dosage and technique must be made for endotracheal instillation of emergency drugs?

59. What initial energy level is recommended electrical countershock during ventricular fibrillation? What is recommended for the second and third shocks?

The Return of Just Say Yes

63. Identify the drug indicated to treat each of the following.

Event	Drug Therapy
A. Ventricular tachycardia	_____
	_____
	_____
B. Pulseless electrical activity	_____
C. Asystole	_____
	_____
D. Poor cardiac contractility	_____
E. Hypotension	_____
F. Hypertension	_____
G. Ventricular fibrillation	_____
H. SVT	_____
I. Coronary artery occlusion	_____
	_____
J. CHF/pulmonary edema (fluid overload)	_____

60. Explain the difference between cardioversion and defibrillation.

Case in Point

We're going to skip the cases and get straight to the board exam questions for once!

NBRC Highlights

The Entry-Level Examination Matrix makes it perfectly clear what you need to know in regard to resuscitation. They even tell you there will be five questions on the subject. If pay attention to this one chapter, you'll get those five questions right!

61. When is electrical pacing indicated?

You must:
A. Recognize when to perform CPR
B. Call for help (Help! Help!)
C. Establish an effective airway
D. Ventilate with the three methods described in Chapter 30 (and watch the chest!)
E. Perform chest compressions
F. Remember to check for a pulse
G. Provide oxygen
H. Ask for blood gases

62. What are the two primary types of pacing?
   A. _____
   B. _____

The Registry Examinations adds much, much more, but again, the matrix is specific.

A. ET instillation of drugs
B. Cardioversion and defibrillation
C. Use capnometry to determine tube placement and adequacy of perfusion
D. Intubation
E. Know your basic drugs, including bicarbonate
F. Initiate and interpret ECG monitoring
G. Check on the pupils (of the eye)

Admittedly, there is a lot to know. I don't think there is any substitute for an ACLS course to complete your knowledge in preparation for work in the ICU or the Registry Examination. (Chapter 30, along with the previous material, will give you most of what you need.)

64. When is the jaw-thrust technique indicated to help maintain an open airway?
    A. When foreign body obstruction is suspected
    B. Following trauma to the head
    C. In cases of suspected neck injury
    D. During most CPR efforts

65. While attempting mask-to-mouth ventilation, an RCP notes that the chest does not rise with each breath. The most appropriate action to take at this time is to
    A. Intubate the patient
    B. Switch to bag-mask ventilation
    C. Use an oxygen-powered breathing device
    D. Give another breath after repositioning the head

66. Where should you check the pulse of an unresponsive infant?
    A. Brachial artery
    B. Carotid artery
    C. Femoral artery
    D. Radial artery

67. Upon entering a hospital room you see a physical therapist administering CPR to a patient who is lying on the floor. Your first action would be to
    A. Move the patient onto the bed
    B. Call for help
    C. Take over chest compressions
    D. Deliver two slow breaths to the airway

68. What is the correct number of rescue breaths to deliver during mouth-to-mouth ventilation of an adult victim?
    A. 10 breaths per minute
    B. 12 breaths per minute
    C. 16 breaths per minute
    D. 20 breaths per minute

69. An unconscious patient begins gagging during your attempt to insert an oropharyngeal airway. The correct action to take at this time would be to
    A. Insert a smaller oral airway
    B. Intubate the patient
    C. Perform the jaw-thrust maneuver
    D. Insert a nasal airway

70. The correct ratio of ventilations to compressions during two-rescuer CPR is
    A. 5:1
    B. 1:15
    C. 1:5
    D. 2:15

71. The ideal airway to use during a resuscitation effort is
    A. An oropharyngeal airway
    B. A nasopharyngeal airway
    C. The fenestrated tracheostomy tube
    D. An oral endotracheal tube

72. A patient is coughing and wheezing after accidentally aspirating a piece of meat. At this time, the RCP should
    A. Do nothing but reassure the patient
    B. Perform the Heimlich maneuver
    C. Deliver five back blows
    D. Call for help

73. Upon entering an ICU room, an RCP observes ventricular fibrillation on the cardiac monitor. The most appropriate treatment for this rhythm is
   A. CPR
   B. Administration of lidocaine
   C. Administration of epinephrine
   D. Electrical countershock

74. During a resuscitation effort, no IV line can be established. The RCP should recommend
   A. Intraosseous infusion of the medications
   B. Endotracheal instillation of the medications
   C. Insertion of a central line
   D. Aerosol administration of the medications

75. The effectiveness of chest compressions in producing circulation can be measured by
   I. Pulse oximetry
   II. Capnography
   III. Transcutaneous monitoring
   IV. Arterial blood gases
   A. I, II only
   B. II, III only
   C. II, IV only
   D. I, II, III, IV

76. A patient has symptomatic atrial fibrillation that does not respond to medications. The treatment of choice would be
   A. Vagal stimulation
   B. Defibrillation
   C. Oxygen administration
   D. Cardioversion

Get the picture? Any question on the subject of resuscitation is fair game. Start by learning the basic rates, depths, and management techniques. Then move on to the advanced material.

Food for Thought

77. Why doesn't anyone want to do mouth-to-mouth resuscitation in the hospital? What are the alternatives?

78. How do you "activate EMS" in a hospital?

79. Who provides emotional support to the family of a resuscitation victim? For the health care providers?

Humidity and Bland Aerosol Therapy

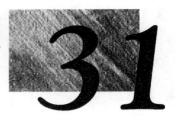

31

I recently traveled to Las Vegas to attend a conference. After the first night in the hotel room I woke up with a dry sore nose. Have you ever traveled to a low-humidity environment and experienced a humidity deficit? Imagine what happens to patients when we give them dry gases to breathe. Or worse, when we bypass the upper airway's natural humidification system. Humidification is a simple thing, really, but then it's often the simple things in life that matter most.

Wet Words

The amount of relative humidity in gas can be measured by a device called a _____. When air does not have enough moisture to meet the normal _____ humidity of 44 mg/L, a humidity deficit is present. This problem may occur when the normal upper airway is bypassed by an endotracheal tube. Secretions may become very thick or _____, resulting in airway obstruction. A _____ is a device that adds gaseous water to inspired air. When you heat a humidifier it can deliver more water to the lungs. An artificial nose, or _____ and _____ exchanger is a simple device that does not require a water-filled chamber. _____, or devices that produce particles of water are also useful for adding moisture to inspired air. An electrically powered device called an _____ nebulizer, utilizes a _____ crystal, and produces a large output of small particles of water for deposition in the lung.

Meet the Objectives

1. How are heat and moisture normally exchanged in your body?

2. List at least four consequences of prolonged inspiration of improperly conditioned gases.
   A. _____
   B. _____
   C. _____
   D. _____

3. Liter flows exceeding what value require humidification?

4. Give one other situation in which you would *always* provide humidification.

5. List the two primary and two secondary indications for humidification.
   A. Primary
      1. _____
      2. _____
   B. Secondary
      1. _____
      2. _____

6. What are the three variables that determine how well a humidifier works?
      A. _____
      B. _____
      C. _____

   Which is most important?

7. Bubble humidifiers are added to what type of oxygen delivery system?

8. What is the typical range for absolute humidity delivered by a bubble humidifier? What does this amount convert to in terms of relative body humidity?
   A. _____
   B. _____

9. What safety device is incorporated into the design of a bubble humidifier?

10. Discuss the primary advantages of passover humidifiers compared to bubble humidifiers.

11. Discuss the principle of operation of each of the following noses.

 A. Condenser humidifier

 B. Hygroscopic condenser humidifier

 C. Hydrophobic condenser humidifier

12. What are four contraindications to using HMEs, according to the AARC CPG on humidification with mechanical ventilation?

 A.

 B.

 C.

 D.

13. Identify three possible risks of using heated humidifiers. (Hint: see Box 31-1 and the CPG!)

    A. _____

    B. _____

    C. _____

14. Identify three hazards associated with water that "rains out," or condenses in humidified breathing circuits.

    A. _____
    _____
    _____

    B. _____
    _____

    C. _____
    _____

15. What specialized breathing circuit circumvents the condensation problem?

16. The AARC recommends what range of alarm settings for electronically controlled heated humidifiers?

17. What specific characteristic is the single most important factor to monitor to determine the effectiveness of a humidification system?

18. Egan describes what really simple way to estimated the performance of an HME or heated-wire circuit without using a hygrometer?

19. What three indications are given in the AARC CPG for bland aerosol administration?

    A.

    B.

    C.

20. Give three examples of bland aerosols.
    A. _____
    B. _____
    C. _____

21. Identify the parts of the ultrasonic nebulizer shown below.
    A. _____
    B. _____
    C. _____
    D. _____
    E. _____
    F. _____
    G. _____

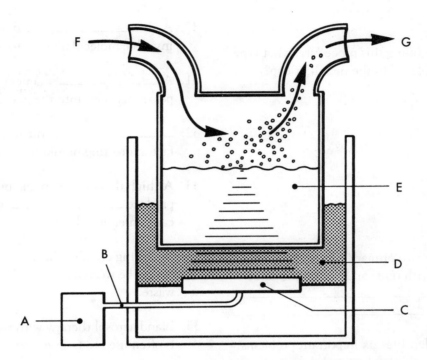

Functional schematic of a typical large-volume ultrasonic nebulizer (USN). (From Barnes TA: *Core textbook for respiratory care practice*, ed 2, Chicago, 1994, Mosby.)

22. What preset variable determines the size of the aerosol particles generated by a USN?

23. What adjustable control determines the actual amount of aerosol produced?

24. Ultrasonic nebulizers are primarily used to accomplish what specific clinical goal/procedure?

25. When performing this procedure, what type of water is placed in the nebulizer cup?

26. Identify the two primary clinical problems associated with tents and body enclosures?
    A. _____
    B. _____

27. Your text identifies six important problems associated with bland aerosol therapy. For each of these problems, give a possible solution or means of prevention.

Problem	Solution
A. Cross-contamination/ infection	_____
B. Environmental safety	_____
C. Inadequate mist	_____
D. Overhydration	_____
E. Bronchospasm	_____
F. Noise	_____

Chapter Highlights

Let's review some basic concepts from Chapter 31. Fill in the blanks.

28. Heat and _____ exchange is done primarily by the _____.

29. Gases delivered to the trachea should be warmed to _____ to _____ degrees C.

30. A _____ is a device that adds invisible molecular water to a gas.

31. A _____ generates and disperses particles into the gas stream.

32. _____ is the most important factor affecting humidifier output.

33. At high flows some bubble humidifiers may produce _____, which can carry infectious bacteria.

34. Breathing circuit _____ must always be treated as _____ waste.

35. Bland aerosol therapy with sterile _____ is often used to treat airway _____.

Case Studies

Use the algorithm on p. 678 of your textbook to choose the right humidity or bland aerosol system.

Case 1

Gunther Snorkelson has fallen into a lake while ice-fishing. He is brought to the Emergency Department with a core temperature of 30° Celsius. Gunther is intubated with a number 8 endotracheal tube. He is unconscious and requires mechanical ventilation.

36. Give two reasons why you can't use an HME with this patient.

A.

B.

37. What humidification system would you recommend?

39. Why is Anthony unable to benefit from an HME?

Case 3

Billy Butler is a 57-year-old man who has undergone coronary artery bypass graft (CABG) surgery. He is being mechanically ventilated pending recovery from the procedure.

40. What humidification system would you recommend?

Case 2

Anthony Marcus is a 32-year-old man admitted to the medical floor with a diagnosis of *Mycoplasma* pneumonia. He is receiving oxygen via nasal cannula at 5 L/min. He complains of a stuffy, dry nose a few hours after admission.

38. What humidification system would you recommend for this patient?

What About Those Board Exams?

Sure enough, you should be able to recommend and administer bland aerosol and humidity therapy. You should know when to change to another system. Selecting, assembling, cleaning and troubleshooting are in there, too. Expect 3 to 5 questions, and especially expect something on HMEs and USNs.

41. An RCP hears a loud whistling sound as she enters the room of a patient receiving oxygen via cannula at 6 L/min. In reference to the humidifier, what is the most likely cause of the problem?
    A. the top of the humidifier is cross-threaded
    B. The humidifier has run out of water
    C. The flow rate is set at less than the ordered amount
    D. There is a kink in the oxygen supply tubing

42. An ultrasonic nebulizer is ordered for sputum induction. Which of the following solutions should be placed in the medication cup to accomplish this goal?
    A. Sterile distilled water
    B. 0.45% NaCL solution
    C. 0.9% NaCL solution
    D. 3% NaCL solution

43. A large-volume, all-purpose nebulizer is set at an FIO_2 of 40% and a flow rate of 10 L/min. to deliver humidified oxygen to a patient with a tracheostomy. The nebulizer is producing very little mist. Which of the following could be done to improve the aerosol output?
    I. Check the water level in the nebulizer
    II. Increase the flow rate to the nebulizer
    III. Drain condensation from the supply tubing
    IV. Turn off the nebulizer's heating system
    A. I only
    B. I, II only
    C. I, III only
    D. I, III, IV only

44. While performing a ventilator check, the RCP observes a large amount of thin, white mucus in the tubing connected to the HME. Which of the following actions should be taken at this time?
    A. Rinse out the HME with sterile water
    B. Suction the mucus from the tubing
    C. Place the patient on a heated humidification system
    D. Replace the HME

45. Sputum induction via USN is ordered. The nebulizer will produce 5 ml of water per minute output on the maximum amplitude setting. The treatment is to last for 15 minutes. How much solution should the RCP place in the nebulizer?
    A. 5 ml
    B. 15 ml
    C. 50 ml
    D. 75 ml

 These questions are only samples! Lots more possibilities in the area of humidification!

Food for Thought

46. The industry standard for adding simple humidification to an oxygen delivery system is a flow rate of greater than 4 L/min. Can you think of any situations in which you might add humidification when the flow rate is lower than 4?

Just for fun (respiratory fun), place yourself on a nasal cannula at 6 L/min (be sure to use a clean one!), or a simple mask at 10 L/min in the laboratory setting. Breathe through your nose for 10 or 15 minutes. How does it feel?

Aerosol Drug Therapy

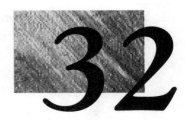

"The pen is mightier than the sword! The case for prescriptions rather than surgery."
Marvin Kitman

Now that you have the drugs, what do you do with them? When I was a student we gave almost all our medications via intermittent positive pressure breathing (IPPB). It was expensive, complicated, time and labor intensive, and most certainly was not customized to the customer! The good news was that we didn't have to know about so many delivery systems. You, of course, are expected to learn a wide variety of ways to deliver aerosolized drugs and find the most cost-effective and therapeutic method of delivery.

Chapter 32 will get you off to a good start on this quest.

Terminology Torture

By now you must have noticed that respiratory care has a language all its own. You won't go far without the passwords. Drug administration is no different, so you need to start by matching the following terms to their definitions.

_____ 1. Aerosol
_____ 2. Atomizer
_____ 3. Baffle
_____ 4. Deposition
_____ 5. Hygroscopic
_____ 6. Inertial impaction
_____ 7. MMAD
_____ 8. Nebulizer
_____ 9. Propellant
_____ 10. Therapeutic index

A. Suspension of solid or liquid particles in a gas
B. Difference between therapeutic and toxic drug concentrations
C. Device that produces uniformly sized aerosol particles
D. Device that removes large particles
E. Device that produces non-uniformly sized aerosol particles
F. Deposition of particles by collision
G. Particles being retained in the respiratory tract
H. Absorbs moisture in the air
I. Measurement of average particle size
J. Something that provides thrust

Characteristics of Therapeutic Aerosols

11. Why is particle size so important in aerosol therapy?

12. What is the primary method of deposition for large, high-mass particles?

13. Particles of 10 microns or larger tend to deposit in what part of the respiratory tract? Where do particles between 5 and 10 microns tend to deposit?

14. In what part of the lung would you like to deposit beta-adrenergic bronchodilator drugs? What particle size is needed to accomplish this goal?

15. Since it is extremely difficult to predict exactly what happens to particles once they enter the lung, what is the most practical way to determine how well you are delivering a drug?

Hazards of Aerosol Therapy

What is the number one hazard of aerosol drug therapy? Why, the drugs themselves, of course!

16. Nebulizers are a great source for nosocomial infections. Describe three of the CDC recommendations for preventing this serious problem.
    A.

    B.

    C.

17. List five aerosolized substances associated with increased airway resistance.

A. _____

B. _____

C. _____

D. _____

E. _____

18. What can you do to prevent bronchospasm from happening?

19. Aerosolizing drugs *always* has the potential for inducing bronchospasm. Describe at least four ways you can monitor this potential problem.

A.

B.

C.

D.

20. What group of patients is most prone to harm from bland aerosols?

21. What is meant by the term "drug re-concentration?" When is this most likely to occur?

Aerosol Drug Delivery Systems

I mentioned earlier that there are a lot of different delivery options available. Naturally, every company claims their system is the best. Let's see if we can figure out which really is the best, using the information in Egan.

Metered-Dose Inhalers

MDIs are the most widely prescribed aerosol drug delivery system, even though they are not completely socially accepted. It's okay to pop your antacids in the boardroom, but most executives will hide their inhalers!

22. What percentage of patients and health care professionals is believed to use MDIs incorrectly?

23. What propellant is used in most MDIs and why is this a problem?

24. What other substances are found in MDIs that may produce clinical problems?

25. What percentage of the drug in an MDI is actually deposited in the lung? Why is there so much variability?

26. What MDI-delivered drugs should always be used with a spacer? Why?

27. Put the following steps of optimal MDI delivery in order.
    A. Hold your breath _____
    B. Breathe out normally _____
    C. Wait 1 minute _____
    D. Shake the canister _____
    E. Hold the MDI two fingers from mouth _____
    F. Slowly inhale as deeply as you can _____

28. What is the difference between a spacer and a holding chamber? Does it matter?

29. How does the recommended breathing pattern differ with a holding chamber from that of a spacer or unassisted MDI?

30. What is a DPI? What's the big deal?

31. How does DPI breathing technique differ from that recommended with an MDI?

32. What patients cannot use DPIs? What warning should every patient receive about using their DPI during an acute episode of bronchospasm?

Small Volume Nebulizers

Small volume nebulizers (SVNs) have been around a long time and are still widely used. They have an amazing number of aliases: mini-neb, acorn neb, hand-held neb, updraft neb, micro-neb, med neb. . .the list seems to go on forever. These devices are indicated when a patient is unable to physically use an MDI or cannot generate sufficient inspiratory flow rates for an MDI.

33. List three potential power sources to drive the SVN.
    A. _____
    B. _____
    C. _____

34. How does an atomizer differ from an SVN? When would you want to use one?

35. What is the optimal flow rate and amount of solution to put in an SVN?
    A. _____
    B. _____

36. What potential problem exists when you deliver an SVN via mask? How can you deal with this problem?

Large Volume Nebulizers

Large volume nebulizers (LVNs) are usually used to deliver bland aerosols. You may want to try one to deliver drugs when a severely obstructed patient does not respond to a single SVN treatment and needs repeated series in a short time.

37. What potential clinical problems may exist with continuous bronchodilator therapy?

38. Why is the SPAG generator unique?

Small Ultrasonic Nebulizers

Small USNs have a lot of advantages: small uniform particles, high output, and they can be used with ventilators.

39. List three advantages and three disadvantages of USNs to deliver medications.

	Advantages	Disadvantages
A.	_____	_____
B.	_____	_____
C.	_____	_____

Case Studies

 Use the algorithms (Figs. 32-15, 32-16) on pages 701 and 703 in Egan to answer the following questions about selection of aerosol drug delivery devices and doses.

Case 1

Bob Bloater is an alert, cooperative 52-year-old male who has been recently diagnosed with chronic bronchitis. He quit smoking (60 pack-year history) 6 months ago, but still has respiratory symptoms. He is in your pulmonary clinic today to receive his PFT results and medications. The physician has ordered Atrovent and Vanceril for Bob.

40. What method of delivery would you recommend for this patient?

41. What other equipment is indicated?

42. What general considerations for patient education would you stress for Mr. Bloater?

43. How will you know if he is able to perform the therapy correctly?

Case 2

Randy Andrews presents in the ER with acute respiratory distress. He is diagnosed with status asthmaticus. This 27-year-old man has high-pitched diffuse wheezes, a respiratory rate of 24, heart rate of 106, and an SpO_2 of 92%. His PEFR is 150 after four puffs of albuterol via MDI.

44. What are the possible options for treating Mr. Andrews at this point?

45. What method of bronchodilator delivery would you recommend for Mr. Andrews?

46. What is meant by "dose-response" assessment?

Case 3

You are asked to deliver a bronchodilator to a patient in the neuro unit. When you arrive to assess the patient, you note that she is obtunded. Breath sounds reveal scattered rhonchi and wheezing in the upper lobes.

47. What method of bronchodilator delivery would you recommend in this situation?

48. What modification will you need to make?

49. Since peak flow is unlikely to be performed, how will you assess the effectiveness of the therapy?

What About Intubated Patients?

Delivering bronchodilators to intubated patients has always been difficult. Much of the drug ends up in the circuit or the endotracheal tube. Assessment of effectiveness can be difficult as well. Both SVNs and MDIs can be used to achieve good results if you follow some guidelines and use the right equipment.

50. SVN dosages should be adjusted when delivered to an intubated patient by what amount?

51. What standard starting dosage is recommended for albuterol by MDI to a ventilator patient?

52. Where should you place the SVN in the ventilator circuit?

53. When should an MDI be activated for a ventilator patient?

54. What adjustments to dilution need to be made with the SVN for ventilator delivery?

What About Those Board Exams?

It will come as no surprise that this information is on your boards. What is unusual is how little of this material is on the test considering the importance and frequency of aerosol drug administration in the clinical setting. One reason is that only recently have good studies been done to provide more scientific conclusions about how best to deliver medications. The matrix specifically mentions MDIs, spacers, and pneumatic-powered nebulizers. Of course peak flow and assessment are included. I could not find continuous nebulization in the matrix! Perhaps it will appear on the new exams that are coming soon.

Asthma has been recently diagnosed in a 16-year-old patient. The respiratory care practitioner is asked to teach the patient how to self-administer Vanceril via MDI. (Questions 55-56)

55. In addition to the inhaler, what other equipment would be indicated?
    I. A spacer device
    II. A pulse oximeter
    III. A peak flow meter
    A. I only
    B. I, II only
    C. I, III only
    D. II, III only

56. After performing the inhalation, the RCP instructs the patient to perform a breath-holding maneuver. The purpose of this maneuver is to
    A. Promote a strong cough
    B. Improve venous return
    C. Improve inertial impaction
    D. Increase medication delivery

57. While attempting to administer albuterol via SVN to a patient who has had a recent CVA, the RCP notes that the patient is unable to hold the nebulizer or keep her lips sealed on the mouthpiece. The RCP should recommend
    A. Switching to an MDI
    B. Utilizing an aerosol mask for delivery
    C. Discontinuing the medication
    D. Subcutaneous administration of the medication

58. An MDI is ordered for a patient who is intubated and being mechanically ventilated and humidified with a heat-moisture exchanger. Which of the following is the most appropriate way to administer the bronchodilator?
    A. Place the MDI in the expiratory limb of the ventilator circuit
    B. Place the MDI between the HME and the endotracheal tube
    C. Recommend changing the delivery method to an SVN
    D. Remove the HME during delivery of the drug

59. An alert adult patient with asthma is receiving bronchodilator therapy via SVN during a hospitalization. What recommendations should the RCP make in regard to this therapy when the patient is ready for discharge?
   A. Recommend MDI instruction
   B. Recommend oral administration of the medication
   C. Recommend training in home use of the SVN
   D. Recommend administration of the drug via IPPB

60. Which of the following devices is most suitable for delivery of virazole (Ribavirin)?
   A. Continuous LVN
   B. Small particle aerosol generator
   C. USN
   D. Atomizer

61. What two inhalational drugs have the greatest occupational risk for RCPs?
   A. _____
   B. _____

62. Describe some of the physical ways to control environmental contamination when delivering medications that have potential side effects for the provider.

63. To what do the acronyms HEPA and PAPR refer?

Food for Thought

Chapter 32 ends with some important material on the subject of protecting the practitioner from continuous exposure to a wide variety of inhaled agents.

Storage and Delivery of Medical Gases

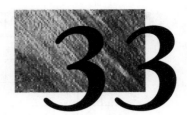

33

> ——— "O Lord, help me to be ———
> pure, but not yet."
> St. Augustine

One thing is certain: every generation of respiratory care students since the dawn of time has had a good laugh at the engineers who thought up the name Pin Index Safety System. And what's up with that American Standard Safety System? Another thing I'm sure of is that we all have to learn more about medical gases than any other mortals on this planet! I have to admit this information has come in handy many times in the clinical setting, and it is good to be an expert when the delivery systems malfunction and no one else knows quite what to do but the RCP!

Gas Powered

There's a little puzzle on p. 280 to help you learn the new terms found in Chapter 33.

Characteristics of Medical Gases

1. Nonflammable gases simply will not burn. Name three gases categorized as nonflammable.
   A. _____
   B. _____
   C. _____

2. Most medical gases will support combustion. Name three gases in this category.
   A. _____
   B. _____
   C. _____

3. Describe the four basic steps of the fractional distillation process. (Don't just list them!)
   A.

   B.

   C.

   D.

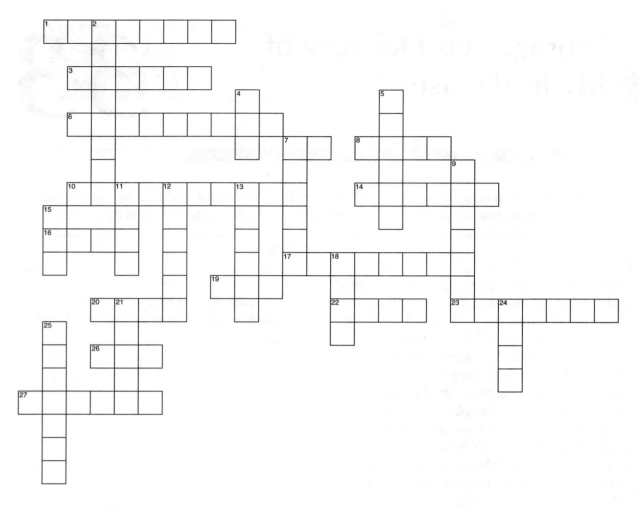

ACROSS

1. Valve that lowers gas pressure
3. _____ dioxide, used to treat hiccups
6. A device that controls both pressure and flow
7. Chemical named for this light gas
8. This meter controls the volume of gas per unit of volume
10. Type of "distillation" that produces oxygen
14. Gas used in treatment of severe asthma
16. Low pressure safety system
17. Pipe with many connections used to link gas cylinders together
19. Gas delivered in a yellow cylinder
20. _____ valves shut off the gas in case of a fire
22. Your mom told you not to say this, but it really is a safety system!
23. Gas delivered in a blue cylinder
26. The "P" in PISS
27. Gas that makes up 20.95% of air

DOWN

2. The "D" in DISS
4. Agency that classifies cylinders
5. Needle _____ adjust the flow in a Thorpe tube
7. Low density gas
9. Fixed orifice, variable pressure measuring or metering device
11. Rear end: also a safety system
12. Variable orifice, constant pressure flow metering device
13. Just say "NO"
15. Agency that sets standards for gas purity
18. Sets standards for design, construction, placement, and use of bulk oxygen systems
21. Gas with only one oxygen molecule
24. Slang term for cylinder
25. Second half of gas made by heating limestone in contact with water

4. What purity level is required for medical grade oxygen?

7. Most medical grade CO_2 is used for what purpose?

5. Describe the two methods used to separate oxygen from air. What concentration is produced by each method?
   A.

8. What is heliox? What is it used for?

   B.

9. What is the primary medical use for nitrous oxide? What are some of the hazards of nitrous oxide administration?

6. Describe the devices used to produce medical grade air for hospital system and for home use.
   A.

10. How is nitric oxide (NO) being used in the neonatal setting?

   B.

11. Describe two possible hazards of using nitric oxide.

12. Give the chemical symbol for each of the following medical gases.

Gas	Symbol
A. Oxygen	_____
B. Air	_____
C. Carbon dioxide	_____
D. Helium	_____
E. Nitrous oxide	_____
F. Nitric oxide	_____

Storing Medical Gases

High-pressure medical gas cylinders have been around for about 100 years. The modern cylinder is the subject of numerous regulations and rules that control manufacture, storage, and transportation of these potentially dangerous steel bottles.

Naturally, you will be expected to have considerable knowledge on this subject even if you don't use it on a daily basis.

13. Identify the cylinder markings on the diagram shown below.

A. _____
B. _____
C. _____
D. _____
E. _____

Typical markings for cylinders containing medical gases. Front and back views are for illustration purposes only; exact location and order of markings may vary.

14. What do the symbols * and + mean when stamped on a cylinder?
   A. *

   B. +

15. Identify the proper color for these gas cylinders (in the United States).

   A. Oxygen _____
   B. Carbon dioxide _____
   C. Nitrous oxide _____
   D. Helium _____
   E. Nitrogen _____
   F. Air _____

16. Since cylinder color is only a guideline, how do you actually determine what gas is in a tank?

17. What is the best way to determine the actual oxygen concentration in a cylinder?

Fill 'Er Up

Cylinders are either filled with gas or liquid. The liquid will either be at room temperature or in a cryogenic state.

18. Name two gases that can be stored in the liquid state at room temperature.

   A. _____
   B. _____

19. Explain why the pressure in a gas-filled cylinder is different than that of a liquid-filled cylinder.

20. Describe the methods for measuring the contents of a gas-filled cylinder and a liquid-filled cylinder.

   A.

   B.

21. Write the formula for calculating the cylinder factor for a gas-filled cylinder.

22. What are the factors for the "E" and "H" oxygen cylinders?

    A.

    B.

23. Now write the formula for calculating duration of flow in minutes.

I promise we'll come back to this and practice these calculations. They are important for clinical practice and for your board exams!

Bulk Oxygen

Try to imagine how much oxygen a large hospital needs every day. If you had 100 patients wearing oxygen at 6 L/min, you would need over 800,000 liters for one day! Ventilators draw much more gas. You could do this with individual cylinders in each room, but imagine how much work that involves. A bulk system, by definition, contains at least 13,000 cubic feet of gas.

24. Describe a gaseous bulk system. Be sure to discuss the manifold, the primary, and reserve banks.

25. Why do most hospitals use a liquid bulk oxygen system?

26. One liter of liquid oxygen will expand into how many liters of gaseous oxygen?

27. What is the critical temperature of oxygen? How is the bulk liquid oxygen maintained at this temperature?

28. What is the normal working pressure for a hospital oxygen piping system?

29. What are zone valves? Give two reasons why you might need to use these valves.

Safety Systems

Safety systems come in two general types: those built into the cylinder valve stem to prevent rupture from high pressures, and indexed systems designed to keep you from giving the wrong gas to a patient.

30. Remember the gas laws? If a cylinder overheats, the pressure will rise. Describe the type of pressure release valve usually found in these cylinders.
    A. Small cylinder

    B. Large cylinder

31. Name the three basic indexed safety systems for medical gases. (Give both names.)
    A. Abbreviated Name _____
       Full name _____
    B. Abbreviated Name _____
       Full name _____
    C. Abbreviated Name _____
       Full name _____

32. A large cylinder of oxygen is described as follows: CGA-540 0.903-14NGORH-Ext. Explain what this means.

33. What type of cylinder uses pins and holes for the safety connection system?

34. What system was established to prevent accidental interchange of low-pressure medical gas connectors? What do they mean by "low-pressure?"

35. What is the purpose of the quick-connect system?

Regulating Pressure and Flow

Since a large cylinder of oxygen may have a pressure as high as 2400 psi, we need to have a way to lower this pressure and control it or our equipment (or the patient) could be harmed.

36. Describe the action of the following devices.
    A. Reducing valve

    B. Flowmeter

    C. Regulator

37. Describe the normal way each of the following is used in respiratory care.
    A. Preset reducing valve

    B. Adjustable reducing valve

    C. Multiple stage reducing valve

38. What two hazards can be created when you open a cylinder attached to a high-pressure reducing valve?

Three categories of flowmeters are used in respiratory care. The next set of questions will test your knowledge of these commonly used devices.

39. What are two advantages and two disadvantages of flow restrictors?
   A. Advantages
      1. ————————————————
      2. ————————————————
   B. Disadvantages
      1. ————————————————
      2. ————————————————

40. Describe the Bourdon flowmeter.

41. What is the chief advantage of the Bourdon type flowmeter?

42. How will indicated flow compare to actual flow when a Bourdon flowmeter meets up with downstream resistance?

43. What do Bourdon gauges actually measure? What do Thorpe tubes measure?
   A. Bourdon

   B. Thorpe

44. Compare indicated flow and actual flow in a compensated Thorpe flowmeter and an uncompensated Thorpe flowmeter when downstream resistance occurs.

45. What happens to the float in a compensated Thorpe tube when you connect it to a 50 psi gas source?

Case Studies

Case 1

A patient is to be transported from the ICU to the imaging department for a CT scan. The patient requires continuous supplemental oxygen at 10 L/min by mask. You will need to provide portable oxygen for the transport. An E cylinder is available.

51. What type of regulator is most appropriate for transport?

52. How long will the cylinder last at the given flow rate if the pressure is 1000 psi?

    Formula: _____
    Calculation: _____

53. When you turn on the cylinder valve, a hissing noise is heard from the regulator. The flowmeter is off, so there must be a leak. What should you check to try to correct the leak?
    A. _____
    B. _____

Mathemagic

I told you we'd come back to the problem of cylinder duration calculations. Obviously this is important, and not just because it is on tests! Let's say you have to transport a patient by plane, or send someone home with oxygen, or just go from the ER to the ICU. Will you have enough gas? Running out in the elevator is not really acceptable!

There are two ways to do this—the board exam precise way and the rule of thumb quick and dirty way. We'll do it the precise way first.

The two most common cylinders you will be using are the small E type and the larger H or K type. Factors are 0.28 and 3.14.

Example: You are sending a patient home by car. The E cylinder is full (2200 psi) and the patient is wearing a cannula at 2 L/min. How long will the oxygen last?
Start by writing out the formula. (You have to know this one.)
Duration = PSI × Factor / Flow Now plug in the numbers.
Calculation: 2200 x 0.28/ 2= 616/2= 308 minutes. How many hours is that? 308/60 = 5.1 hours

Now for the quick and dirty way. 0.28 is roughly 1/3. One third of 2200 is 700. 700 divided by 2 = 350 minutes, divided by 60 minutes in the hour = 5+ hours. You can see how you could get into trouble with this . . .? Of course if the patient is taking a 30-minute trip home, it would hardly matter. Be sensible when you take short cuts! (*By the way, everyone knows about short cuts. If you use this on the boards you could get burned.*)

Speaking of Board Exams?

You won't see too many questions on the material in Chapter 33. Cylinder duration is one common question, and usually involves duration of an E or H cylinder. Here are some typical questions for you to try.

54. An H cylinder of oxygen is being used to deliver oxygen to a patient in a subacute care facility where no piped in oxygen is available. The cylinder gauge shows a pressure of 1000 psi. The patient is receiving oxygen at 5 L/min by cannula. Approximately how long will the cylinder gas last at this flow rate?
    A. 1 hour
    B. 8 hours
    C. 10 hours
    D. 628 hours

55. An RCP notices that a flowmeter plugged into the wall outlet continues to read 1 L/min even though it is not turned on. What is the most appropriate action at this time?
   A. Replace the flowmeter
   B. Include the extra liter in any calculations
   C. Disassemble the flowmeter and replace the "O-rings"
   D. Do nothing, this is not an unusual situation

56. An RCP has to transport a patient via air from the island of Maui to Honolulu. The patient is being manually ventilated with an oxygen flow set at 10 L/min. The cylinder gauge reads 2000 psi. How long will the cylinder last?
   A. 42 minutes
   B. 56 minutes
   C. 1 hour
   D. 10 hours

57. When a respiratory care practitioner unplugs a Thorpe-type flowmeter, a huge leak occurs from the wall outlet. What action should the RCP take at this time?
   A. Shut off the gas to the room with the zone valve
   B. Shut off the bulk oxygen system
   C. Plug the flowmeter back into the outlet
   D. Call maintenance to fix the outlet

Food for Thought

58. What would happen if nitrous oxide leaked in the ER or OR setting?

59. What would you do if the bulk system at your hospital failed?

60. What protective gear is appropriate when opening a valve on a high-pressure cylinder?

Medical Gas Therapy

34

"I like the dreams of the future better than the history of the past."
Thomas Jefferson

My first job in respiratory therapy was that of oxygen technician. I was excited by the thought of being responsible for all those cannulas, masks, and humidifiers. We've come a long way since then, but medical gas therapy is still a cornerstone of respiratory care. Of course we think of oxygen as a drug now, and things have changed a lot in our understanding of administering this powerful medication.

The modern RCP must have a much firmer grasp of the goals and objectives of medical gas therapy than I did when I made my first patient rounds 20 years ago.

Tank Jockey

Let's try something different in the war of the words. My students always have a hard time with the spelling of medical terms. Check your ability by circling the correct spelling for this gas jargon.

1. canulla   cannula
2. reservore   reservoir
3. lasitude   lassitude
4. diaphramatic   diaphragmatic
5. retanopathy   retinopathy

6. hypoxemia   hypoxemea
7. toxicity   toxisity
8. infarction   infraction
9. displasia   dysplasia
10. pendent   pendant
11. concentration concintration
12. entranement   entrainment
13. wye   why

Please Pass the Gas

We're not just going to slap the mask on their faces—any old knob twirler could figure out how to do that part of the procedure. Let's start by reviewing the reasons for giving oxygen and how to clinically recognize those needs.

14. What is acute hypoxemia?

15. What are the threshold criteria for defining hypoxemia in adults and newborns according to the AARC? Give two laboratory values.
    A. Adults (and children)
        1. _____
        2. _____
    B. Newborns
        1. _____
        2. _____

16. Specifically, what effect does oxygen have on patients with COPD and chronic hypoxemia (besides treating hypoxemia!)
    A. COPD (and ILD)

    B. Chronic hypoxemia

17. Describe the two compensatory mechanisms of the cardiopulmonary system when faced with hypoxemia.
    A.

    B.

18. In what acute cardiac condition is oxygen therapy especially important?

19. What effect does hypoxemia have on the pulmonary blood vessels? What are the long-term consequences of this effect?

20. State the three basic ways to determine if a patient needs oxygen.
    A. _____
    B. _____
    C. _____

21. List six common acute situations in which hypoxemia is so common that oxygen therapy is usually provided.
    A. _____
    B. _____
    C. _____
    D. _____
    E. _____
    F. _____

22. Give two signs of mild and severe hypoxia for each of the following systems.
    A. Respiratory
        1. Mild ————————————————
        2. Severe ———————————————
    B. Cardiovascular
        1. Mild ————————————————
        2. Severe ———————————————
    C. Neurological
        1. Mild ————————————————
        2. Severe ———————————————

What Could Go Wrong?

There are four great big problems associated with oxygen therapy (besides burning down the hospital!). Naturally, you have to know them.

▶ *Toxic Talk*

23. Oxygen toxicity affects what two organ systems?
    A. ————————————————————
    B. ————————————————————

24. The harm caused by oxygen is influenced by what two factors?
    A. ————————————————————
    B. ————————————————————

25. Describe the effects of breathing excessive oxygen on the lung tissue.

26. What is meant by a "vicious cycle" in reference to oxygen toxicity?

27. While every patient is unique, what general rules can be applied to prevent oxygen toxicity?

28. When should oxygen be withheld from a hypoxic patient to avoid the consequences of toxicity?

▶ *I feel depressed . . .*

29. What specific type of COPD patient is likely to experience depression of ventilatory drive while breathing oxygen?

30. Give two explanations for this effect.
    A.

    B.

31. When should oxygen be withheld from a hypoxic COPD patient to avoid depressing ventilation?

RFL or ROP, it's all the same to me!

32. Describe how blood oxygen causes blindness.

33. What age group is likely to develop ROP?

34. How can you reduce the risk of ROP?

Absorbing Information

35. Describe how oxygen can cause atelectasis.

36. What groups of patients are at increased risk for absorption atelectasis?

37. How can you reduce the risk of absorption atelectasis?

Oxygen Delivery Systems

Now that you know why to give a patient oxygen and some of the hazards of administration, it's time to learn how to make the proper selections from the complex choices offered in oxygen delivery systems.

38. The three basic categories are low-flow, high-flow, and reservoir. Match the category to the description below.

Category	Description
A. Low-flow _____	1. Always exceeds patient's inspiratory needs
B. Reservoir _____	2. Provides some of patient's inspiratory needs
C. High-flow _____	3. May meet needs if no leaks occur

Low-Flow

39. Why do you think the nasal cannula is the most commonly used low-flow system?

40. When should you attach the cannula to a bubble humidifier?

41. What maximum flow does the text suggest for newborns?

Experiment

If you have access to a cannula, humidifier, and some medical oxygen, I think you should find out what it feels like to be a patient! First, attach the cannula to a flowmeter with the nipple adaptor (or "Christmas tree" if you like that term better). Insert the prongs in your nose and set the flow to 1 L/min. Try that for 1 minute. Increase the flow by 1 L/min. Continue this until you get to the 8 L/min maximum suggested by the text. Try again with a humidifier.

Questions

How well could you feel the gas at 1 L? What implication does this have for patient care? When did the flow start to become noticeable? When did it become uncomfortable? What happened to the humidifier as the flow rates exceeded 5 L/min?

42. What is the primary advantage of using a transtracheal oxygen catheter?

43. Why does the range of FIO_2 delivered by nasal cannulas vary so much?

44. Since you can't tell exactly how much oxygen the patient is receiving at any given moment, how can assess the effects of administering the drug?

45. What are the advantages and disadvantages of reservoir cannulas?
    A. Advantages

    B. Disadvantages

46. In what setting are reservoir cannulas usually used?

Reservoir

47. Use Table 34-3 to help you find the information about oxygen masks.

Mask	FiO_2 Range	Advantage	Disadvantage
A. Simple			
B. Partial			
C. Non-rebreathing			

48. What is the primary difference between the partial rebreathing and non-rebreathing (NRB) masks?

49. How can you tell if a non-rebreathing mask has an adequate flow rate?

50. Give a solution for each of these common problems with reservoir masks.

Problem	Solution
A. Confused patient removes mask	_____
B. Humidifier pop-off activated	_____
C. Mask causes claustrophobia	_____
D. Bag collapses on inspiration	_____
E. Bag fully inflated on inspiration	_____

Experiment

Get a non-rebreather (NRB), a simple mask, a bubble humidifier, a nipple adapter, and a flowmeter. Make sure you have *2 valves* for the exhalation ports of the non-rebreather. *First*, try the simple mask without a humidifier. Set the flowmeter at 2 L/min and breathe from the simple mask for a few breaths. Now take deep breaths. Set the flowmeter at 10L/min and try again. *Next*, set up the NRB. Repeat the experiment. Breathe as deeply as you can and adjust the flowmeter until the bag doesn't collapse. *Try* the mask with one expiratory flap valve in place and with two. *Finally*, attach the bubble humidifier, set the flow at 10, and put on the mask. Now increase the flow rate to 15, then flush.

Questions

How did it feel to breathe on the simple mask at a low flow rate? What happened when you tried the NRB at a low flow? How did mask performance vary when you used two valves? What difference did the humidifier make?

High-Flow

Air-entrainment systems are commonly used to provide high-flow oxygen because they are simple and inexpensive to operate. Oxygen is directed through a small tube, or jet, which creates a very high forward velocity. Air is entrained into the system, which dilutes the oxygen and increases the total flow rate.

51. Describe the effects of varying the jet size or entrainment port opening on FiO_2 and total flow rate.

Factor	Increased Size	Decreased Size
A. Jet		
1. FiO_2	_____	_____
2. Flow	_____	_____
B. Port		
1. FiO_2	_____	_____
2. Flow	_____	_____

52. Fill in the air-to-oxygen ratios for the following oxygen concentrations.

    A. 100%   _____
    B. 60%   _____
    C. 40%   _____
    D. 35%   _____
    E. 30%   _____
    F. 24%   _____

53. What is the common name for an air entrainment mask (AEM)?

54. Why does the AEM have larger openings on the side of the mask than a simple oxygen mask?

55. What effect does raising the delivered flow from the flowmeter have on the FiO_2 delivered by an AEM?

56. Air-entrainment devices are classified as high-flow. For what FIO_2 settings is this usually true?

57. How do you boost the total flow when using an AEM?

58. Why is this not possible with an air-entrainment nebulizer?

59. There are four devices used to deliver gas from an air-entrainment nebulizer to the patient. Choose the device that fits each of the following patients. (Some have two.)

Patient	Aerosol Appliance
A. Tracheostomy tube	_____
	_____
B. Endotracheal tube	_____
	_____
C. Intact upper airway	_____
	_____

60. Describe an easy way to tell if an air-entrainment nebulizer is providing sufficient gas to meet the patients needs.

61. Give one example of a specialized flow generator that produces an aerosol and one example that produces dry gas.
   A. Aerosol: _____
   B. Dry: _____

62. What effect does downstream resistance to flow have on FIO_2 and total flow delivered by an entrainment system?

Experiment

You will need an AEM , and oxygen analyzer, and an air-entrainment jet nebulizer with a length of corrugated tubing. **First**, set the AEM at 40% with a flow of 5 L/min of oxygen. Analyze the FIO_2 (detach the mask and put the analyzer tee on). Increase the flow to 8 L/min. Analyze again. **Next**, set up the nebulizer. Use 40% and a flow of 10. Analyze the output. Increase the flow to 12 and analyze again. **Now** pour enough water into the tube to partially occlude it. Analyze. **Add** enough water to completely occlude the tubing. Analyze. **Finally**, drain out the water. Try to increase the flowmeter setting past 15.

What is the effect of altering flow rate on the AEM? What is the effect of water (resistance) in the tubing of a jet nebulizer? What happened when you tried to increase the flow? Why?

Mathemagic

Oxygen-to-air entrainment ratios and total flow from air-entrainment devices are more of the universal clinical and board exam expectations that countless students have struggled with. The way I see it, you have three choices. Memorize the ratios for each FiO$_2$, learn the algebraic formula, or learn the magic box. **You must learn and master this information!**

▶ If you like the first method, you must memorize in every detail Table 34-7 on page 754 of Egan. READ the fine print.

Or

Look at the Mini-Clini on page 753. A three-step method is provided for calculating the ratio and the subsequent total flow. Let's try one.

A patient is receiving oxygen at 40% via a Venti-mask with the flowmeter set at 8 L/min. What is the ratio of oxygen-to-air? What is the total flow.

Step 1:Compute the ratio

Liters of Air	(100-40)
Liters of O$_2$	(40-21)

Liters of Air	(60)
Liters of O$_2$	(19)

Liters of Air	3
Liters of O$_2$	1

Step 2: Add the ratio parts
3 + 1 = 4

Step 3: Multiply the sum of the parts times the oxygen flow rate
4 × 8= 32 L/min total flow.

Now you try.

63. What is the oxygen-to-air entrainment ratio and total flow for a patient who is receiving 60% oxygen via an entrainment nebulizer with the flowmeter set at 10 L/min?
   A. Step 1: Compute the ratio
      Formula: _____
      Calculation: _____
      Reduce answer to get ratio: _____
   B. Step 2: Add the parts _____
   C. Step 3: Multiply the sum of the parts times the O$_2$ flow rate _____

The "magic box" is my personal favorite. Retry the sample problem above for the patient on 40%. Pretty nifty. The only problem with this method is that you substitute 20 (instead of 21) to make the math easy. At percentages below 40, your answers will start to vary from the algebraic method. You can solve this by using "21" for low percentages, and "20" for 40% or more.

▶ *Practice with your chosen method until you can solve for every FiO$_2$. There is no way out of this!*

Blenders

Oxygen blenders are another kind of "magic box." The blender requires a 50 psi input of air and oxygen. When you twirl the knob to set the FiO$_2$, you are actually adjusting a proportioning valve. Turning toward a high percentage of oxygen makes the opening for oxygen larger and the opening for air smaller. 100% closes the air side and only lets oxygen out. Vice versa for turning the knob toward 21%. The blender is a very handy device. It gives you high flow rates or 50 psi to power equipment at any FiO$_2$ you desire.

64. Describe the three-step process for confirming the proper operation of a blender.

A.

B.

C.

Put that Child in a Box!

The opening scene of the venerable "Marcus Welby MD" television show depicted a man in an oxygen tent. You may see this being done on soap operas as well. Nowadays, enclosures are a simple way to deliver oxygen to infants and children.

65. What is the major problem with oxygen tents?

66. What is the highest FIO_2 you can expect to deliver with a tent?

67. Why is a hood the best method for delivering oxygen to an infant?

68. What minimum flow must be set for a hood? Why?

69. What harmful consequence occurs when flow rates into the hood are too high?

70. What effect will cold air flowing into the hood have on a premature infant?

71. What is the best way to control oxygen delivery to an infant inside an incubator?

72. What is the primary benefit of the infant incubator?

HBO

Life under pressure: that's hyperbaric oxygen, or HBO. We can administer oxygen to the patient at 2 or 3 atmospheres (ATA) to treat several acute and chronic problems. Originally designed for decompression sickness in divers, HBO operates according to Boyle's Law. RCPs often work with patients who require this mode of oxygen administration, and it is also common for RCPs to work in hyperbaric units.

73. Compare the monoplace and multiplace hyperbaric chambers.
    A. Monoplace
        1. O_2
        2. Patient
        3. Staff
    B. Multiplace
        1. O_2
        2. Patient
        3. Staff

74. List three acute and three chronic conditions where hyperbaric oxygen is indicated.

	Acute	Chronic
A.	_____	_____
B.	_____	_____
C.	_____	_____

75. Under what circumstances is HBO indicated in cases of carbon monoxide poisoning?

What Else Could There Be?

76. Two other therapeutic gases are administered by RCPs. Give indications for each.

	Gas	Indications
A.	NO	_____
		_____
B.	Helium	_____
		_____

77. What other gas is always mixed with helium? What is the most common combination?

78. What physical property of helium results in decreased work of breathing?

79. Helium is so diffusible that special balloons are used to hold it. What type of gas delivery device is used to administer helium to patients who are not intubated?

Case Studies

Case 1

Abraham Dink, a 58-year-old college professor, is admitted for chest pain and possible MI. ECG monitoring reveals sinus tachycardia. The chest pain has been decreased by administration of nitroglycerin. Respirations are 20 per minute, and SpO_2 on room air is 94%.

80. What is your assessment of this patient's oxygenation status?

81. What is your recommendation in regard to administration of supplemental oxygen?

Case 2

Rolly Clemens has been admitted for exacerbation of his COPD. He is receiving oxygen at 2 L/min via nasal cannula. The pulse oximeter shows a saturation of 94% while Mr. Clemens is at rest. The nurse calls you to ask for your assistance in evaluation of Rolly's dyspnea during ambulation.

82. What changes occur in breathing pattern during exercise?

83. How are low-flow oxygen devices affected by changes in breathing pattern?

84. How would you assess dyspnea on ambulation for a patient wearing oxygen?

Case 3

Linda Loo is recovering from surgery following a head injury. She is trached and requires supplemental oxygen at 60% via T-piece. The flowmeter is set at 12 L/min. Each time Linda inhales, the mist exiting the T-piece disappears.

85. Air-entrainment nebulizers are considered high-flow delivery systems. Discuss this in terms of the disappearing mist.

86. What should be added to the T-piece to help deal with this problem?

87. Describe a common method of increasing the delivered flow when administering high FIO_2 levels via air-entrainment nebulizers.

88. What is the oxygen-to-air entrainment ratio for 60%?

89. What is the total flow in the system described in this case?

Board Exam Broadside

There must be some reason why this chapter has gone on forever. The NBRC will expect you to know about all types of delivery systems and when to use them. You should know when oxygen is indicated and recognize and minimize potential hazards and complications. The Entry-Level Exam will have a minimum of eight questions based on the topic of "conducting therapeutic procedures to achieve adequate arterial and tissue oxygenation." Heliox administration is covered on the Registry Exams. Nitric oxide and HBO are not currently on the tests, but I would not be surprised to see these therapies in the near future. Pour yourself another cup of coffee and answer the following questions.

90. During a suctioning procedure a patient experiences tachycardia with PVCs. Which of the following could be responsible for this response?
    A. Inadequate vacuum pressure
    B. Lack of sterile technique during the procedure
    C. Fear of the suctioning procedure
    D. Inadequate preoxygenation

91. A patient with a history of CO_2 retention is receiving oxygen at 6 L/min via nasal cannula. He is becoming lethargic and difficult to arouse. In regard to the oxygen delivery, what change would you recommend?
    A. Change to a 40% venturi mask
    B. Maintain the present therapy
    C. Change to a partial rebreathing mask
    D. Reduce the flow to 2 L/min and obtain an ABG

92. A newborn requires oxygen therapy. Which of the following methods of delivery would you select?
    A. Partial rebreathing mask
    B. Oxygen hood
    C. Venturi mask
    D. Oxygen tent

93. A patient is receiving oxygen therapy from an NRB mask with a flow rate of 10 L/min. The RCP observes the bag deflating with each inspiration. What action is indicated in this situation?
    A. Replace the mask with a cannula
    B. Immediately perform pulse oximetry
    C. Increase the flow to the mask
    D. Change to a venturi mask

94. A patient is to receive a mixture of helium and oxygen. Which of the following delivery devices would be appropriate?
    A. Nasal cannula
    B. Oxygen tent
    C. Venturi mask
    D. Nonrebreathing mask

95. An 80/20 mixture of helium and oxygen is administered. The oxygen flowmeter is set at 10 L/min. What is the actual flow delivered to the patient?
    A. 10 L
    B. 14 L
    C. 16 L
    D. 18 L

96. A patient is receiving 40% oxygen via an AEM with the flowmeter set at 8 L/min. What is the total flow delivered to the patient?
    A. 24 L/min
    B. 32 L/min
    C. 40 L/min
    D. 48 L/min

97. Water has accumulated in the delivery tubing of an aerosol system. This will result in all of the following except
    A. Increased FIO_2
    B. Decreased aerosol output
    C. Increased flow rate
    D. Increased backpressure in the system

98. A patient requires a flow rate of 40 L/min to meet his inspiratory demand for gas. He is to receive oxygen via a venturi mask set at 24%. What is the minimum setting on the flowmeter to produce the appropriate flow?
    A. 1L/min
    B. 2L/min
    C. 3L/min
    D. 4L/min

Food for Thought

99. Why does common use of the term "100% non-rebreather" create a clinical problem?

100. Why would an AEM be preferred over an air-entrainment nebulizer for a patient who has asthma?

Lung Expansion Therapy

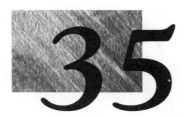

35

1. Atelectasis: "When you don't take deep breaths . . ."

Postoperative complications are dreaded by everyone involved: surgeons, nurses, third-party payers, and yes, even patients. Postoperative pulmonary complications have been recognized as a problem for as long as surgery has been around and we RCPs have been at the forefront of the battle against atelectasis and retained secretions for many years. Anesthesia, pain, medications, and preexisting lung disease are the enemy. Fortunately, we have a powerful arsenal of lung expansion devices and treatments on our side.

2. Incentive spirometer (IS):
   A. "The purpose of this treatment is to . . ."

   B. "This device will . . ."

Word Power

One of the problems associated with lung expansion therapy is to explain the goals, procedures, and equipment so the patient can understand. For each of the following terms or treatments, give a simple, short explanation in lay terms that even your kid brother could understand. (I'll help you get started, but you don't have to use my words if you don't need to.)

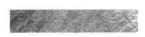

3. Sustained maximal inspiration (SMI): "I want you to take . . ."

4. Intermittent positive pressure breathing (IPPB):
   A. "Your doctor has ordered a breathing treatment that will . . ."

   B. "This machine will . . ."

5. Continuous positive airway pressure (CPAP):
   A. "This treatment will . . ."

B. "I am going to put a mask on your face . . ."

In fact, maybe you should try out your explanations on friends or family members to see if they make sense!

Meet the Objectives

6. What is the definition of atelectasis?

7. What is resorption atelectasis and when is it likely to occur?

8. What causes passive atelectasis?

9. Why are postoperative patients at highest risk for development of atelectasis?

10. Explain why hypoxemia may result when FRC decreases in the first 48 hours after surgery.

11. What specific group of post-operative patients is at highest risk?

12. Name two other types of patients who have increased likelihood of developing atelectasis. Explain why.
    A.

    B.

13. Explain how each of the following signs may help provide clues that atelectasis is present.
    A. History

    B. Breath sounds

    C. Respiratory rate

    D. Heart rate

    E. Chest film

14. All modes of lung expansion therapy increase lung volume by increasing the transpulmonary pressure gradient by what two methods?

    A. _____

    B. _____

15. List three indications, two contraindications, and two hazards of incentive spirometry.

    A. Indications

       1. _____

       2. _____

       3. _____

    B. Contraindications

       1. _____

       2. _____

    C. Hazards

       1. _____

       2. _____

16. By whom and in what year was IPPB first introduced? (Oops! Sorry I went into sputum bowl mode for a minute!)

17. Like IS, IPPB is used to treat atelectasis. Specifically, when would IPPB be indicated as compared with IS?

18. What is the one absolute contraindication to IPPB?

19. List five additional partial contraindications.

    A. _____

    B. _____

    C. _____

    D. _____

    E. _____

20. Name two common complications of IPPB administration.

    A. _____

    B. _____

21. Discuss the four factors that probably contribute to the beneficial effects of CPAP.

22. Name two contraindications to CPAP therapy.

    A. _____

    B. _____

23. The text suggests three major complications of this therapy. Discuss each of the following problems.
    A. Hypoventilation

    B. Barotrauma

    C. Gastric distention

24. What alarm system is essential for monitoring patients receiving CPAP?

Chapter Highlights

25. Atelectasis is caused by persistent _____ with _____ tidal volumes.

26. Patients who have undergone upper _____ or _____ surgery are at the greatest risk for atelectasis.

27. A history of _____ disease or _____ are additional risk factors.

28. _____ is not associated with atelectasis unless the patient also has pneumonia.

29. Patients with atelectasis usually demonstrate _____ _____ breathing.

30. The most common problem associated with lung expansion therapy is the onset of respiratory _____, which occurs when the patient breathes _____.

Case Studies

Use the protocol found in Fig. 35-8 on page 787 of the textbook to help answer the following questions.

Case 1

John Babbit is an alert, 34-year-old male admitted for a cholecystectomy. John smokes two packs of cigarettes per day. Following surgery, the doctor asks for your recommendation for therapy to prevent lung complications.

31. Discuss potential risk factors for atelectasis in this case.

32. What therapy would you recommend for prevention of atelectasis for Mr. Babbit?

Case 2

Maria Contraire is immobilized following hip replacement. Mrs. Contraire is a 70-year-old, 5'2" tall female. Her predicted inspiratory capacity is 1.8 L. She is performing incentive spirometry at 400 ml per breath. Breath sounds reveal bilateral basilar crackles.

33. What is the minimum acceptable volume for this therapy?

34. What treatment would you recommend at this time?

Case 3

Marcy Strongarm is an obese, confused 54-year-old female. She is recovering from a CABG (open-heart surgery). Marcy has persistent atelectasis with mild hypoxemia that has not responded to incentive spirometry. Her radiograph shows an elevated left hemi-diaphragm with air bronchograms in the left base.

35. What is the significance of the elevated diaphragm and air bronchograms seen on the chest film?

36. What treatment would you recommend? Why?

What About Those Board Exams?

Lung expansion techniques such as incentive spirometry and IPPB are important parts of the Entry-Level Examination. The equipment, breathing circuits, and techniques are included. You should expect a minimum of 3 to 5 questions. It is especially important to review IPPB in depth. Since this modality is not as commonly used and is more complicated than IS, it is easy to miss the details required on the exams. One or two questions about CPAP are also likely. PEEP will not show up until the Written Registry Exam, and we'll save that for the next chapter.

37. A patient complains of a "tingling" feeling in her lips during an incentive spirometry treatment. The RCP should instruct the patient to
    A. Breathe more slowly
    B. Take smaller breaths
    C. Continue with the treatment as ordered
    D. Exhale through pursed lips after each breath

38. Which of the following alarms are a vital part of the system when setting up CPAP therapy for treatment of atelectasis?
    A. Exhaled volume
    B. High respiratory rate
    C. Pulse oximetry
    D. Low pressure

39. During administration of IPPB therapy, the practitioner observes the system pressure rise above the pressure set to end the inspiration. The RCP should instruct the patient to
    A. "Help the machine give you a deep breath"
    B. "Inhale slowly along with the machine"
    C. "Exhale gently and normally"
    D. "Exhale through pursed lips after each breath"

40. A patient is having difficulty initiating each breath with an IPPB machine. The practitioner should adjust the
    A. Pressure limit
    B. Peak flow
    C. FiO_2
    D. Sensitivity

41. Which control is used to increase the volume delivered by an IPPB machine?
    A. Pressure limit
    B. Peak flow
    C. FiO_2
    D. Sensitivity

42. Continuous positive airway pressure is used to increase which of the following?
    A. Functional residual capacity
    B. Peak expiratory flow rate
    C. FEV_1
    D. Arterial CO_2 levels

43. An IPPB machine cycles on with the patient effort, but does not shut off. The most likely cause of this problem is
    A. The pressure is set too low
    B. The sensitivity is set incorrectly
    C. There is a leak in the system
    D. The patient is not blowing out hard enough

44. How should you instruct a patient to breathe during incentive spirometry?
    A. "Exhale gently, then inhale rapidly through the spirometer"
    B. "Inhale deeply and rapidly through the spirometer"
    C. "Exhale until your lungs are empty, then inhale and hold your breath"
    D. Exhale normally, then inhale slowly and deeply and hold your breath"

45. How often should a patient be instructed to use their incentive spirometer after they are taught to perform the procedure correctly?
    A. 10 breaths, four times per day
    B. 6 to 10 breaths every hour
    C. 10 to 20 breaths every 2 hours
    D. 6 to 8 breaths TID

46. A patient who has had surgery for an abdominal aortic aneurysm suffers from arrhythmias and hypotension after surgery. The physician asks for your recommendation for lung expansion therapy. The best choice in this situation would be
    A. IS
    B. IPPB
    C. PEEP
    D. CPAP

47. When adjusting the flow rate control on an IPPB machine, the RCP would be altering the
    A. Maximum pressure delivered by the device
    B. The effort required to initiate a breath
    C. The volume delivered by the machine
    D. The inspiratory time for a given breath

I'll stop torturing you now, but I could go on and on. To get good at lung expansion therapy you will need to get out the equipment and practice in the lab. All of these treatments can be delivered to classmates in practice sessions until you are skilled with the devices, the coaching, and the breathing circuits.

Food for Thought

48. Your textbook refers to using vital capacity or inspiratory capacity as important indicators in lung expansion therapy, especially incentive spirometry. How can you determine the predicted inspiratory capacity?

Bronchial Hygiene Therapy

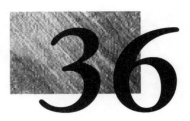

36

2. ARDS

Bronchial hygiene. Well, it sounds better than "pulmonary toilet," which was the catch phrase when I was a student. After medical gas administration, playing with sputum is what makes our profession famous (or infamous). I distinctly remember my early clinical experience of asking a man to "cough it up" while I turned my head away to gag. That was before I got used to that lovely rattling sound. Join me now, for the halls are alive with the sound of mucus, and we've got work to do.

3. AD

Acronyms Again?

After you've read Chapter 36, you will have noticed a lot of acronyms. Let's get those out of the way before we dive into bronchial hygiene. Write the definition for each of these mystical medical markings.

4. CF

1. ACB

5. CPT

6. CPAP

7. EPAP

8. FET

9. HFCC

10. HZ

11. ICP

12. IPV

13. MI-E

14. PDPV

15. PEP

16. PIE

Airway Clearance

Normal lungs generate a modest amount of mucus from the goblet cells, glands, and Clara cells. The mucociliary escalator whips that stuff up and out in no time. You hardly even notice. Of course, things go wrong—that's where we come in.

17. Name the four phases of the normal cough. Give two examples of impairments for each.

Phase	Impairments
A. _____	_____
	_____
B. _____	_____
	_____
C. _____	_____
	_____
D. _____	_____
	_____

18. Compare the effects of full and partial airway obstruction by retained secretions.

19. Name at least three conditions that may cause internal obstruction or external compression of the airway lumen.
    A. _____
    B. _____
    C. _____

20. Name two obstructive lung diseases that result in excessive secretion of mucus and impairment of normal clearance.
    A. _____
    B. _____

21. List four neurological or musculoskeletal conditions that impair cough.
    A. _____
    B. _____
    C. _____
    D. _____

Bronchial Hygiene: Goals and Indications

Obviously, getting the gunk out of the lungs is the main idea, but there's more to it, of course! The big picture is made up of acute conditions, chronic disorders, prevention, and assessment.

22. Name four acute conditions where bronchial hygiene is indicated.
    A. _____
    B. _____
    C. _____
    D. _____

23. Explain why these techniques are not useful in treating most cases of pneumonia or asthma.

24. Discuss bronchial hygiene therapy for chronic lung conditions.

25. Describe the two well-documented preventive uses of this type of therapy.
    A.

    B.

26. In order to determine the need for bronchial hygiene therapy, you would assess the patient and the medical record. Give a brief explanation of the significance of each factor listed below.

Factor	Significance
A. History	_____
B. Airway	_____
C. Chest radiograph	_____
D. Breath sounds	_____
E. Vital signs	_____

Bronchial Hygiene: Approaches to Therapy

There are five general noninvasive approaches to managing secretion problems. Within each general approach are several choices. You will need to customize therapy for each patient based on cost, effectiveness, clinical condition, and ability to participate in therapy.

Postural Drainage

27. Kinetic therapy has many pulmonary benefits. Name two non-pulmonary benefits.
    A. _____
    B. _____

28. Name four advantages of frequent turning for the critically ill patient.
    A. _____
    B. _____
    C. _____
    D. _____

29. List two absolute and two relative contraindications to turning.
    A. Absolute
       1. _____
       2. _____
    B. Relative
       1. _____
       2. _____

30. What does the textbook mean by "plumbing problems?"

31. Describe dependent positioning. Compare positions for unilateral pneumonia, ARDS, lung abscess, and lung contusion.

32. How long should you wait to schedule postural drainage after a patient eats? Why?

33. What is the minimum *range* of time for effective application of postural drainage therapy?

34. Give two recommended interventions for each of the complications of postural drainage listed below.

    Complication   *Interventions*
    A. Hypoxemia

    B. Increased ICP

    C. Acute hypotension

    D. Pulmonary bleeding

    E. Vomiting

    F. Bronchospasm

    G. Cardiac arrhythmias

35. Discuss cough in relationship to postural drainage.

36. How long does it take to determine the effectiveness of postural drainage? If therapy is effective, how often should you reevaluate?

37. Describe five factors that must be documented after each postural drainage treatment.
    A.

    B.

    C.

    D.

    E.

38. Compare percussion and vibration as techniques to loosen secretions.

39. Compare manual and machine methods of percussion and vibration.

Exercise: Learn those pesky positions!

I wish I could tell you an easy way to learn the positions for chest drainage. Here are some suggestions. Photocopy Fig. 36-3. Cut out each position and cut off the heading that names the position. Tape the picture to the front of a 3 × 5 index card and the title (lung segment) to the back. My students find this an effective way to make flash cards, and it works well as a visual learning tool.

Maybe you are more of a kinetic learner. Get a partner (two partners works better) and a hospital bed (this could be in the lab or the medical center, for instance). One person should name a lung segment. Position your victim in what you think is the correct position. Now check the position to see if you got it right. This way you will physically learn the positions and have to move someone around, add pillows, and so on. Since there are about 12 different positions for the 18 lung segments, you will need to spend 30 to 45 minutes on this exercise. I think you will

need to repeat this at least 2 to 3 times before you have the positioning and related segments rock solid in your memory. I am sure this will pay off when you get tested. If you don't have a partner use a mannequin.

Coughing Techniques

40. How would you position a patient (ideally) for an effective cough?

41. Standard directed cough must frequently be modified. Give three examples of patients who may need modified cough techniques.
   A. _____
   B. _____
   C. _____

42. What is splinting?

43. What special form of cough assistance is used with patients who have neuromuscular conditions?

44. Describe the forced expiratory technique (FET).

45. Describe the 3 repeated cycles of the ACB technique.

    A.

    B.

    C.

46. What is the primary problem with autogenic drainage?

47. Describe the two cycles of MI-E in terms of time and pressure.

Positive Airway Pressure

48. PEP is a popular way to help mobilize secretions. What are the four indications for PEP according to the AARC CPG on page 808 of the text?

    A. _____

    B. _____

    C. _____

    D. _____

49. What type of monitoring is essential regardless of the equipment used to deliver positive airway pressure to help mobilize secretions?

High-Frequency Compression/Oscillation

50. Describe the two general approaches to oscillation.

51. What do you think are the primary problems with vests and shells?

52. State at least four of the benefits or advantages of the flutter valve as a secretion management tool.

A.

B.

C.

D.

Mobilization and Exercise

Early mobilization and frequent position changes are standards of care in preventing pulmonary complications after surgery or trauma.

53. Describe the benefits of adding exercise as a mobilization technique.

54. What should you specifically monitor when exercising patients with lung problems?

Case Studies

Use the algorithm (Fig. 36-13) on page 813 to assist you in answering the following questions.

Case 1

Dr. Abraham Dock is a 60-year-old professor who has had a colon resection for an intestinal tumor. He is receiving incentive spirometry to help expand his lungs. You are asked to assess Dr. Dock for retained secretions. Auscultation reveals coarse rhonchi bilaterally in the upper lobes. A few scattered crackles are heard in the bases. SpO_2 on room air is 94%. The patient states he is unable to cough up anything "because it hurts too much."

55. What technique could you use to decrease the pain associated with cough in a postoperative patient?

56. What cough techniques are options for this patient?

Case 2

Mabel Horowitz is a 75-year-old woman with bronchiectasis who states she coughs up "cups of awful mucous every day" She is admitted with a diagnosis of pneumonia.

57. What therapy is indicated while Mabel is in the hospital?

As you provide the therapy, you find out that Mrs. H is a widow who lives alone. She takes albuterol treatments via SVN when she has difficulty breathing.

58. What therapy alternatives could you recommend for home use?

What Does the NBRC Say?

The Entrance-Level Exam matrix has this to say:

> "Achieve removal of bronchopulmonary secretions
> a. instruct and encourage proper coughing
> b. perform postural drainage
> c. perform percussion and or vibration "

As I mentioned in Chapter 35, recommending and initiating PEP therapy is found on the Written Registry Exam. Currently, flutter, AD, ACB, pulsating vests, MI-E, and IPV are not found on the boards. Since the NBRC is in the process of testing revised exams as I write this, you can be pretty sure that PDPV will have to share the hygiene spotlight with some of the new kids on the block.

Here's a sample of what you can expect on the current exams.

59. During the initial treatment, a PEP device is set to deliver a pressure of 15 cm H_2O. The patient complains of dyspnea and can only maintain exhalation for a short period. Which of the following should the RCP recommend?
    A. Decrease the PEP level to 10 cm H_2O
    B. Increase the PEP level to 20 cm H_2O
    C. Discontinue the PEP therapy
    D. Add a bronchodilator to the PEP therapy

60. A patient is lying on her left side, one quarter turn toward her back, with the head of the bed down. What division of the lung is being drained?
    A. Lateral segments of the right lower lobe
    B. Right middle lobe
    C. Left upper lobe, lingular segments
    D. Posterior segment of the right upper lobe

61. A patient is receiving postural drainage in the Trendelenburg position. The patient begins to cough uncontrollably. What action should the RCP take at this time?
    A. Encourage the patient to use a huff cough
    B. Administer oxygen therapy
    C. Administer a bronchodilator
    D. Raise the head of the bed

62. In explaining the goal of PEP therapy to a patient, it would be most appropriate to say
    A. "This will help prevent pneumonia."
    B. "This will increase your intrathoracic pressure."
    C. "This will help you cough more effectively."
    D. "This will prevent atelectasis."

63. A COPD patient with left lower lobe infiltrates is unable to tolerate a head-down position for postural drainage. What action would you recommend?
    A. Perform the drainage with the head of the bed raised
    B. Do not perform the therapy until 2 hours after the last meal
    C. Administer a bronchodilator prior to the postural drainage
    D. Notify the doctor and suggest a different secretion management technique

64. Patient cooperation is an important part of which of the following procedures?
    I. Postural drainage
    II. Directed cough techniques
    III. Airway suctioning
    IV. Positive Expiratory Pressure (PEP)
    A. I and II only
    B. II and IV only
    C. I, III, IV only
    D. I, II, and IV only

Food for Thought

65. How does hydration affect secretion clearance? What respiratory therapy modality can augment hydration?

66. Your text mentions never clapping directly over the spine or clavicles. Can you think of other places you should not clap? Use your imagination! (Could you get fired for clapping on certain parts of the anatomy?) So where *exactly* should you clap?

Respiratory Failure and the Need for Ventilatory Support

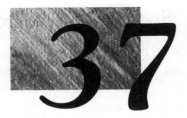

37

"There's no success like failure, and failure's no success at all."
Bob Dylan

Chapter 37 is short, sweet and essential to your understanding of why patients need mechanical ventilation. Strategies for choosing modes for interfacing the patient with the machine are introduced. When you understand the material in this chapter, you will be ready to tackle the very complex and difficult subject of mechanical ventilation and critical care.

Acronyms

Here's a really short sweet crossword puzzle to help you get over your fear of small words.

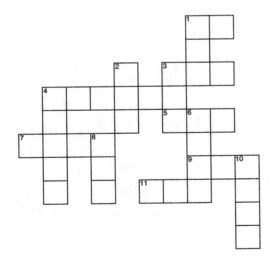

ACROSS

1. Preset minimum rate, patient can trigger breaths with set volumes
3. Maximum voluntary ventilation
4. Inability to maintain normal oxygen delivery to the tissues
5. Mode of ventilatory support designed to augment spontaneous breathing
7. Ventilatory support which patient breathes spontaneously at an elevated baseline
9. Measure of the output of respiratory muscles in cm H_2O pressure
11. Ventilator mode that uses high respiratory rates

DOWN

1. Another name for AC
2. Opposite of MIP
3. Also called NIF and MIF
4. Respirarory failure indicated by CO_2 greater than 50 in an otherwise healthy individual
6. Mode of support where spontaneous breaths are allowed between patient-triggered machine breaths
8. Mode of support in which breaths are delivered at a preset inspiratory pressure
10. Pressure above atmospheric during exhalation of a mechanical ventilator breath

So, what could go wrong?

1. Complete this sentence: "Put simply, respiratory failure is the . . ."

2. What is the blood gas criteria for respiratory failure?
   A. PaO_2

   B. $PaCO_2$

3. What is "true respiratory failure?"

Let's Review

Egan lists six causes of hypoxemia. Of these, decreased FIO_2, diffusion defect, and perfusion/diffusion impairment are not commonly seen in the acute care setting. V/Q mismatch, shunt, and hypoventilation are common.

- V/Q mismatch is usually a result of poorly ventilated areas that still get blood flow. *A typical example would be bronchospasm.*
- Shunt occurs when there is no ventilation at all. *A typical example would be pneumonia or ARDS.*
- Hypoventilation occurs in an essentially normal lung when CO_2 displaces O_2. *A typical example would be a drug overdose.*
- It's not too hard to tell these babies apart.
- V/Q mismatch responds to oxygen therapy.
- Shunt does not respond to oxygen therapy.
- Hypoventilation present with a normal A-a gradient and responds to. . .ventilation!

4. What is the classic blood gas presentation of acute hypoxemic respiratory failure due to V/Q mismatch or shunt? (Remember this one, it will show up to haunt you on the boards!)

5. What is the relationship between $PaCO_2$ and alveolar ventilation?

6. Egan states that there are 3 major disorders responsible for acute hypercapnic respiratory failure (Type II). Give 2 examples of disorders representative of each category.
   A. Decreased ventilatory drive
      1. _____
      2. _____
   B. Respiratory muscle fatigue/failure
      1. _____
      2. _____
   C. Increased work of breathing
      1. _____
      2. _____

7. Give an example of a condition that could cause greatly increased CO_2 production.

8. How does the body compensate for chronically elevated carbon dioxide levels associated with COPD or obesity hypoventilation syndrome?

9. What happens to the normal blood gas classification of respiratory failure in patients with chronic respiratory failure?

10. Identify the five most common factors that lead to acute-on-chronic failure.
    A. _____
    B. _____
    C. _____
    D. _____
    E. _____

11. What are the four main treatment goals for this group of patients?
    A. _____
    B. _____
    C. _____
    D. _____

12. The complications from treating acute respiratory failure are as life-threatening as the failure itself. Identify the likely causes of these pulmonary complications.
    A. Emboli

    B. Barotrauma

    C. Infection

13. Give one example of each of these non-pulmonary complications of life in the ICU.
    A. Cardiac

    B. Gastrointestinal

    C. Renal

14. List three more complications associated with prolonged visits to the unit.
    A. _____
    B. _____
    C. _____

Mechanical Ventilation

15. What is the goal of mechanical ventilation?

16. Your board exams will expect you to identify these classic criteria for mechanical ventilation. Remember that no one criteria mandates ventilation (except apnea).

Mechanism	Critical Value
A. $PaCO_2$	_____
B. pH	_____
C. VC (ml/kg)	_____
D. MIP	_____
E. MVV	_____
F. VE	_____
G. VD/VT	_____
H. $P(A\text{-}a)O_2$ on 100%	_____
I. P/F ratio	_____

I'm not kidding. You *really* need to learn these values!

17. Oxygenation indices like P/F ratio and A-a gradient are useful in determining the severity of failure. What is the limitation of these methods?

18. Why is it useful to consider pH when evaluating CO_2 levels to determine the need to intubate and ventilate a patient?

19. Identify the two common causes of decreased ventilatory drive.
    A. _____
    B. _____

20. Name four other less common potential causes of decreased drive.
    A. _____
    B. _____
    C. _____
    D. _____

21. Respiratory *muscle weakness* is most likely to occur in what patient group?

22. Name three conditions that frequently lead to respiratory *muscle fatigue*.
    A. _____
    B. _____
    C. _____

23. List three objective tests that can be performed to assess respiratory muscle strength at the bedside.
    A. _____
    B. _____
    C. _____

24. What will the blood gas show (one more time!) in full-blown ventilatory failure?

25. What is the cardinal sign of increased work of breathing?

Strategies

26. State the modes of support that are indicated for each of the following causes of respiratory failure.
    A. Rapidly reversible hypoxemic failure
    _____

    B. Slowly reversible hypoxemic failure
    _____
    _____

    C. Acute alveolar hypoventilation
    _____
    _____

    D. Chronic alveolar hypoventilation
    _____
    _____

    E. Altered mental status
    _____
    _____

    F. Acute muscle fatigue
    _____
    _____

    G. Chronic muscle fatigue
    _____
    _____

27. Give two strategies for preventing overdistention of alveoli in ARDS.
    A. _____
    B. _____

28. What mode of ventilation is most commonly used to guarantee minute ventilation in patients with acute alveolar hypoventilation?

29. In terms of blood gases, what is the treatment goal for ventilation of patients with chronic hypoventilation?

33. What is the target $PaCO_2$ in these cases?

34. What is the chief concern regarding use of PEEP to increase oxygenation in patients with acute head injuries?

30. Why are PSV and noninvasive ventilation contraindicated in patients who have altered mental status due to drugs or head injury?

35. Air-trapping, or hyperinflation, as a result of obstructive lung disease (COPD, asthma) causes what two complications in mechanically ventilated patients?
   A. _____
   B. _____

31. Patients who require intubation for respiratory muscle fatigue (not weakness!) generally need what type of support (and for how long) to rest their muscles?
   A. Type of support: _____
   B. For how long?: _____

36. How are tidal volume and flow rate manipulated to reduce complications in mechanically ventilated COPD patients?
   A. Tidal volume

Special Cases

32. How does hyperventilation result in reduced ICP in head injury?

   B. Flow rate

37. What surprising technique was found by MacIntyre to reduce auto-PEEP?

42. Proportional assist ventilation is unique because...

Weird Ways to Ventilate

38. Ventilating each lung separately (ILV) is potentially useful in what three conditions?
    A. _____
    B. _____
    C. _____

39. High-frequency ventilation is usually applied in what two conditions?
    A. _____
    B. _____

40. What is the primary use of pressure assist ventilation (PAV)?

41. Describe airway pressure release ventilation (APRV).

Chapter Highlights

43. Acute respiratory failure is identified by a $PaCO_2$ greater than _____ mm Hg and /or a PaO_2 less than _____ mm Hg in an otherwise healthy individual (at sea level, of course).

44. _____ respiratory failure is usually due to V/Q mismatch or intrapulmonary _____.

45. _____ respiratory failure results from inadequate drive, respiratory muscle _____, or excessive work of _____.

46. Chronic respiratory failure may be represented by ABG's demonstrating _____ with evidence of metabolic compensation or _____ reflecting chronic hypoxemia.

47. The _____ status of the patient is the most important factor determining the need for ventilator support.

48. Excessive _____ is the most common cause of respiratory muscle fatigue.

49. Only patients with rapidly reversible conditions should undergo _____ ventilation in the acute setting.

50. The goal of therapy in acute hypercapnic respiratory failure is to guarantee a set _____ ventilation.

Case Studies

Case 1

Wendy Baldo is an alert, anxious 25-year-old woman who presents in the emergency department complaining of chills, fever, and shortness of breath. An arterial blood gas is drawn on room air with these results:

pH	7.45
$PaCO_2$	32 mm Hg
PaO_2	50 mm Hg
HCO_3	23 mEq/L

51. Interpret this blood gas.

52. What is the A-a gradient?

53. What type of respiratory failure is present?

54. What do you recommend for initial respiratory treatment?

Case 2

Anne Town is a 27-year-old brought to the emergency department by paramedics following a drug overdose. She is obtunded. Blood gases are drawn on room air:

pH	7.24
$PaCO_2$	60 mm Hg
PaO_2	65 mm Hg
HCO_3	26 mEq/L

55. Interpret this blood gas.

56. What is the A-a gradient?

57. What type of respiratory failure is present?

58. What is the appropriate initial respiratory treatment in this case?

Case 3

Danny Lang is an alert 56-year-old man with a history of COPD. He presents in the emergency department complaining of dyspnea, which has worsened over the last few days. A blood gas is drawn on room air:

pH	7.28
$PaCO_2$	70 mm Hg
PaO_2	50 mm Hg
HCO_3	32 mEq/L

59. Interpret this blood gas.

60. What is the A-a gradient?

61. What type of respiratory failure is present?

62. What initial respiratory treatment is indicated?

What Does the NBRC Say?

The information presented in Chapter 37 forms a fundamental basis for our understanding of respiratory failure. It is highly complex, combining blood gases, pathophysiology, and more. The NBRC is passionate about your understanding of this material and will present you with many similar situations. Assess. Interpret. Recommend. Treat. Modify. Wow! When you are working on these problems, always start by interpreting the ABG. Do this in the context of the patient's history. COPD should raise a red flag that suggests you think hard before you interpret or act. Here are some examples.

63. An RCP is asked to evaluate a lethargic 50-year-old woman who is in respiratory distress following abdominal surgery. She is breathing spontaneously, on a 50% air-entrainment mask, at 32 breaths per minute. ABG results show:

pH	7.28
$PaCO_2$	55 mm Hg
PaO_2	60 mm Hg
HCO_3	26 mEq/L

Based on this information what would you recommend?
A. Intubation and mechanical ventilation
B. Increase the FIO_2 to 1.0
C. Administer IPPB
D. Administer bronchodilator therapy via SVN

64. An alert, anxious 60-year-old man with a history of CHF presents in the ER with respiratory distress. Auscultation reveals bilateral inspiratory crackles. He has peripheral edema. ABG results drawn on a partial rebreathing mask show:

pH   7.45
$PaCO_2$ 35 mm Hg
PaO_2 40 mm Hg
HCO_3 23 mEq/L

The most appropriate therapy for improving oxygenation would be
A. Intubation and mechanical ventilation
B. Administer oxygen therapy via non-rebreathing mask
C. Administer oxygen therapy via CPAP
D. Administer bronchodilator therapy via SVN

65. An adult male is being mechanically ventilated immediately after surgery for a closed-head injury. Settings are:

Tidal volume   700 ml
Rate   10
Mode   AC
FIO_2 .40
PEEP   0

ABGs show:

pH   7.37
$PaCO_2$ 44 mm Hg
PaO_2 86 mm Hg
HCO_3 24 mEq/L

Which of the following ventilator changes would you recommend at this time?
A. Increase the FIO_2
B. Decrease the Volume
C. Increase the rate
D. Increase the PEEP

66. An adult patient is being mechanically ventilated following respiratory failure. Settings are:

Tidal volume   800 ml
Rate   12
Mode   AC
FIO_2 .60
PEEP   2 cm H20

ABGs show:

pH   7.37
$PaCO_2$ 41 mm Hg
PaO_2 43 mm Hg
HCO_3 22 mEq/L

Which of the following ventilator changes would you recommend at this time?
A. Increase the FIO_2
B. Decrease the volume
C. Increase the rate
D. Increase the PEEP

67. A patient with a history of hypercapnia and COPD is intubated and placed on the ventilator following respiratory failure. Twenty-four hours later the patient is alert and breathing spontaneously.

Settings are:

Tidal volume   800 ml
Rate   12
Mode   AC
FIO_2 .30
PEEP   0 cm H20

ABG's show:

pH   7.48
$PaCO_2$ 41 mm Hg
PaO_2 60 mm Hg
HCO_3 30 mEq/L

Which of the following ventilator changes would you recommend at this time?
A. Decrease the FIO_2
B. Decrease the Volume
C. Change to Pressure controlled ventilation (PCV)
D. Change to Synchronized intermittent mandatory ventilation (SIMV)

68. A 77-year-old man with COPD is admitted with acute bronchitis. Room air blood gas results show:

pH   7.52
PaCO$_2$ 45 mm Hg
PaO$_2$ 40 mm Hg
HCO$_3$ 36 mEq/L

What intervention would be appropriate at this time?
A. CPAP with 24% oxygen
B. 28% air entrainment mask
C. Nasal cannula at 5 L/min
D. Simple mask at 8 L/min

69. CPAP is indicated for treatment of patients with
A. Respiratory failure secondary to shunting
B. Apnea
C. Ventilatory failure with hypercapnia
D. Hypoxemia secondary to V/Q mismatch

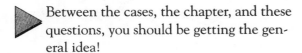

Between the cases, the chapter, and these questions, you should be getting the general idea!

Food for Thought

Remember Table 37-2, the one about measurable indications for ventilatory support? I didn't forget about that one. Your boards expect you to know this information, as part of the decision to intubate and ventilate, or as part of the decision to wean.

70. What clinical situations or condition suggests using ABGs to evaluate the need to intubate and ventilate? Compare this with situations better assessed by measures like VC and MIP.

We'll come back to this again in Chapter 42 when we talk about weaning.

Ventilatory Modes and Functions

"Just bag 'em till I get there."
Florida Society for RC T-Shirt

CMV PSV PCV AMV MMV VAPS ZEEP NEEP PEEP Bleep . . . Brain reeling. Neuronal meltdown. Must try to understand Chapter 38 . . . must remain conscious . . . Once upon a time there were only three modes of ventilation. Control, assist-control, and the new kid, IMV. Ventilators were driven by pistons or bellows and an occasional light bulb glowed or buzzer sounded when there was a problem. Volume-cycled, pressure-limited was just exactly what it sounded like. Times have changed. Ventilators cost more than new cars and microprocessors have permitted engineers to fulfill their wildest dreams. Whether or not the explosion of technology in ventilator design has improved health care has yet to be determined, but you will have to try to make sense of it anyway.

Ventilator Verbiage

Match these definitions to the key terms in the beginning of the chapter.

_____ 1. Ventilator design that incorporates hydrodynamic principles.

_____ 2. Providing all the minute ventilation requirements with the machine.

_____ 3. Relationship between inspiratory and expiratory time during ventilation.

_____ 4. Inspiratory technique used in estimating airway resistance and compliance.

_____ 5. Breath initiated or ended by the machine.

_____ 6. Providing only part of the ventilation requirements with the ventilator.

_____ 7. Pressure above the baseline in the expiratory phase of a machine breath.

_____ 8. The way the ventilator senses the patient's effort.

_____ 9. Breath initiated and ended by the patient.

A. Spontaneous breath
B. Fluidic
C. I:E ratio
D. Partial ventilatory support
E. Mandatory breath
F. Sensitivity control
G. Full ventilatory support
H. Positive end expiratory pressure
I. Inflation-hold maneuver

How Ventilators Work

10. What is a ventilator?

11. Describe the desired output of the ventilator in terms of the patient.

12. Identify three settings where ventilators use DC back-up power sources.
    A. _____
    B. _____
    C. _____

13. How are most modern intensive care ventilators powered?

14. Identify one setting where electrical power is undesirable.

15. When compressed gas is used as the drive mechanism, this force is adjusted to a working level by a reducing valve. Give examples of approaches for gas delivery once the pressure is reduced.
    A. Puritan-Bennett 7200

    B. Siemens Servo 900C

    C. Engstrom Erica IV

16. The output control valve opens and shuts to deliver gas to the patient. Proportional valves don't just turn flow on and off. What else can they do?

17. Name five ventilators that use proportional valves.
    A. _____
    B. _____
    C. _____
    D. _____
    E. _____

18. What are the three variables that ventilators control?
    A. _____
    B. _____
    C. _____

19. Give an example where the ventilator changes the control variable between breaths.

20. Identify the five types of control circuits used in ventilators.
    A. _____
    B. _____
    C. _____
    D. _____
    E. _____

21. State two advantages of fluidic control circuits.
    A. _____
    B. _____

22. Describe the basic purpose of the following phase variables.
    A. Trigger variable

    B. Limit variable

    C. Cycle variable

    D. Baseline variable

23. Why is controlled ventilation rarely used anymore?

24. Give one advantage and one disadvantage for the two methods of patient triggering.
    A. Pressure
       1. Advantage
       2. Disadvantage
    B. Flow
       1. Advantage
       2. Disadvantage

25. Identify the modes that these statements describe.
    A. Pure time triggering: _____
    B. Pure patient triggering: _____
    C. Patient *and* time triggering: _____

26. Define the term "limit variable."

27. What are the two common modes that employ pressure limiting?
    A. _____
    B. _____

28. What is the most common type of ventilatory support for infants?

29. Volume-limited breaths with inflation hold are usually used for what purpose?

30. Define the term "cycle variable."

31. What is the most common application of pressure-cycling?

32. Explain the difference between pressure-limiting and pressure-cycling.

33. What is the usual cycling parameter for pressure support ventilation?

34. Define the term "baseline variable."

35. What baseline variable is used on all modern ventilators?

36. Explain what is meant by these acronyms.
   A. ZEEP

   B. NEEP

   C. PEEP

37. Why are threshold resistors the most desirable mechanisms for generating PEEP?

38. Identify four devices used to generate PEEP.
   A. _____
   B. _____
   C. _____
   D. _____

39. Explain the difference between CPAP and PEEP. (Draw a picture if you are at a loss for words.)

40. Define spontaneous and mandatory breaths. Give another term for each.
   A. Spontaneous

   B. Mandatory

41. Define the phrase "mode of ventilation."

42. Explain the basic pattern of ventilation represented by each of these terms.
   A. CMV

   B. CSV

   C. IMV

See Table 38-3 on p. 850 of the text. These are the most common modes in use today.

43. To start learning this material, you need to write out the name for each acronym and list the control variables.
   A. CMV
      1. Name _____
      2. Control variables _____
   B. A/C
      1. Name _____
      2. Control variables _____
   C. AMV
      1. Name _____
      2. Control variables _____
   D. IMV
      1. Name _____
      2. Control variables _____
   E. SIMV
      1. Name _____
      2. Control variables _____
   F. CPAP
      1. Name _____
      2. Control variables _____
   G. PCV
      1. Name _____
      2. Control variables _____
   H. PC-IMV
      1. Name _____
      2. Control variables _____
   I. PCIRV
      1. Name _____
      2. Control variables _____
   J. APRV
      1. Name _____
      2. Control variables _____
   K. MMV
      1. Name _____
      2. Control variables _____
   L. VAPS
      1. Name _____
      2. Control variables _____
   M. BiPAP
      1. Name _____
      2. Control variables _____

Many modern ventilators are capable of displaying waveforms graphically so you can apply them clinically. For example, if you see that expiratory flow does not return to baseline before the next breath starts, you know that the patient is not able to exhale completely. You can then adjust the ventilator to allow complete exhalation, or try to treat the problem (by giving a bronchodilator, for example). I know only two ways to help you learn waveforms. One method of learning this difficult subject is to practice drawing the waveforms. The other way is to go to a ventilator in the classroom or lab setting. Attach the ventilator to a test lung, turn on the graphics, and adjust the ventilator to deliver different settings and look at the waveforms that are produced. It will help you if an instructor is handy to guide you through this procedure! Once you learn to identify the various waveforms, you can move on to the next step, which is to learn the problem pictures, what they mean clinically, and how to fix the problem. Egan covers this area in Chapter 41.

44. Draw these flow patterns.
   A. Rectangular

   B. Ascending ramp

   C. Descending ramp

   D. Sinusoidal

45. What is the goal of a ventilator alarm?

46. Use your text to identify examples of clinical conditions that could activate the following alarms.
A. Loss of electrical power

B. Ventilator inoperative

C. High peak airway pressure

D. Low peak airway pressure

E. High baseline pressure

F. Low baseline pressure

G. Low exhaled tidal volume

H. High minute volume

I. Low minute volume

J. Low respiratory rate

I'm not even going to touch Table 38-6 on pp. 856 to 857. The value of this table is simple. If you are working with specific ventilators in the lab or clinical setting, you should know the capabilities of the machine you are using. You will want to use Table 38-6 as a reference when you are learning about a particular machine.

Clinical Application of Ventilator Modes

47. When is controlled ventilation the preferred mode of ventilatory support?

48. Give a clinical example.

49. Pressure or volume may be used as the control variable in controlled ventilation. What happens to volume and airway pressure when compliance drops?

Control variable	Volume	Airway Pressure
A. Pressure	_____	_____
B. Volume	_____	_____

50. How well do patients tolerate controlled ventilation? How will we minimize patient effort in this mode if the patient fights the ventilator?

51. What is the primary indication for assist-control ventilation?

52. What is a potential harmful effect of assist-control ventilation in COPD patients?

53. Use the formulas in Table 38-8 on Page 860 to calculate these I:E ratios.
    A. Rate of 10, inspiratory time 1 second.
       1. Total cycle time: _____
       2. I:E ratio: _____
    B. Rate of 15, inspiratory time 1 second
       1. Total cycle time: _____
       2. I:E ratio: _____
    C. Rate of 20, inspiratory time 2 seconds
       1. Total cycle time: _____
       2. I:E ratio: _____

54. Identify the two general uses of IMV (SIMV).
    A.

    B.

55. Compare mean pleural pressures for IMV and CMV.

56. What are the two methods for supplying fresh gas for spontaneous breaths in IMV?
    A. _____
    B. _____

57. What is the biggest drawback of an external continuous flow IMV circuit?

58. What type of humidifier is preferred for use with IMV to minimize work of breathing?

59. What type of triggering is preferred for use with IMV to minimize work of breathing?

60. What type of breathing pattern results in an unacceptable level of alveolar ventilation with MMV?

61. Describe the 3 primary indications for PSV.
    A.

    B.

    C.

62. Identify two other modes where PSV is used to augment spontaneous breaths.
    A. _____
    B. _____

63. When is CPAP an appropriate primary mode of ventilation?

64. Name two ways to apply CPAP to the airway.

A. _____
   _____

B. _____
   _____

65. What is the difference between BiPAP and CPAP?

66. Identify the two main indications for BiPAP.

A. _____

B. _____

Case Studies

Case 1

Dane Lopez, a 21-year old patient, is placed on a ventilator following a head injury. The physician desires to control this patient's ventilation to achieve a specific CO_2 level in the arterial blood.

67. What trigger adjustment is required to initiate this mode?

68. What would you recommend if the patient's breathing pattern is out of synch with the ventilator?

Case 2

Martha Gomes is a 35-year-old woman with a neuromuscular disease. She is placed on a Puritan-Bennett 7200 ventilator in CMV mode. The ventilator is set for assist-controlled volume cycled ventilation at a rate of 10, but the machine is triggering at a rate of 28. Martha looks pretty scared.

69. What is the most likely cause of the excess ventilator triggering?

70. What other mode of ventilation could you use to solve this problem?

What Does the NBRC Say?

The following modes of ventilation are listed in the examination matrices.

    IMV
    SIMV
    PSV
    CPAP
    BiPAP(Registry only)
    PCV
    CMV
    PC-IRV
    APRV

For the more common traditional modes you are expected to be able to recommend, initiate, adjust, and so on; in other words, everything. For BiPAP, APRV, PC-IRV, and PCV you will just need to know the basics. What is the mode, when is it indicated—that kind of stuff.

71. A patient with ARDS is being ventilated with the following settings:

Mode	AC
Vt	800
Rate	14
FiO$_2$	80%
PEEP	15 cm H$_2$O

Peak pressures are unacceptably high while oxygenation remains poor. Which of the following changes may be beneficial in this situation?
A. Change the PEEP to 20 cm H$_2$O
B. Increase the FiO$_2$ to 100%
C. Initiate PCIRV
D. Place the patient on BiPAP

72. A patient is being ventilated in SIMV mode. The patient is making spontaneous efforts with tidal volumes of 150 ml. What modification would you recommend?
A. Initiate PEEP
B. Initiate PSV
C. Change to PCIRV mode
D. Change to IMV mode

73. A patient with COPD and CO$_2$ retention is intubated following respiratory failure. The physician states that she wants to avoid overventilation and air-trapping. Which of the following modes would you recommend?
A. SIMV
B. AC
C. CPAP
D. APRV

74. A patient in the early stages of ARDS is intubated. The physician states that he wishes to minimize the possibility of volutrauma or barotrauma. Which of the following modes would you recommend?
A. AC
B. SIMV
C. CPAP
D. PCV

75. An 80 kg (176 lb) patient is being ventilated in pressure control mode. During a ventilator check, the therapist notes that the compliance has decreased from 40 ml/cm H$_2$O to 35 ml/cm H$_2$O. What effect will this change in compliance have on the patient's ventilator system?
A. No effect
B. Increased peak airway pressure
C. Decreased mean airway pressure
D. Decreased tidal volume

Food for Thought

Not all modes are used in all parts of the country. What are your hospitals using? Does practice vary between community hospitals and the trauma center? A good starting point for the new practitioner is to learn about the modes that are most commonly used in current practice where you live and where you do your clinical training. For example, if you are being assigned to do clinical in a small hospital where CMV and AC are the main modes, don't go in with the idea that you will implement PC-IRV. Instead, learn as much as you can about the art of using CMV. The best RCPs can make the best of whatever mode is used in their institution while acting as resources for the nurses and physicians. They pull the other modes out of their bag of tricks when the opportunity arises. But only after making themselves experts. Introducing a new ventilator or new mode of ventilation is fraught with hazards if in-service training doesn't come along with the changes.

Physics and Physiology of Ventilatory Support

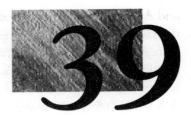

39

Mechanical ventilation can be a life-sustaining procedure. But it is not natural. There are physiologic consequences to applying positive pressure to the lungs and chest. For better or for worse, we're currently married to this technology and you will need to understand what happens when you connect the patient to the machine.

Word Power

There aren't too many new words to learn in Chapter 39. Look up their definitions in your glossary and write them out next to the six words I've listed below.

1. Barotrauma: ———————————
   ————————————————————

2. Compressed
   volume: ————————————————

3. Intrinsic PEEP: ——————————
   ————————————————————

4. Trans-respiratory pressure gradient:
   ————————————————————

5. Ventilator asynchrony: ——————
   ————————————————————

6. Work of breathing: ———————
   ————————————————————

Meet the Objectives

7. Describe how inspiration is accomplished with positive pressure ventilation.

8. Describe the desired effects of positive pressure breathing on each of the following. Explain how each effect is accomplished.
   A. Alveolar ventilation

   B. Acid-base balance

   C. Work of breathing

9. Identify two potential benefits of controlled CMV.
   A. _____
   B. _____

10. Identify two potential harmful effects of controlled CMV.
   A. _____
   B. _____

11. Name two advantages of IMV.
   A. _____
   B. _____

12. Pediatric patients require small tidal volumes. How can you achieve a low compressed volume in this setting?
   A.

   B.

   C.

13. What is the primary reason for using PC-CMV?

14. PC-IRV is implemented when high FiO_2 and high PEEP fail to improve oxygenation in severe cases. What is the mechanism for improvement with this mode? What effect could this have on oxygen delivery? Why?
   A. Mechanism

   B. Oxygen delivery

15. What actually seems to be improved by the application of APRV?

16. What is PSV designed to accomplish?

17. Egan says that PSV will result in four bene-
ficial effects. Name them.
   A. _____
   B. _____
   C. _____
   D. _____

18. What is the effect of CPAP on ventilation?

19. Identify the important physiologic effect of CPAP.

20. Bilevel CPAP was originally developed for treatment of obstructive sleep apnea. It has also been shown to be useful in acute care settings. Name two.
   A. _____
   B. _____

21. What is the most common combination of ventilation modes in current use?

22. What is believed to be the benefit of decelerating flow waveforms?

23. You were taught that a slow deep breath improves the distribution of ventilation. Why don't we use this pattern with ventilator patients?

24. Give one benefit and one drawback to the inflation-hold maneuver.
   A. _____
   B. _____

25. Describe three beneficial physiologic effects of PEEP.
   A. _____
   B. _____
   C. _____

26. PEEP is normally not very good for COPD patients. When should it be used?

27. Identify five detrimental effects of PEEP.
    A. _____
    B. _____
    C. _____
    D. _____
    E. _____

28. Air-trapping during PPV has many names. List three.
    A. _____
    B. _____
    C. _____

29. Identify two conditions that have high risk for developing serious air-trapping while on the ventilator.
    A. _____
    B. _____

30. How can you manipulate the trigger variable to reduce work of breathing?

31. PSV is widely used to decrease work of breathing. Besides adjusting the ventilator, what can the clinician do to reduce work of breathing?

Amazingly enough, positive pressure ventilation affects almost every important organ system in the body! Lungs, heart, kidney, liver, and the gut. And you thought you would just put the patient on the ventilator!

32. Compare distribution of gas in the lung for spontaneous and positive pressure ventilation.

33. Where does the majority of blood flow in the lung end up during positive pressure ventilation?

34. Hyperventilation is commonly associated with positive pressure ventilation! Describe at least three harmful consequences of hyperventilation.
    A.

    B.

    C.

35. Both tidal volume and positive pressure can damage delicate lung tissue. Identify the values for these two areas where damage is more likely to occur.

A. Tidal volume

B. Alveolar pressure (not airway pressure!)

36. What percentage of critically ill ventilator patients is likely to experience some form of barotrauma?

37. List three examples of pulmonary barotrauma.

A. _____

B. _____

C. _____

38. Compare the effects of spontaneous and positive pressure ventilation on cardiac output.

39. PPV might improve cardiac function in what type of disease?

40. What do high peak pressure, long inspiratory time, and PEEP all have in common?

41. Compare the cardiovascular effects of positive pressure in patients with compliant lungs, noncompliant lungs, and noncompliant chest walls. Give examples of these conditions.

A.

B.

C.

42. Normal patients can easily compensate for moderate increases in airway pressure. What patients are especially sensitive to the cardiovascular effects of PPV?

43. Explain the mechanism behind the drop in urine output in ventilated patients.

Chapter Highlights

Fill in the blanks, thanks.

44. Positive physiologic effects of PPV include improved _____ and ventilation, and decreased _____ of breathing.

45. No single _____ pattern has been demonstrated to be more physiologically effective than another.

46. Research indicates better ventilator synchrony with the _____ pattern than the _____ pattern.

47. _____-triggering appears to be a better choice than _____-triggering when it is available on the ventilator.

48. PEEP is applied to restore _____ in restrictive disease and _____ the airways in obstructive disease.

49. PEEP allows the RCP to decrease the _____, thereby avoiding the complications of _____ toxicity.

50. Positive pressure ventilation is detrimental to the V/Q ratio primarily by shifting _____ to areas that are less _____.

51. PPV may decrease venous _____ and cardiac _____.

52. PPV may cause hepatic and gastrointestinal malfunction primarily due to decreased _____ of those _____ beds.

Case Studies

Part 1

Willie Wilson, a trauma patient, is stabilized after a motor vehicle accident. Willie is intubated and transported to the ICU where you place him on ventilator. As soon as you put him on the machine, his blood pressure falls dramatically.

53. What should you do immediately?

54. What is the most likely cause of hypotension in a trauma patient who has been placed on positive pressure ventilation?

Part 2

Two days later, Willie has developed poor lung compliance and hypoxemia associated with non-cardiogenic pulmonary edema (ARDS). He is being ventilated on A/C, 12, 900, +15 cm H_2O PEEP, and FIO_2 70%. Blood gases show: pH, 7.37, $PaCO_2$, 38, PaO_2, 55. Peak inspiratory pressure is 60 cm H_2O, plateau pressure is 50 cm H_2O.

55. There are two serious problems here. Identify them.

A. Serious problem no. 1

B. Serious problem no. 2

56. What change(s) in ventilator strategy would you suggest?

What Does the NBRC Say?

Not much, actually. Nothing new, that is. Of course you need to be able to recognize the harmful effects of PPV. If the patient develops a pneumothorax, you would assess, recognize, and recommend treatment. Chapter 39 reviews each of the common modes of ventilation, and the board exams are quite clear that you should be familiar with them, as I mentioned in Chapter 38. Let's move on.

Food for Thought

57. If the newest modes of ventilation are not proven to alter patient outcomes, why should we use them?

58. Patients on ventilators have a high incidence of GI bleeding. Chapter 39 suggests two possible ways to deal with this problem. What are they? Are there others? Why is GI bleeding such a big deal to RCPs?

Initiating and Adjusting Ventilatory Support

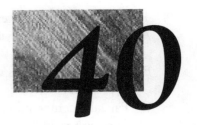

"Paralyze resistance with persistence."
Woody Hayes

It's relatively easy to learn how to make changes in ventilator settings. "Knob twirlers" are what we call people who know how to make adjustments but don't understand why or what the consequences will be. Chapter 40 is an excellent tool to help you to understand the specific strategies and changes used to provide quality mechanical ventilation.

Case Studies

We're nearing the end of this book. At this point, I think you would benefit from less traditional workbook questions and fill-in problems. Let's go right to the cases and find out if you understand how to initiate and adjust ventilatory support.

Case 1

Yvonne Robertson is a 5'5" tall, 60 kg (132 lb), young woman who was beaten up by her boyfriend. She is unconscious, has broken ribs, and facial injuries. The emergency department physician elects to intubate Ms. Robertson because of her mental status and injuries.

1. What size ET tube would be appropriate for an adult female?
   A. 6.0 mm inside diameter
   B. 7.0 mm outside diameter
   C. 7.5 mm inside diameter
   D. 8.0 mm inside diameter

2. In the emergency setting, how will you assess proper tube placement?
   I. Auscultate the chest
   II. Auscultate the epigastrium
   III. Attach an exhaled CO_2 monitor
   IV. Observe chest wall motion
   A. I, II only
   B. I, III only
   C. II, III, IV only
   D. I, II, III, IV

After the intubation is completed, a large amount of bloody secretions are suctioned from the airway. The physician requests an ABG at this point. Results show:

pH	7.47
$PaCO_2$	33 mm Hg
PaO_2	55 mm Hg
HCO_3	24 mEq/L

Vital signs are:

HR	115
BP	125/75
RR	26
T	37

A chest film is taken which reveals the tip of the endotracheal tube to be 6 cm above the carina. The physician notes four adjacent rib fractures on the left side and no sign of a pneumothorax.

3. What action would you recommend in regard to the ET tube placement?
   A. Advance the tube 2-3 cm
   B. Withdraw the tube 2-3 cm
   C. Maintain current placement
   D. Remove the tube and insert a PTL airway

4. The ABG results are interpreted as
   A. Metabolic alkalosis with severe hypoxemia
   B. Respiratory alkalosis with moderate hypoxemia
   C. Partially compensated respiratory alkalosis with mild hypoxemia
   D. Partially compensated metabolic alkalosis with moderate hypoxemia

5. Select an appropriate method of oxygen delivery for this patient.
   A. Venturi mask set at 28% FIO_2
   B. 10 cm H_2O CPAP with 100% oxygen
   C. 40% FIO_2 delivered by a heated aerosol T-piece
   D. Face tent with cool mist set to deliver 60% oxygen

Ms. Robertson is transported to radiology where a CT shows no intracranial bleeding, then to the ICU for observation. Two hours later, you are called by the RN to assess the patient due to an increased level of respiratory distress. Paradoxical chest wall motion is observed. Auscultation reveals coarse rhonchi bilaterally, with decreased breath sounds in the left lower lobe. Another ABG is drawn. Results show:

pH	7.35
$PaCO_2$	50 mm Hg
PaO_2	50 mm Hg (40% FIO_2)
HCO_3	26 mEq/L

Vital signs are:

HR	130
BP	145/90
RR	30
T	37

The physician requests that you initiate mechanical ventilation.

6. Which of the following settings would you recommend?
   A. SIMV, VT 600, 50%, Rate 10, PEEP 3 cm H_2O
   B. A/C, VT 900, 40%, Rate 8, PEEP 0
   C. CPAP, +10 cm H_2O, 100%
   D. PCIRV, 2:1 ratio, 35 cm H_2O, Rate 14

7. Multiple adjacent fractured ribs with paradoxical breathing indicates the presence of
   A. ARDS
   B. Acute obstructive disease
   C. Flail chest
   D. Pneumothorax

8. What type of humidification would you recommend for this patient?
   A. Heated wick humidifier set at 32 degrees C
   B. HME
   C. Heated pass-over humidifier
   D. Bubble humidifier

One week later, Ms. Robertson is alert and weaning is initiated. When the rate is decreased to 5, however, the patient's spontaneous respiratory rate rises to 30 and tidal volumes drop to 200 ml.

9. To help resolve this problem you might recommend initiation of
   A. CMV
   B. A/C
   C. PSV
   D. APRV

Case 2

Diana Olivera is a 5' 2" tall, 50 kg (110 lb), 65-year-old woman with a history of COPD. Paramedics bring her to the emergency department for treatment of dyspnea. She is wearing a nasal cannula set at 2 L/min. ABGs are drawn. Results show:

pH	7.30
$PaCO_2$	70 mm Hg
PaO_2	45 mm Hg
HCO_3	34 mEq/L

Vital signs are:

HR	100
BP	100/70
RR	28
T	39

Noninvasive positive pressure breathing is attempted with bi-level ventilation, but the patient is unable to tolerate the mask and fights the system. A decision is made to intubate and initiate mechanical ventilation. Mrs. Olivera is given a small amount of sedation and intubated nasally with a 6.5 mm ID tube. Settings are:

Mode	SIMV
Rate	8
VT	500 ml
FiO_2	28%
PEEP	0
Peak flow	20 LPM
Sensitivity	1.5 cm H_2O below baseline

10. How long should you wait before drawing an ABG to assess the results of these settings?
   A. 5 minutes
   B. 10 minutes
   C. 20 minutes
   D. 30 minutes

11. What is the maximum desirable plateau pressure during mechanical ventilation?
   A. 15 cm H_2O
   B. 25 cm H_2O
   C. 35 cm H_2O
   D. 45 cm H_2O

During your first ventilator check the following observations are made:

PIP	45 cm H_2O
Plateau	35 cm H_2O
Set rate	8
Total rate	34
Exhaled VT	490 ml
Spont VT	120 ml
I:E ratio	1:3

12. What high-pressure alarm limit should you set?
   A. 35 cm H_2O
   B. 45 cm H_2O
   C. 55 cm H_2O
   D. 65 cm H_2O

13. What value should you set for the low minute ventilation alarm?
   A. 3.5 L
   B. 6.0 L
   C. 7.2 L
   D. 8.0 L

14. Which of the following would result in a lower work of breathing for this patient?
   I. Addition of mechanical dead space
   II. Initiation of PSV
   III. Changing to flow-triggering
   IV. Addition of PEEP
   A. I, II only
   B. II, III only
   C. I, III only
   D. II, III, IV

15. What action should you take to increase the I:E ratio?
   A. Increase the peak flow
   B. Increase the tidal volume
   C. Increase the set rate
   D. Increase the FiO_2

16. According to Egan, what is the desired I:E ratio for COPD patients to provide sufficient time for exhalation and prevent auto-PEEP?
   A. 1:1
   B. 1:2
   C. 1:4
   D. 1:8

Case 3

Lynette Cooler is a 5'6" tall woman who weighs 100 kg (220 lb). She is in the ICU following surgery for multiple injuries sustained in a motor vehicle accident. She has an arterial line and a pulmonary artery catheter in place. Her chest radiograph shows bilateral infiltrates consistent with ARDS. The ET tube is in good position.

Current ventilator settings are:

Mode	Assist-controlled CMV
VT	1000
Rate	12
FiO$_2$	.70
PEEP	5 cm H$_2$O
Peak flow	60 L/min
Sensitivity	1.0 cm H$_2$O below baseline

17. What is this patient's approximate ideal body weight?
   A. 50 kg
   B. 60 kg
   C. 80 kg
   D. 100 kg

18. What set tidal volume would you recommend to prevent further lung injury?
   A. 500 ml
   B. 700 ml
   C. 900 ml
   D. Maintain current setting

The following data are obtained:

HR	110, NSR with occasional PVCs
BP	110/75 mm Hg
SpO$_2$	88%
PA	38/8 mm Hg
PCWP	12 mm Hg
CO	5.8 L/min
SvO$_2$	59%

19. With regard to the patient's oxygenation, what action would you recommend?
   A. Increase the FiO$_2$
   B. Increase the PEEP
   C. Add mechanical dead space
   D. Maintain current settings

A PEEP trial is conducted with the following results:

PEEP	Cs	PaO$_2$	CO
5	22	57	5.8
10	25	66	5.7
15	30	72	5.9
20	35	77	5.2
25	32	85	4.8

20. What PEEP level would you recommend?
   A. 5
   B. 10
   C. 15
   D. 20
   E. 25

Ms. Cooler continues to deteriorate over the next two days. Her compliance and PaO$_2$ have decreased, while PIP has increased to 60 cm H$_2$O to maintain a normal PaCO$_2$.

21. Which of the following ventilator modes could be considered as alternatives?
   I. PCIRV
   II. SIMV
   III. APRV
   IV. PSV
   A. I, III only
   B. II, III only
   C. II, IV only
   D. I, IV only

22. Which of these techniques are used with ARDS to reduce lung injury or improve oxygenation?
   I. Expiratory retard
   II. Prone positioning
   III. Permissive hypercapnia
   IV. Unilateral lung ventilation
   A. I, II only
   B. II, III only
   C. I, II, III
   D. II, III, IV

Case 4

Melodee Flavor is a respiratory student who fell down the stairs while reading Egan and suffered a closed-head injury. Melodee is 5'4" tall and weighs 60 kg. ICP and blood pressure are elevated. She is being ventilated with these settings:

Mode	Control
Rate	8
VT	900
FiO$_2$	.30
PEEP	0

Blood gases on these settings are:

pH	7.40
$PaCO_2$	40
PaO_2	55
HCO_3	24

23. This blood gas should be interpreted as
    A. Normal with moderate hypoxemia
    B. Respiratory alkalosis with mild hypoxemia
    C. Compensated respiratory acidosis with severe hypoxemia
    D. Compensated metabolic alkalosis with moderate hypoxemia

24. With regard to the oxygenation, what change would you suggest?
    A. Increase the PEEP
    B. Increase the rate
    C. Change to APRV
    D. Increase the FiO_2

25. With regard to the ventilation, what change would you suggest?
    A. Increase the rate
    B. Increase the tidal volume
    C. Change to SIMV
    D. Add mechanical dead space

26. What is the formula for calculating the minute ventilation needed to produce a desired change in $PaCO_2$?
    A. New VE= Current VE * (Desired $PaCO_2$/Current $PaCO_2$)
    B. New VE= Current $PaCO_2$ * (Current VE/Desired $PaCO_2$)
    C. New VE= Desired $PaCO_2$ * Current VE
    D. New VE= Current VE * (Current $PaCO_2$/Desired $PaCO_2$)

27. What rate would you suggest for this patient if the desired $PaCO_2$ is 30 mm Hg?
    A. 8
    B. 10
    C. 14
    D. 16

What Does the NBRC Say?

The Entry-Level Examination Matrix is quite clear on this subject. You should be able to:

Initiate and adjust ventilators when settings are specified
Initiate and adjust IMV, SIMV, and PSV
Select appropriate tidal volume, minute volume, and respiratory rate

You should also know when to modify:

FiO_2
Tidal volume
Alarms
Mechanical dead space
PEEP
Sensitivity
Inspiratory flow
Mode

The list goes on. The Written Registry Exam adds more difficult questions and:

PCV
Mask ventilation
APRV
IRV
Bi-level ventilation

They may also ask questions found on the Entry-Level Exam at a higher difficulty level. So even if you don't do APRV at any place in your state, you still need to know the basic idea. Remember that these exam matrices change approximately every 5 years, and the last one was 1994!

Food for Thought

28. What is the single most common ventilator strategy currently in use in the United States?

29. What are the common ventilator modes (and adjuncts like PEEP, PSV, etc) where you are training or working?

30. Describe the important general considerations for ventilating patients with obstructive lung disease.

Monitoring and Management of the Patient in the ICU

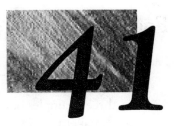

41

Truer words were never spoken. ICU monitoring has reached a level of complexity that is as dazzling as it is expensive. The amount of data available to the critical care clinician is staggering. The key to success in this endeavor is to combine appropriate information gathering with sound clinical assessment. You can't learn that from a book! What you can learn from this book are: normal values, waveforms, terms, and the most common problems and situations you will encounter. When you go out into the clinical setting you can learn to apply this new information. I'm going to make you work hard in this chapter, but then you are near the end of the book and you need to put this all together.

Monitoring Match

Match these key terms to the definitions that follow.

_____ 1. Afterload
_____ 2. Asynchronous
_____ 3. Cardiac tamponade
_____ 4. Dicrotic notch
_____ 5. Normovolemic
_____ 6. Paradoxical breathing

_____ 7. Preload
_____ 8. Pulsus paradoxus
_____ 9. Respiratory alternans
_____ 10. Thermistor

A. Pressure the ventricle has to contract against
B. Pressure stretching the ventricle at the onset of contraction
C. Breathing pattern in which rib cage and abdomen do not move outward together
D. Sign of valve closure seen in the descending limb of a pulse waveform
E. Compression of the heart caused by blood, fluid, or gas under the pericardium
F. Normal fluid volume in the blood vessels
G. Inspiratory pattern in which the abdomen moves out while the chest moves in
H. Abnormal drop in pulse pressure with each inspiratory effort
I. Alternating use of diaphragm and accessory muscles to breathe
J. Electric device used to measure temperature or flow through impedance

General Patient Assessment

11. Identify three body fluids that are frequently cultured when the patient develops a fever.
    A. _____
    B. _____
    C. _____

12. Give two examples of elevated body temperatures that are not associated with infection.
    A. _____
    B. _____

13. List three examples of conditions that could cause weakening of the pulse during inspiration.
    A. _____
    B. _____
    C. _____

14. Why should you check the pulse manually even when it is displayed on the ECG monitor?

15. Name four common respiratory causes of tachypnea in the ICU patient.
    A. _____
    B. _____
    C. _____
    D. _____

16. Identify three non-respiratory causes of tachypnea.
    A. _____
    B. _____
    C. _____

17. How often should chest films be taken during the critical period of a patient's illness?

18. Identify at least two pathologic changes the RCP should look for in the chest film.
    A. _____
    B. _____

19. Explain why assessment of the following hematologic data is useful to RCPs.
    A. Hemoglobin

    B. WBC and differential

20. Identify the two simple non-invasive ways to monitor fluid balance.
    A. _____
    B. _____

21. What lung condition is a patient likely to develop who is taking in more water than is being eliminated?

Physiologic Monitoring

 See Table 41-4 on p. 927.

22. Oxygen exchange at the lung is most frequently monitored by what test?

23. In what patient population is transcutaneous PO_2 monitoring utilized?

24. Identify the two types of oximeters used in clinical practice.
    A. _____
    B. _____

25. What is the most serious clinical limitation of using pulse oximetry to assess the respiratory status?

26. Explain how pulse oximeters can result in tissue injury.

27. Give the general rule for estimating shunt when a patient is breathing 100% oxygen.

28. The most accurate and reliable measure of pulmonary oxygenation efficiency is direct calculation of shunt. State the classic shunt equation.

29. What is DO_2? How is it calculated?

30. State the classic Fick equation.

31. List the normal, abnormal, and critical values for PvO_2 and SvO_2.

	Normal	Abnormal	Critical
A. PvO_2	_____	_____	_____
B. SvO_2	_____	_____	_____

32. What is the gold standard for assessing the adequacy of ventilation?

33. Where should you place the spirometer to measure minute ventilation?

34. What is the difference between arterial and end-tidal CO_2 in normal subjects? Ventilated subjects?
    A. Normal

    B. Ventilated

35. Identify four special applications of the capnometer.
    A. _____
    B. _____
    C. _____
    D. _____

36. Efficiency of ventilation is assessed by measuring physiologic dead space. State the modified Bohr equation.

37. List the normal, ventilator, and critical values for dead space to tidal volume ratio.

Normal	Vent Pt.	Critical
_____	_____	_____

38. State the normal value for exhaled minute volume.

39. What is the difference between dynamic and effective compliance?

40. What is the normal range for effective compliance?

41. Resistance calculations on ventilated patients should be performed with the inspiratory flow set to what pattern?

42. List the normal, ventilator, and abnormal values for airway resistance.

    Normal   *Vent Pt.*   *Abnormal*

43. Work of breathing measurements in spontaneously breathing patients requires measurement of what pressure and placement of what additional device?
   A. Pressure

   B. Device

44. Compare NIF and VC in terms of the type of patient mental status or level of cooperation required for successful measurements.

45. What is the maximum duration of the NIF procedure?

46. Describe the two NIF measurement techniques. Give one advantage and one disadvantage for each.
   A. Technique 1
      1. Advantage: _____

      2. Disadvantage: _____

   B. Technique 2
      1. Advantage: _____

      2. Disadvantage: _____

Mathemagic

A lot of important math problems were presented in the last section of Chapter 41. Before we go on to the dreaded *hemodynamics* section, I want to make sure you can do the math.

Shunt

You will at best have to recognize the classic shunt equation. At worst, be able to calculate it (even though we use computers in the clinical setting). Let's see if you can estimate shunt using the formula from p. 929.

Let's do it together first.

A patient is breathing 100% oxygen. The PaO_2 is 200. What is the estimated shunt? $PAO_2 = (760$ minus $47) \times 1\text{-}PaCO_2$ (assume 40). Assume 673 for PAO_2. Now plug the numbers into the formula. 673-200 = a 473 mm Hg difference between A and a. If there is a 5% shunt for each 100 mm Hg difference, the estimated shunt is 473/100 × 5, or 24%.

Your turn.

47. A patient is breathing 100% oxygen. Pb is 747 (conveniently), $PaCO_2$ is 47, and PaO_2 is 300. Estimate the shunt.
   A. $PAO_2 =$ _____
   B. A-a = _____
   C. Shunt = _____

Fick

Fick was *the* physiologist. You can use his equation to calculate cardiac output or oxygen consumption. This isn't used much in the clinical setting, but can be on your boards. You'll find the Fick equation on p. 930. Let's do one together.

What is cardiac output for a patient who has a VO_2 of 250, a CaO_2 of 19, and a CvO_2 of 14?

Plug the numbers into the formula:

QT (total perfusion or cardiac output) = $VO_2/CaO_2 - CvO_2 \times 10$ or. . .
QT = $250/19 - 14 \times 10 = 250/ 5 \times 10 = 250/50 = 5$ L/min.

48. What is cardiac output for a patient who has an oxygen consumption of 200 ml/min, an arterial content of 20 volume %, and a venous content of 16 volume %?
    A. Formula

    B. Calculation

    C. Answer

49. What is the VE for a patient who has a respiratory rate of 8 and a tidal volume of 400?
    A. Formula

    B. Calculation

    C. Answer

You could rearrange this to calculate oxygen consumption if you knew the cardiac output. For example, what is the oxygen consumption for a patient who has a cardiac output of 4L/min, CaO_2 of 17, and CvO_2 of 13?

$VO_2 = 4 \times 17 - 13$ or 160 ml/min.
You can keep on rearranging all you like.

Minute ventilation

That was fun, now try an easy one. Exhaled minute ventilation is respiratory rate × tidal volume. $VE = f \times VT$. For example, a patient has a respiratory rate of 12 and a tidal volume of 500, so the exhaled minute ventilation is 6000 ml or 6 L. (p. 932)

Bohr

Egan is correct in giving you the precise version of the modified Bohr equation on p. 935. You need to be careful to be accurate and include all factors when performing this procedure on ventilated patients. The board exams are kinder, and only ask you to recognize the main equation: $VD/VT = PaCO_2 - PECO_2/PaCO_2$. First we'll calculate the physiologic dead space to tidal volume ratio, then use it in combination with minute volume. For example, what is the dead space to tidal volume ratio for a patient who has an arterial CO_2 of 40 and an exhaled CO_2 of 30? 40-30/40 = 10/40, or 25%. Normal.

50. Your turn. Calculate VD/VT for a patient who has an arterial CO_2 of 40 and an exhaled CO_2 of 20.
   A. Formula

   B. Calculation

   C. Answer

Now let's combine this with the minute volume equation to calculate alveolar minute ventilation. Let's use respiratory rate of 12, tidal volume of 500, $PaCO_2$ of 40 and $PECO_2$ of 30. The new formula says: $VA = f(VT- VD)$. Dead space is 25%. So multiply the tidal volume $\times$ .25 to get the dead space volume. 500 x .25 = 125 ml. Now plug in the numbers. VA = 12(500-125) or 12 $\times$ 375= 4500 ml.

51. Calculate alveolar minute ventilation for a patient who has a rate of 10, tidal volume of 500, arterial CO_2 of 40, and end-tidal CO_2 of 28.
   A. Formula

   B. Calculation

   C. Answer

Expect some combination of this material on your board exams!

VD/VT Nomogram

As clinicians, we know a patient has an elevated dead space when they have a high minute volume with a normal to high $PaCO_2$. It may be easier and cheaper to use a nomogram to estimate VD/VT. You'll find the classic nomogram on p. 936 (Fig. 41-6)

It's easy to use. For example, if a patient has a CO_2 of 40 and a VE of about 18 L, the dead space is 75%. I just lined up the CO_2 at the bottom with the VE and came down the line where the values intersected.

52. If a patient had an arterial CO_2 of 50, and a minute volume of 15 L, what is the percentage of dead space?

Compliance

Like dead space, compliance calculations are simplified on the board exams.

We'll do it both ways here. First, static effective compliance the simple way.

A patient has an exhaled volume of 600 ml. The plateau pressure is 35 and the PEEP is 5. Compliance is $600/35 - 5$ or $600/30 = 20$ ml/cm H_2O. You try:

53. Calculate static effective compliance for a patient who has an exhaled volume of 1000, plateau pressure of 35, PEEP of 10.
   A. Formula

   B. Calculation

   C. Compliance

In clinical practice it is important to subtract the compressed volume. A comparison will make this clear. The first patient had a volume of 600 and compliance of 20. But, if the PIP was 40 cm H_2O and the circuit expansion factor is 5 ml/cm H_2O, then the volume lost to expansion is 200 ml (factor × PIP)! The new compliance calculation is:

$(600-200) / (35-5)$ or $400/30 = 13$ ml/cm H_2O! You try:

54. Calculate compliance for a patient who has a tidal volume of 800, PIP 50, plateau 35, PEEP 5. The circuit factor is 4 ml/cm H_2O.
   A. Formula

   B. Calculation

   C. Compliance

Resistance

A look at the difference between PIP and plateau pressure is useful for clinical estimates of airway resistance as well. First, you need to use a square or constant flow pattern on most modern ventilators. Next, you need to determine the flow rate in liters per second, not liters per minute.

Here is an example:

Calculate resistance for a patient who has a PIP of 50 cm H_2O, plateau of 40 cm H_2O, and flow rate of 60 L/min. 60 L/min converts to L/second this way: 60 L/min divided by 60 seconds per minute = 1 L/ sec. Now calculate:

PIP-Plateau/ Flow = 50-40/1 = 10 cm H_2O per liter per second. Now your turn.

55. Calculate airway resistance for a patient who has a peak pressure of 50 cm H_2O, plateau pressure of 40 cm H_2O, flow rate of 30 L/min.
   A. Convert flow to liters per second

   B. Resistance formula

   C. Calculation

   D. Airway resistance is:

If you are doing patient care, you may not have to calculate to see that resistance or compliance has changed. Look at the difference between peak pressure and plateau pressure. If the difference has increased and all else is stable, then the resistance has also increased. Some ventilators will perform compliance and resistance calculations for you. The manual calculations will give slightly different answers than the ventilator.

Policy will determine the way you do the numbers at any particular hospital.

Remember, if the patient is actively breathing spontaneously, it will be very difficult to make accurate calculations. These are really intended for full ventilatory support.

Assessment of Hemodynamics

We're here at last. The dreaded hemodynamics. I'll break it down into small pieces: indications, complications, normal values, equipment, waveforms. You can do it! Let's start with invasive arterial monitoring.

The Art Line

56. Identify the three main sites for arterial cannulation in adults.
   A. _____
   B. _____
   C. _____

57. What are the two indications for an indwelling arterial line?
   A. _____
   B. _____

58. List the normal values for these systemic arterial parameters.
    A. Systolic *

    B. Diastolic

    C. Mean

    D. Pulse pressure

59. How long can the art line stay in place before the risk of infection is increased?

60. What action should you take if you suspect a clot in the line?

61. A "damped or dampened" pressure is a lower than normal reading with a flattened tracing. Name four possible causes of a damped tracing and how to fix them.
    A. _____
    B. _____
    C. _____
    D. _____

62. What is usually the cause of abnormally high or low readings from an art line?

*Note the two different values in Egan. Use 90 mm Hg for the low end.

Equipment

One more area you need to become familiar with is the basic parts of the system. Take a look at this picture.

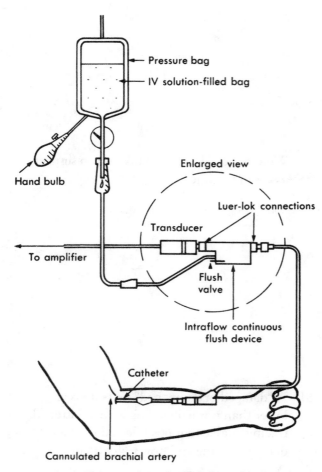

Use of pressurized IV fluid bag and Intraflow flush device for optimal maintenance of arterial catheter patency. Stop-cocks may be placed on each side of the flush device for room air reference and blood sampling. (From Schroeder JS, Daily EK: *Techniques in bedside hemodynamic monitoring*, St Louis, 1976, Mosby.)

Starting at the top, you see a *pressurized IV bag* that may also contain heparin to help reduce the chance of clotting. The main thing is the pressure. Without it, blood from the patient could back up into the system, and we wouldn't be able to *flush*, or wash out blood back into the artery. The *transducer* converts the arterial pressure waveform to an electronic signal that can be sent to the amplifier and displayed on the monitor.

Special *stiff, or noncompliant, IV tubing* connects from the transducer and continuous flush device to the catheter that is in the artery. This tubing prevents the arterial pressure wave from being damped as it passes up to the transducer (just like when ventilator tubing expands as a breath passes through it we lose some in the expansion).

There now, that wasn't too bad.

Flow-directed, Balloon-tipped, Pulmonary Artery Catheter . . . Let's Just Call it a Swan

Dr. Swan and Dr. Ganz are credited with developing this nifty tube for looking at the pressures inside the heart and lungs. So many people still call it a "Swan" or "Swan-Ganz" catheter. Pulmonary artery catheter is more generic. Pulmonary artery monitoring is a complex subject, but you can make it much simpler if you start by learning certain basic pieces of information.

63. Identify the two most common insertion sites for a pulmonary artery catheter. (From here on I'm going to call it a PAC for short.)

    A. _____

    B. _____

64. Name five conditions that suggest insertion of a PAC.

    A. _____

    B. _____

    C. _____

    D. _____

    E. _____

65. Let's look at the catheter itself. Identify the labeled parts.

    A. _____

    B. _____

    C. _____

    D. _____

    E. _____

    F. _____

    G. _____

    H. _____

    I. _____

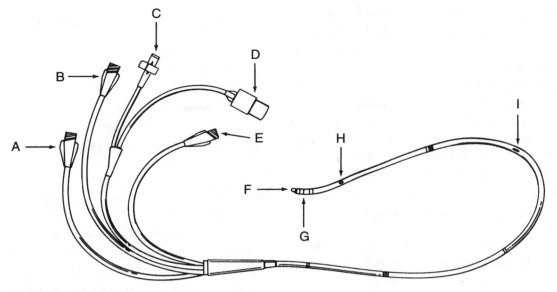

The quadruple-channel pulmonary artery catheter. (From Martin L: *Pulmonary physiology in clinical practice*, St Louis, 1987, Mosby.)

Pneumopnugget: A picture is not the best way to learn this, but it's okay. Either get a catheter from one of your instructors or look at one in the ICU that is in a box, then in a patient. You really should learn to identify the parts.

66. Now label the following four waveforms.
   A. _____
   B. _____
   C. _____
   D. _____

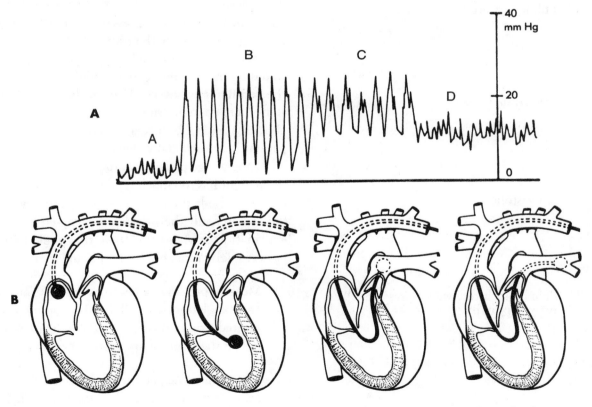

A, Pressure tracings. **B,** Pulmonary artery catheter position in heart. (From Martin L: *Pulmonary physiology in clinical practice*, St Louis, 1987, Mosby.)

Pneumopnugget: These are the four patterns seen on insertion and during normal monitoring. Very useful. Just like in ECGs there are abnormal patterns too, but don't worry about them yet. Each of the normal waveforms corresponds to an anatomic location. So if, for example, the catheter is supposed to be in the pulmonary artery, but you see a right ventricular waveform, you know something is wrong (maybe it is pulled back too far). Or, if the waveform appears wedged when it isn't supposed to be, perhaps the catheter has migrated too far forward.

67. List the normal values for these parameters.
    A. Central venous pressure (CVP)

    B. Right atrial pressure (RA)

    C. Pulmonary artery

       1. Systolic

       2. Diastolic

    D. Pulmonary artery wedge pressure (PWP, PCWP, PAWP)

What Does it All Mean?

Interpretation of PAC readings is a complex subject. I want you to learn some of the basics, so I will deliberately be simplifying. A glance at Box 41-3 will give you a good idea of how many things can alter CVP readings alone. Right atrial pressure and CVP are often used interchangeably. CVP represents preload to the right side of the heart. It can be a good indicator of the fluid volume status of the patient. It could also tell us if there is a backup in the system between the right atrium and the left atrium, like pulmonary hypertension, a blood clot, heart failure, or a defect in the tricuspid valve. The wedge pressure does much the same for the left side. Under normal circumstances it shows us the left ventricular preload. Considered along with CVP, it helps decide the fluid balance. If both CVP and PWP are low, you should consider hypovolemia.

Here is where the RCP must really think. Since both values are measured inside the chest, and positive pressure ventilation increases intrathoracic pressure, it is possible for the ventilator to affect the readings. The pressure tracings will move up and down with positive pressure breaths, so you may be able to detect this by watching the tracing increase and decrease as the ventilator cycles. But PEEP makes a constant increase in pressure, and PEEP levels above 10 cm H_2O, especially in hypovolemic patients, can artificially elevate the values, especially the wedge pressure. A high value means the patient has too much fluid, so someone might conclude the patient needs to lose some fluid when really they are dry. A complete explanation of what to do about this would keep us here a long time, but here are some ideas:

1. Measure pressure values from the PAC at end exhalation. You will need to run off a printed strip to do this, since the digital values on the monitor are averaged.

2. Do not take the patient off the ventilator to measure values, especially if the patient is on a high level of PEEP.

3. Correct the PAC values if the patient is on a high level of PEEP. This is not simple—remember that the degree of pressure transmitted depends on lung compliance as well...so learn more about this before you try it.

You can use the catheter to look at other things besides overall fluid balance. Diagnosis of certain conditions is aided by information from the PAC. Table 41-12 provides a look at some of these conditions. For example, compare ARDS to left-ventricular failure. The pulmonary artery pressure may increase in both conditions, the radiograph shows infiltrates, and breath sounds may reveal crackles. Both patients have hypoxemia and decreased lung compliance. But, the failing left ventricle causes the wedge pressure to go up where ARDS does not. Combine this with patient history and other assessments, and you get the big picture. Certain other values can be measured besides pressure, so let's look at those next.

68. List the normal values for these parameters.
    A. Cardiac output (CO)

    B. Cardiac index (CI)

    C. Systemic vascular resistance (SVR)

    D. Pulmonary vascular resistance (PVR)

With the Swan, cardiac output is measured via thermodilution. This is very helpful information, especially in the administration of drugs that support cardiac function, or if you want to know if changes in the ventilator are affecting the heart. The problem is, cardiac output is not personal enough. For example, you would expect a sumo wrestler to have a bigger cardiac output than an elderly female, but both would be technically within the normal range at 5 L/min of output. If you divide the output by the body surface area, you derive cardiac index, and this is more useful, because everyone should have the same range for cardiac index. Anyone who drops below 2.5 is in trouble!

Another useful calculation is vascular resistance. It's just like airway resistance (PIP − plateau/flow), only now we want to know how much pressure drop occurs when we push the blood through the vessels. Let's look at the pulmonary vascular resistance formula, since you might have to calculate this on your boards.

$$PVR = MPAP - PAWP/CO$$

If we have a patient with a mean pulmonary artery pressure of 12 mm Hg, PAWP of 4 mm Hg, and cardiac output of 4 L/min we get $12 - 4/4 = 2$ mm Hg/L/min for the resistance. Sometimes this number is multiplied by 80 to convert it to dynes. Either way, PVR is normally quite low.

69. What common respiratory problem results in vasoconstriction, or elevated vascular resistance in the pulmonary vessels?

70. Calculate PVR for a patient who has a mean pulmonary artery pressure of 15 mm Hg, PAWP of 5 mm Hg, and CO of 5 L/min.

Sometimes you need to be able to calculate mean arterial pressure so you can work the resistance problem. Remember that MAP = systolic pressure + (2 × diastolic)/3.

71. Calculate mean pulmonary artery pressure if systolic pulmonary artery pressure is 25 mm Hg and diastolic pulmonary artery pressure is 10 mm Hg.

▶ **Remember** to learn the basics and normal values. When you are looking at the data, think about where in the heart or lungs the pressure is being measured. That will help give you a clue about what part of the system has become abnormal. To increase your expertise you will have to go to the clinical setting and look at the patient data from the PAC and learn interpretation at the bedside.

Management of the Patient-Ventilator System

I think that checking the system every 2 hours is sort of a national average (not a standard of care), but I have worked at hospitals where formal checks were made every hour, and some where it was only done every 4 hours. What you do during the check also varies widely according to where you work. For example, sometimes you don't routinely analyze FIO_2, you use the pulse oximeter to see what is going on with the patient. Analysis is only done when the ventilator is tested. There are lots of possibilities of just how to do this procedure, the main point is to ensure patient safety through early identification of potential problems.

72. Identify the four key components of a P-V system check.
    A. _____
    B. _____
    C. _____
    D. _____

73. Describe the two methods used to detect auto-PEEP.
    A.

    B.

74. What does Egan mean by an OVP?

75. What actions can you take to minimize potential complications associated with removing the patient from the ventilator during a circuit change or system check?

76. Disconnecting a patient who is attached to a ventilator that generates high system flows can result in increased risk to the patient and RCP by what mechanism?

77. List five clinical observations you think are especially important to make during a P-V system check.

A. _____

B. _____

C. _____

D. _____

E. _____

78. Describe (or draw a picture of) the abnormal waveforms associated with each of the following:

A. *Pressure* waveform when inadequate flow is present

B. *Pressure-volume loop* when overdistention occurs

C. *Flow-volume loop* when a bronchodilator is needed

79. Troubleshooting revolves around what three general problem areas?

A. _____

B. _____

C. _____

80. Use Table 41-13 to help you identify common problems.

Possible Problem   *Corrective Action*
A. Sudden increase in PIP
   1.

   2.

B. Gradual increase in PIP
   1.

C. Sudden decrease in PIP
   1.

   2.

D. Decreased minute/tidal volume
   1.

   2.

E. Increased respiratory rate
   1.

   2.

81. Use Box 41-9 to help you identify four patient-related causes of sudden respiratory distress.
    A. _____
    B. _____
    C. _____
    D. _____

82. List four ventilator-related causes of sudden respiratory distress.
    A. _____
    B. _____
    C. _____
    D. _____

83. Regardless of the source of the problem, what is always the first priority?

84. If there is any doubt as to the cause or solution of a problem, what action should you take?

85. As a last resort, when all other options have been ruled out, it may be necessary to sedate or paralyze the patient. Give examples of drugs in the following classes:
    A. Tranquilizing agents
       1. _____
       2. _____
       3. _____
    B. Narcotic analgesics
       1. _____
       2. _____
    C. Neuromuscular blocking agents
       1. Long-term: _____
       2. Short-acting: _____

Board Exams

After reviewing several practice exams I have concluded that you could see up to 10 questions on any given Written Registry Exam on hemodynamic monitoring alone! The material in this chapter could include even more.

Let me be specific:

Review the chart...
- Cardiac output, PCWP, PAP, CVP
- Shunt studies
- Fluid balance (I and O)
- Dead space to tidal volume ratio

Recommend...
- Shunt studies
- Insertion of arterial or central venous lines
- Cardiac output

Perform and /or interpret bedside procedures...
- VD/VT
- Shunt
- Pulmonary capillary wedge pressure
- Mixed venous sampling
- P(A-a) O_2
- Lung compliance
- Cardiac output
- C(a-v) O_2
- Airway resistance

Assemble and check equipment for proper function
- Hemodynamic monitoring devices: Swan-Ganz, arterial catheters
- Ventilators

Modify mechanical ventilation . . . in every way imaginable.

So you can clearly see that the information in Chapter 41 is vital. Since whole textbooks are devoted to hemodynamic monitoring or ventilator management, Egan cannot possibly give you everything you need. It is a great place to start, and clearly summarizes the main points. Chapter 41 will make an excellent reference when you go to prepare for the tests. Here are some sample questions.

86. A 42-year-old patient with a cervical spine injury is being mechanically ventilated in control mode. As you enter the room, the low-pressure alarm is sounding. The patient is connected to the ventilator, but you do not see his chest moving. Your first action would be to
   A. Manually ventilate the patient with the resuscitation bag
   B. Check the alarm settings
   C. Observe the exhaled volumes
   D. Manually ventilate the patient with the mechanical ventilator

87. After insertion of a Swan-Ganz catheter via the left subclavian vein, a patient's compliance quickly drops. The high-pressure alarm on the ventilator is activated. Breath sounds are absent over the left chest and the trachea is deviated to the right side. The patient appears extremely anxious. What action should the RCP take?
   A. Use a capnometer to assess ventilation noninvasively
   B. Recommend administration of Versed
   C. Call for a portable chest radiograph
   D. Recommend a chest tube

88. A 38-year-old woman with a diagnosis of myasthenia gravis is being mechanically ventilated. As you enter the room the high-pressure alarm is sounding. The patient appears anxious. Auscultation reveals coarse bilateral rhonchi. What action should you take at this time?
   A. Manually ventilate the patient
   B. Check the alarm setting
   C. Recommend sedation
   D. Suction the patient

89. An 89-year-old woman with emphysema is being mechanically ventilated. The high-pressure and high-rate alarms are being activated. Breath sounds are clear but diminished. Pulse oximetry and vital sign values are within normal limits. The patient is very agitated and her respiratory rate is 32. What are your recommendations?
   A. Administer Valium
   B. Increase the alarm limit
   C. Suction the patient
   D. Call for a portable chest radiograph

90. The data below are reported for a patient:

PCWP	18 mm Hg
PAP	40/24 mm Hg
CI	1.9 L/min/M$_2$

   These data suggest which of the following?
   A. Non-cardiogenic pulmonary edema
   B. Cardiogenic pulmonary edema
   C. Pulsus paradoxus
   D. Hypovolemia

91. When properly placed, the distal tip of the Swan-Ganz catheter will be located in the
    A. Left atrium
    B. Right atrium
    C. Right ventricle
    D. Pulmonary artery

Questions 92 through 94 refer to the following situation. A patient is intubated and placed on the ventilator after she develops respiratory failure following a hip replacement surgery. The following values are recorded:

$PaCO_2$	50 mm Hg
PaO_2	60 mm Hg
FiO_2	.40
$PECO_2$	10 mm Hg
Tidal volume	800 ml
Respiratory rate	20

92. These data indicate a dead space to tidal volume ratio of
    A. 20 %
    B. 40%
    C. 60%
    D. 80%

93. What is the exhaled minute volume?
    A. 8 L
    B. 12 L
    C. 16 L
    D. 20 L

94. What is the alveolar minute volume?
    A. 3.2 L
    B. 11.2 L
    C. 12. 8 L
    D. 16.0 L

95. The following information is recorded for a patient:

VO_2	200 ml/min
CaO_2	16 vol %
CvO_2	12 vol %

What is the cardiac output?
    A. 2 L/min
    B. 3 L/min
    C. 4 L/min
    D. 5 L/min

96. The hemodynamic data below are recorded for a patient who is being mechanically ventilated.

Cardiac output	3.5 L/min
PAP	18/8 mm Hg
PWP	6 mm Hg
CVP	2 mm Hg
HR	125/min

These data probably indicate
    A. Hypovolemia
    B. Pulmonary hypertension
    C. Fluid overload
    D. Pulmonary embolism

97. A pressure waveform obtained from a radial artery catheter is dampened. Possible causes of this problem include all of the following except
    A. An air bubble in the tubing
    B. A blood clot on the tip of the catheter
    C. The transducer elevated above the heart
    D. Use of standard IV tubing

Food for Thought

There was an editorial in the journal *Respiratory Care* a few years ago entitled something like this: "The Pulmonary Artery Catheter—It Goes in Through Your Arm and You Pay Through the Nose." I want you to think about three questions in relationship to this idea. First, do you think it is important to use top-of-the-line technology in every setting?

Second, if your loved one was ill, what would you want for them? Third, do you think the average person understands the complexity of "the high cost of medicine?"

Discontinuing Ventilatory Support

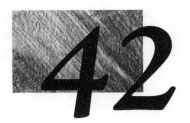

> "I'm losing."
> **Reported as the last words**
> **of Frank Sinatra**

It's relatively easy to initiate mechanical ventilation, and some patients are equally easy to get back off again. Unfortunately, there is no magic number that tells you a patient will be successfully weaned or removed from support. You will have to customize the job for each patient. Sometimes this task takes all your skills and resources to accomplish. Sometimes, it can't be done.

First Things First

1. What is the purpose of mechanical ventilation?

2. What can ventilators do? What can't they do?

3. List three situations in which the ventilator can be discontinued without gradual weaning.
   A. _____
   B. _____
   C. _____

4. Identify four groups of patients who may need weaning.
   A. _____
   B. _____
   C. _____
   D. _____

5. What are the three general categories of patients being considered for removal from ventilatory support?
   A. _____
   B. _____
   C. _____

Reasons for Ventilator Dependence

6. Patients may require mechanical ventilation for what three general reasons?
   A. _____
   B. _____
   C. _____

7. State the four factors that determine total ventilatory workload.
   A. _____
   B. _____
   C. _____
   D. _____

8. What do fever, shivering, agitation, trauma, and sepsis have in common?

9. List two causes of increased dead space ventilation.
   A. _____
   B. _____

10. Name four common causes of decreased lung compliance.
    A. _____
    B. _____
    C. _____
    D. _____

11. Name four causes of decreased chest wall compliance.
    A. _____
    B. _____
    C. _____
    D. _____

12. State three causes of increased airway resistance.
    A. _____
    B. _____
    C. _____

13. Why are artificial airways implicated in increased airway resistance?

14. Give examples of conditions that adversely affect ventilatory capacity.
    A. CNS drive
       1. _____
       2. _____
       3. _____
       4. _____
    B. Muscle strength
       1. _____
       2. _____
       3. _____
       4. _____

15. Once ventilatory muscles are fatigued, how long should they be rested prior to any attempt at weaning?

Okay, so now you have this giant shopping list of things that could make removal from the ventilator difficult. Sometimes one thing, like reduced drive to breathe from drugs, is the problem. That's easy to solve. You can give an antidote (such as Narcan for heroin or morphine), cleanse the blood (dialysis, for example), or just wait for the effects to wear off (anesthesia, for instance). Or, you might run into something a little more complicated, such as a depressed COPD patient with CHF who has a small ET tube, bronchospasm, malnutrition, CO_2 retention, and electrolyte disorders along with the lung infection that put him on the ventilator in the first place. That's a lot of issues to be resolved prior to weaning.

Patient Evaluation

Careful, systematic assessment is an especially important part of your approach to ventilator discontinuance.

16. What is the first thing you should evaluate whether you are considering weaning or taking the patient off the ventilator?

17. What are the three questions you should ask?

    A.

    B.

    C.

Once the patient is stable and things are looking up, you can take a look at the weaning indexes. I told you (Chapter 37) these things would return to haunt you.

Do they work? Like everything else, sometimes. Even though indexes have limitations, we still need to gather the information because it helps quantify the patient's overall status.

18. Your board exams will expect you to identify these classic criteria for weaning from mechanical ventilation. Remember that no one criterion mandates that you wean or don't wean!

Measurement	Critical Value
A. $PaCO_2$	_____
B. pH	_____
C. VC (ml/kg)	_____
D. Spont VT	_____
E. Spont rate	_____
F. VE	_____
G. MVV	_____
H. MIF (NIF, MIP)	_____
I. VD/VT	_____
J. P (A-a)O_2 on 100%	_____
K. P/F ratio	_____
L. PaO_2	_____
M. Qs/Qt	_____
N. FiO_2	_____

Another giant menu to memorize, then apply to clinical. (If it seems overwhelming, break it down into small pieces, learn a few at a time.)

19. Describe the breathing patterns that may cause problems with weaning or discontinuance.

20. Physical assessment of respiratory muscles may be useful. Describe what you are looking for in this area.

21. What is airway occlusion pressure? Tell us all about it.

22. Rapid shallow breathing index may be an accurate, early predictor of weaning outcomes. Calculate the index for a patient who has a spontaneous rate of 25 with a spontaneous volume of 350 ml. What is the criteria for success?
    A. Calculation

    B. Criteria

23. Give the PaO_2 and FIO_2 values that should be met prior to weaning.
    A. PaO_2

    B. FIO_2

24. What is the effect of excessive carbohydrate administration?

25. Identify the critical values for confirming cardiovascular stability?

Measurement	Values inconsistent with weaning
A. Heart rate	_____
B. Systolic pressure	_____
C. Diastolic pressure	_____
D. Hemoglobin	_____
E. Cardiac Index (CI)	_____

26. Describe the two ways that renal function may affect weaning.
    A.

    B.

27. Describe the ideal CNS status you'd like to see.

28. How is ability to be weaned different from ability to be extubated?

Preparing the Patient

A quick glance at Box 42-5 on p. 974 should amuse you—or scare you. The RCP should start by optimizing those parts of the patient's medical condition they have direct control over, and focus on psychologic and environmental factors they can influence.

29. Name two drug therapies the RCP can utilize to reduce airway resistance.
    A. _____
    B. _____

30. How else can the RCP improve conditions in the airway?

31. What time of day should weaning activities be conducted?

32. What percentage of patients may develop "ICU psychosis" or other psychologic disturbances after a few days in the unit?

33. How could the RCP help the patient get adequate sleep?

34. Describe the environmental considerations that may improve patient well-being.

35. What three methods does Egan identify for helping patients communicate?
    A. _____
    B. _____
    C. _____

Weaning Methods

When the original problem is resolving, the indexes look good, and you've optimized as many factors as possible, you must get down to the business of discontinuing the ventilator. Rapidly or slowly, you have several methods to choose from.

36. Why do some clinicians prefer to use low levels of pressure support ventilation?

37. What advantages does CPAP mode offer?

38. Describe the specific advantage both CPAP and PSV have in terms of safety.

39. What is the typical minimum length of time for a spontaneous breathing trial?

40. How should you position the patient prior to the trial breathing period?

Rapid discontinuance works really well on patients who have been on the ventilator for a short period of time. A post-operative patient, an OD who is now awake, that sort of thing. Wouldn't it be nice if more patients fell into this category? For the more difficult customer, you have two choices.

41. Describe the T-piece (T tube) trial for gradual weaning.

42. What FiO$_2$ is ideal for T-piece weaning?

43. What happens at night?

44. Describe the variation of this method where the patient is kept on the ventilator.

45. What are the biggest drawbacks to T-piece weaning?

46. Compare T-piece to IMV weaning.

47. Why do you think IMV (SIMV) is the predominant weaning method in the United States?

48. How can you overcome the increased work of breathing associated with demand flow systems?

49. What are the typical initial settings when SIMV is used for full ventilatory support?
   A. Tidal volume: _____
   B. Respiratory rate: _____

50. What is the typical amount the rate is adjusted at any one time in SIMV weaning?

51. When is partial support an unwise ventilator strategy?

52. Describe pressure support ventilation (PSV).

53. What is PSV max?

54. From what level of PSV may a patient be extubated?

55. Egan gives a formula for estimating the level of pressure support needed to overcome work of breathing. Calculate the level needed for a patient who has a PIP of 50 cm H_2O, plateau pressure of 30 cm H_2O, a ventilator flow rate of 60 L/min, and a spontaneous inspiratory flow rate of 30 L/min. (You can look at the Mini Clini on p. 980 for help.)
    A. Formula: _____
    B. Calculation: _____
    C. Answer: _____

Other institutions set PSV to achieve a desired tidal volume, either in milliliters or milliliters per kilogram. Another way to set PSV is to increase the pressure until spontaneous rate drops to a desirable level.

Instead of placing the patient on a T-piece, some ventilators allow you to use CPAP, or spontaneous modes. By allowing spontaneous breathing at an elevated baseline, oxygenation and lung volumes are maintained while auto-PEEP and work of breathing is minimized.

56. What is another advantage for the RCP in using CPAP mode for trials?

57. What do clinical studies show regarding the proven effectiveness of one method of weaning over another?

58. Describe mandatory minute ventilation.

59. What specific patient population would be at risk when using MMV?

60. MMV systems compare spontaneous minute ventilation to desired minute ventilation. How do they adjust the ventilation delivered by the machine?

61. What is the main advantage of flow-triggering over pressure-triggering?

62. VERSUS and VAPS are new methods of approaching ventilation. What is the basic idea behind these modes?

63. Discuss the role of NIPPV in weaning.

67. Give the expected and excessive changes for each of the following parameters.

Parameter	Expected	Deleterious
A. Respiratory rate		
B. PaO_2		
C. $PaCO_2$		
D. Heart rate		
E. Blood pressure		

The NBRC will expect you to know these changes well. So do your instructors.

(So does the patient!)

▶ Table 42-5 summarizes the pros and cons of the various weaning methods.

Monitoring the Patient

64. What are the two easily monitored and reliable indicators of patient progress during weaning?
    A. _____
    B. _____

65. What is the single best index of ventilation?

Extubation

Weaning and extubation are separate issues. We know this, but other clinicians may not be as clear, so the RCP has to be a strong advocate in the decision to remove or maintain the artificial airway.

68. What is the most important thing to remember about the presence of the artificial airway in terms of weaning? What can be done about it?

66. What is the simplest way to monitor oxygenation during weaning?

69. What is the minimum ability required for personnel performing routine extubation?

70. What is the minimum ability required for personnel performing high-risk extubation?

71. What are common patient complaints following extubation?

72. Describe the cuff leak test.

73. Identify the appropriate treatment for post-extubation stridor.
    A. Mild

    B. Moderate

    C. Severe

74. What patients are at risk for aspiration following extubation? How can you minimize the risk?

Failure to Wean

As much as we all want to get the patient off the vent, it doesn't always work.

75. Identify two common causes of weaning failure for each of the following areas.
    A. Oxygenation
       1. _____
       2. _____
    B. Ventilation
       1. _____
       2. _____
    C. Cardiovascular
       1. _____
       2. _____

76. The ICU is no place for the long-term ventilator patient. It's too expensive, and the staff is not usually trained to deal with the issues. What are the alternate care sites?

77. Refer to Table 42-8 in the text. Identify strategies for each of the following problems.

A. Anemia _____

_____

B. Tube-related WOB _____

_____

C. Bronchospasm _____

_____

D. Secretions _____

_____

E. Dyspnea _____

_____

F. Muscle fatigue _____

_____

G. Hemodynamics _____

_____

H. Infection _____

I. Metabolic _____

_____

J. Nutrition _____

_____

K. Exercise _____

_____

L. Psychologic _____

_____

M. Sleep _____

_____

_____

N. Pain _____

_____

Many of these techniques are useful once the patient is removed from the ICU and placed in an alternate site. A skilled, multidisciplinary approach is needed for the chronic ventilator patient. In the end, some patients will remain on the machine for life.

78. Who should be involved in the decision to terminate life support?

79. Who does Egan suggest perform the actual termination?

Case Studies

Case 1

Melba T. is an alert 61-year-old placed on the ventilator for respiratory failure for her CHF and COPD. 24 hours later, the physician asks for your recommendation regarding weaning. Breath sounds reveal coarse crackles in both bases. Pedal edema is present as well. The following information is obtained.

Spont RR	28
Spont VT	0.2 L
MIF	−18 cm H_2O
VC	0.6 L
HR	116
BP	90/60
pH	7.33
$PaCO_2$	35 mm Hg
PaO_2	65 (on FIO_2 0.5)
Cardiac Index	2.3

80. What is your assessment of her respiratory status?

81. Has the primary problem been resolved?

82. What is the rapid shallow breathing index?

83. Explain your recommendation regarding initiating weaning? If you recommend weaning, also recommend the method.

84. What is your assessment of his respiratory status?

85. Has the primary problem been resolved?

86. What is the rapid shallow breathing index?

Case 2

Ed McM. is a 61-year-old placed on the ventilator following open heart surgery. 12 hours later the patient is awake and the physician asks for your recommendation regarding weaning. The following information is obtained.

Spont RR	14
Spont VT	0.2 L
MIF	−35 cm H_2O
VC	1.2 L
HR	116
BP	90/60
pH	7.37
$PaCO_2$	35 mm Hg
PaO_2	85 (on FIO_2 0.35)

87. Explain your recommendation regarding initiating weaning? If you recommend weaning, also recommend a technique.

Case 3

E. Benedict is a 61-year-old placed on the ventilator following an acute episode of Guillain-Barre syndrome. Three weeks later the patient is regaining strength and movement in his limbs. The physician asks for your recommendation regarding weaning. The following information is obtained.

Spont RR	22
Spont VT	0.22 L
MIF	−20 cm H_2O
VC	1.0 L
HR	116
BP	90/60
pH	7.38
$PaCO_2$	37 mm Hg
PaO_2	70 (on FIO_2 0.40)

88. What is your assessment of his respiratory status?

89. Has the primary problem been resolved?

90. What is the rapid shallow breathing index?

91. Explain your recommendation regarding initiating weaning? If you recommend weaning, also recommend a technique.

What Does the NBRC Say?

I guess it's clear from the amount of questions I've put in this chapter that weaning and discontinuance are important topics. But is weaning really specified in the exam matrices? The Entry Level Exam matrix states that you should "Initiate and modify weaning procedures" but includes this in the larger categories of achieving adequate ventilation or modifying therapeutic procedures/care plan. The Written Registry Matrix specifically mentions extubation, but not weaning. The key to understanding this subject is in the way mechanical ventilation is applied. Modes such as PSV, SIMV, IMV, CPAP, and PEEP are frequently cited in different areas of these test preparation tools. This makes it difficult to know exactly how many questions on weaning will be on an individual test. It could vary from a few (2 to 3) to many (5 to 7)! Here are some examples for your thinking pleasure.

92. Which of the following would you evaluate prior to initiating T-piece weaning?
   I. PaO_2
   II. Gag reflex
   III. Spontaneous respiratory rate
   IV. Minute ventilation
   A. I, II only
   B. I, III only
   C. II, III, IV only
   D. I, III, IV only

93. A patient being assessed for readiness to wean has the following values:

pH	7.36
PaCO$_2$	42 mm Hg
PaO$_2$	67 mm Hg (FIO$_2$ 40%)
MIP	−25 cm H$_2$O
Pulse	105
Respirations	20
Vital Capacity	12 ml/kg

What action should the RCP recommend at this time?
A. Initiate a T-piece trial
B. Continue with mechanical ventilation
C. Initiate breathing exercises to strengthen ventilatory muscles
D. Repeat the vital capacity maneuver

94. Which of the following indicates a readiness to wean?
A. Spontaneous rate of 28
B. Spontaneous tidal volume of 200 ml
C. Negative inspiratory force of 18 cm H$_2$O
D. Minute volume of 8 L/min

95. An alert patient is being mechanically ventilated. Settings are:

Mode	SIMV
Rate	2
Tidal volume (set)	800
FIO$_2$	.30
PEEP	5 cm H$_2$O

ABG results 30 minutes after initiating these settings are:

pH	7.37
PaCO$_2$	38 mm Hg
PaO$_2$	75 mm Hg

What should the RCP recommend at this time?
A. Increase the set rate to 4
B. Discontinue mechanical ventilation
C. Decrease the PEEP to 0 cm H$_2$O
D. Decrease the FIO$_2$ to .21

96. A 70-year-old, 70 kg (154 lb) patient with a history of COPD is being mechanically ventilated. The patient is alert, but making no spontaneous efforts.

Mode	AC
Rate	12
Tidal volume (set)	800
FIO$_2$	.40
PEEP	3 cm H$_2$O
pH	7. 51
PaCO$_2$	38 mm Hg
PaO$_2$	95 mm Hg
HCO$_3$	36 mEq/L

Which of the following should the RCP recommend?

  I. Change to SIMV mode
 II. Decrease the FIO$_2$
III. Decrease the set rate
IV. Decrease the PEEP
A. I, II only
B. I, III only
C. I, II, III only
D. I, III, IV only

97. A patient is being ventilated in the SIMV mode with a rate of 8, volume of 800, and FIO$_2$ of 0.40. ABG results show:

pH	7.47
PaCO$_2$	33 mm Hg
PaO$_2$	88 mm Hg
HCO$_3$	23 mEq/L

What action should the RCP recommend in response to these findings?
A. Increase the tidal volume
B. Increase the FIO$_2$
C. Change to A/C mode
D. Reduce the rate

98. A patient on SIMV experiences difficulty each time you try to reduce the rate below 6. The patient becomes tachypneic with a rate of 28 and a spontaneous volume of 200. Which of the following modifications would be *least* useful in this situation?
    A. Pressure support ventilation
    B. T-piece weaning
    C. PEEP
    D. Flow-by or flow-triggering

It's not too difficult to wean patients on paper. If you know your *values!* Watch out for COPD patients who are being over-ventilated or over-oxygenated by the machine.

Food for Thought

99. What would happen to a flow-triggering system if a gas-powered nebulizer was placed in line?

100. What is the single best approach to weaning?

Neonatal and Pediatric Respiratory Care

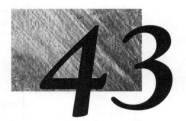

Whether you dream of working with this special population, or in a community hospital where you will need the skills and knowledge periodically, or just want to do well on your boards, you will find Chapter 43 is just what the doctor ordered. It's a comprehensive and comprehensible overview of the care and feeding of children who can't breathe. I'll warn you right now that this is a very long chapter, packed with a huge amount of information.

Word Power

I guess you've noticed that I think medical terminology is important, and that I like crossword puzzles. A final puzzle to help you build your pediatric terminology is on p. 398.

1. During what stage and week of development is alveolar capillary surface area considered sufficient enough to support extrauterine life?
   A. Stage: _____
   B. Week: _____

2. What is the primary organ of gas exchange for the fetus?

3. Describe the umbilical cord blood vessels.

4. The fetus lives in a relatively hypoxic environment. What is considered to be a major factor that enables the fetus to survive under these conditions?

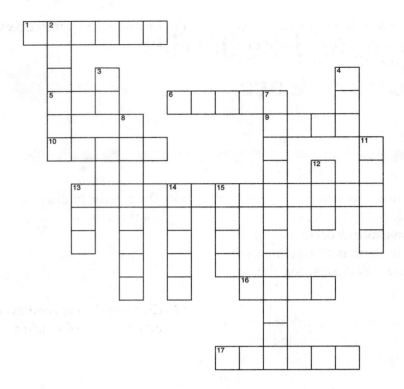

ACROSS

1. Four part cardiac disorder
5. Baby hemoglobin
6. This hole connects the right and left atria
9. Persistent hypertension
10. Premature babies are prone to this breathing pattern
13. Inflammation of the small airways
16. Mysterious fatal disorder of newborns
17. _____ fibrosis, a lethal genetic disorder

DOWN

2. Common obstructive disease of chidren
3. Short for 65 roses
4. Rapid breathing that comes and goes
7. Life-threatening infection of airway cartilage
8. Fetal doo-doo
11. Flaring means distress
12. Neutral thermal environment
13. Lung disease in IRDS and ventilator survivors
14. Viral upper airway infection that results in a barking cough
15. Infant respiratory distress syndrome

5. About half of the blood entering the right atrium is shunted to the left atrium via what structure?

6. Why is fetal pulmonary vascular resistance so high?

7. What percentage of blood entering the pulmonary artery actually flows through the lungs? Where does the rest of the blood go?

8. Describe the events that occur in the first few breaths after birth in terms of transpulmonary pressure, blood gases, and circulatory changes.

9. Compare the development of lung structures in newborns, children, and adults.

	Newborn	Child	Adult
A. number of alveoli	_____	_____	_____
B. Surface area	_____	_____	_____
C. TLC	_____	_____	_____

Children Aren't "Little Adults"

10. Let's compare the head and upper airway of adults and babies.

Anatomy	Baby	Adult
A. Head	_____	_____
B. Tongue	_____	_____
C. Nasal passages	_____	_____
D. Larynx	_____	_____
E. Narrow point	_____	_____
F. Dead space	_____	_____
G. Airways	_____	_____

11. Describe the breathing pattern of preterm infant.

12. Compare the metabolism of a healthy infant to that of an adult.

13. What is considered a normal tidal volume and respiratory rate for a newborn?

14. Why do infants experience severe hypox-emia more readily than adults?

18. The fetus can be assessed by a variety of methods. Discuss each of the following tests.
    A. Ultrasonography

    B. Amniocentesis

Assessing the Newborn

15. Assessment of the newborn begins with maternal history. Identify three conditions that are likely to result in a baby that is small for its gestational age.
    A. _____
    B. _____
    C. _____

    C. Fetal heart rate monitoring

16. Identify five maternal factors likely to lead to premature delivery.
    A. _____
    B. _____
    C. _____
    D. _____
    E. _____

    D. Fetal blood gas analysis

17. What maternal condition is likely to result in an infant that is large for its gestational age?

19. What L/S ratio indicates lung maturity? When does this usually occur?

20. What is the relationship between fetal scalp gases and arterial blood gases?

21. When are Apgar scores taken?

22. You really need to learn the Apgar scoring system, so...

Sign	0	1	2
A. Heart rate	_____	_____	_____
B. Respiration	_____	_____	_____
C. Muscle tone	_____	_____	_____
D. Reflex	_____	_____	_____
E. Color	_____	_____	_____

(You could make up some kind of mnemonic to help you remember the 5 signs, such as "Heart Rate Must Really Count," if it helps you.)

23. What term is used to describe the following weeks of gestation?
    A. Before 38 weeks: _____
    B. 38 to 42 weeks: _____
    C. After 42 weeks: _____

24. Name the two common systems used for assessing gestational age based on physical characteristics and neurologic signs.
    A. _____
    B. _____

25. Explain the abbreviations and identify the weights that correspond to the following terms.
    A. VLBW

    B. LBW

    C. AGA

    D. LGA

26. Why does anyone care about birth weight and gestational age?

27. State the normal range for a full-term infant's vital signs.
   A. Heart rate: _____
   B. Respiratory rate: _____
   C. Blood pressure: _____

28. Describe the usual way to take an infant's heart rate.

29. Infants in respiratory distress typically exhibit one or more of these five signs. Explain the significance of each sign.
   A. Nasal flaring

   B. Cyanosis

   C. Expiratory grunting

   D. Retractions

   E. Paradoxical breathing

30. What scoring system is used to grade the severity of underlying lung disease?

31. What are the two usual sources for arterial blood in infants?
   A. _____
   B. _____

32. Name two alternate sources.
   A. _____
   B. _____

32. List the ABG values for preterm and term infants at birth and 5 days.

Parameter	Preterm	Term	5 Days
A. pH	_____	_____	_____
B. PaCO$_2$	_____	_____	_____
C. PaO$_2$	_____	_____	_____

What's the Big Idea?

33. At what temperature does cold-stress occur in newborns?

34. Identify five harmful consequences of cold-stress or hypothermia in babies.
   A. _____
   B. _____
   C. _____
   D. _____
   E. _____

35. What is meant by neutral thermal environment?

36. What is the usual range of ambient temperature needed to maintain NTE?

37. How are sick infants usually fed?

38. What is a major source of colonization by staphylococcus and streptococcus in newborns?

Respiratory Care Techniques

Basics

39. Considering the hazards, we need to agree on the safe limits for oxygen therapy. Give the accepted ranges for these parameters.
    A. PaO_2 _____ to _____
    B. FiO_2 _____ to _____
    C. SpO_2 _____ to _____

40. Hyperoxia is associated with ROP and BPD in some infants. What do these acronyms stand for?
    A. ROP: _____
    B. BPD: _____

41. Name two other factors associated with ROP.
    A. _____
    B. _____

42. What is meant by the "flip-flop phenomenon?"

43. Name three factors that should be continuously monitored when administering oxygen to infants.
    A. _____
    B. _____
    C. _____

44. Compare the use of the following oxygen delivery devices.
    A. AEM
       1. Age _____
       2. Advantage _____
       3. Disadvantage _____
    B. Cannula
       1. Age _____
       2. Advantage _____
       3. Disadvantage _____

B. Cannula
    1. Age _____
    2. Advantage _____
    3. Disadvantage _____
C. Incubator
    1. Age _____
    2. Advantage _____
    3. Disadvantage _____
D. Hood
    1. Age _____
    2. Advantage _____
    3. Disadvantage _____
E. Tent
    1. Age _____
    2. Advantage _____
    3. Disadvantage _____

45. Name four conditions where secretion retention is common in children.
    A. _____
    B. _____
    C. _____
    D. _____

46. Identify one other situation where bronchial hygiene therapy may be useful.

47. Since infants can't cough on command, how will you get the mucus out once it is mobilized?

48. How long should you wait after feedings to perform postural drainage on infants and small children?

49. How can you help prevent hypoxemia during head-down positioning?

50. Give three hazards of overheating or under-heating gases administered to newborns.
    A. Overheating
      1. _____
      2. _____
      3. _____
    B. Underheating
      1. _____
      2. _____
      3. _____

51. How is application of the nasal cannula different for adults and kids in terms of humidification?

52. Identify three reasons why continuous nebulization is usually avoided in infants.
    A. _____
    B. _____
    C. _____

53. How would you deliver a bronchodilator to a newborn?

54. How would you deliver an MDI to an infant?

55. What is the dosage range for albuterol delivered by SVN?

56. What is the dosage range and frequency for racemic epinephrine?
    A. Dose: _____
    B. Frequency: _____

57. What is the dosage and treatment schedule for Ribavirin?
    A. Dose: _____
    B. Treatment schedule: _____
    _____

58. Identify the correct ET tube size and suction catheter size for these kids.

Age/weight	ET	Length (oral)	Suction
A. < 100 g	_____	_____	_____
B. 1000-2000	_____	_____	_____
C. 2000-3000	_____	_____	_____
D. >3000g	_____	_____	_____
E. 2 years	_____	_____	_____
F. 6 years	_____	_____	_____

59. State the two formulas for calculating tube size.
    A. _____
    B. _____

60. Estimate the correct tube size for a 4-year-old using the first formula.

61. Estimate the correct tube size for a child who is 122 cm tall.

62. Which laryngoscope blade is usually used for infant intubation?

63. What is the main difference between infant or pediatric ET tubes and adult tubes?

64. What are the recommended vacuum pressures for suctioning infants and children?
    A. Infants: _____
    B. Children: _____

65. How should you preoxygenate newborns to avoid hyperoxia?

Neonatal Resuscitation

66. What is the first step of resuscitation immediately after delivery?

67. What action should be taken if meconium is visible in the larynx?

68. Identify the criteria for performing chest compressions after delivery.

More Advanced Questions

69. Play with baby's FRC by applying CPAP. What is the specific indication for CPAP?

70. Name four signs of respiratory distress that suggest using CPAP.
    A. _____
    B. _____
    C. _____
    D. _____

71. Discuss adjustment of CPAP in infants.

72. CPAP is usually administered to an infant via what type of delivery system?

73. Give the range of tidal volumes for children and infants for mechanical ventilation.
    A. Children: _____
    B. Term infants: _____
    C. Low birth weight infants: _____

74. PIP should be limited to what maximum value in term infants and children?

75. Give the rule of thumb for maximum PIPs in preterm infants.

76. Identify the inspiratory time ranges that should be set for these age groups.
    A. Low birth weight infants: _____
    B. Term infants: _____
    C. Toddlers: _____
    D. Children: _____

77. Mean airway pressure is an important indicator of the degree of mechanical ventilation needed to achieve what therapeutic goal?

78. Why would it be common to observe lower exhaled than inhaled volumes in pediatric patients?

79. Describe how to reduce the following parameters during weaning.
    A. FiO_2

    B. PEEP

    C. Rate

80. What ventilator settings suggest evaluation for extubation?
    A. Set rate: _____
    B. PIP: _____
    C. FiO_2: _____
    D. PEEP: _____

81. Describe the leak test for upper airway edema.

82. Infants are usually extubated from what rates? Why?

88. What does ECMO do?

89. Describe the two basic forms of ECMO.
    A. VA

83. List four clinical indications for initiating HFV.
    A. _____
    B. _____
    C. _____
    D. _____

    B. VV

84. Identify the three common characteristics of high-frequency ventilation.
    A. _____
    B. _____
    C. _____

85. What are the three most common types of HFV?
    A. _____
    B. _____
    C. _____

90. Give three examples of neonatal conditions where ECMO is being used after conventional medical therapies fail.
    A. _____
    B. _____
    C. _____

86. Oxygenation in HFV is adjusted through what two parameters?
    A. _____
    B. _____

New Kids on the Block

87. CO_2 elimination depends mainly on what factor?

91. What is meconium? What does presence of meconium in amniotic fluid suggest?

92. What type of obstruction occurs in meconium aspiration? What are the consequences?

93. How should you manage the airway in meconium aspiration?
   A. During delivery

   B. After delivery

94. How many infants are affected by RDS in the United States each year?

95. What is the major factor in the development of RDS?

96. Why does RDS result in elevated pulmonary vascular resistance?

97. Definitive diagnosis of RDS is usually made by chest radiographs. Describe the chest film of an infant with RDS.

98. What are the traditional treatments for RDS?

99. Surfactant administration has been successful in both prophylactic and rescue treatment of RDS. How is the surfactant administered?

100. Describe the two surfactant preparations used in the United States.

A.

B.

101. What is Type II RDS and what factors lead to its development?

102. What is the treatment for Type II RDS?

103. What two factors indicate that apnea is abnormal in an infant?

A. _____

B. _____

104. Identify the possible causes of apnea (besides prematurity) in infants.

Cause	Signs	Investigate
A. Infection		
B. Oxygenation		
C. Maternal		
D. Environmental		

105. What drugs can be helpful in treating apnea of prematurity?

106. What should you do to stimulate breathing if you observe an apneic incident?

107. BPD is a chronic pulmonary condition thought to be caused by what three factors?

A. _____

B.

_____

C.

_____

108. Describe the pathophysiologic changes associated with BPD.

109. Identify three respiratory care treatments used with BPD kids.

A. _____

B. _____

C. _____

110. Name the two treatments for PDA.

A. _____

B. _____

111. Most congenital defects require what type of intervention?

Sudden Infant Death Syndrome

SIDS is the leading cause of death in infants less than 1 year of age in the United States, with about 7,000 deaths each year. Diagnosis isn't made until a previously healthy baby dies unexpectedly.

112. What is the cause of SIDS?

113. Describe the typical profile of a baby who dies of SIDS.

114. What sleeping position is strongly linked with SIDS?

115. Identify the four infant characteristics often seen near the time of death.

A. _____

B. _____

C. _____

D. _____

116. Once an at-risk infant is identified, what can be done to try to prevent a SIDS death?

Case Studies

Bronchiolitis, croup, epiglottitis, asthma, cystic fibrosis, and pneumonia are all serious and relatively common pediatric respiratory disorders that you should be able to recognize and differentiate from each other.

Case 1

A mother brings her previously healthy one-year-old to the emergency department. She states that her baby had a cold 2 days ago, but he still has a slight fever and has been coughing. The mother became concerned when she heard audible wheezing. A treatment with albuterol in the emergency department has had no effect. Vital signs are essentially normal, except for a slight elevation in respiratory rate. The chest radiograph shows mild hyperinflation with no signs of consolidation. Pulse oximetry shows a saturation of 94%.

117. What diagnosis is most likely?

118. How can a diagnosis of RSV be ruled out?

119. The physician decides to send mom and baby home. What treatment would you recommend?

121. What aerosolized medication should be delivered?

122. How would you deliver oxygen to this child?

Case 2

A 3-year-old is brought to the emergency department with respiratory distress and a barking, seal-like cough. The child has been sick for several days with a low-grade fever and stuffy nose. Examination reveals moderate inspiratory stridor and retractions.

The pulse oximeter shows a saturation of 88% on room air. A lateral neck film identifies subglottic narrowing with a "steeple sign."

120. What is the most likely diagnosis?

Case 3

A 5-year-old is brought to the emergency department with labored breathing and a high fever. Examination reveals marked inspiratory stridor. The child is listless and dad says he has had a sore throat. When you talk to the boy, he responds very quietly with short answers. A lateral neck radiograph identifies a "thumb sign."

123. What is the most likely diagnosis?

124. What organism is usually responsible for this condition? How could you confirm?

125. What is the immediate treatment for this condition? Who should perform the intervention and where?

126. What shouldn't be done?

Case 4

Grandma brings her son's 2-year-old in to the clinic because "his breathing just isn't right." She states "This boy is coughing all the time. Besides, he isn't growing very well, and when I kiss him his skin tastes salty!"

127. How would Ïyour diagnosis be confirmed?

128. What dietary modifications are needed in cystic fibrosis?

129. Name five respiratory treatments aimed at decreasing airway obstruction.
   A. _____
   B. _____
   C. _____
   D. _____
   E. _____

130. What new drug can be aerosolized to thin the secretions?

Case 5

Every spring, little Donna Hopper starts to cough. She won't play with the other kids during PE at school because she says it makes it hard to breathe. This year she was hospitalized for a particularly bad episode. Asthma is diagnosed, and Donna is started on albuterol via SVN at home. Her father doesn't want her to take steroids because he heard they could stunt her growth.

131. What method would you recommend for Donna to use for delivery of beta agonists?

132. How would you go about convincing her father that inhaled steroids are okay?

Case 6

Kevin Chunk is a 4-year-old who presents in the emergency department with a high fever, cough, and dyspnea. His parents say the problem came on suddenly. Kevin is listless and weak. The chest radiograph shows consolidation in his right lower lobe. His WBCs are elevated with a high neutrophil count.

133. What is the most likely diagnosis?

134. Do you think the problem is viral or bacterial? Support your answer.

135. What are the primary treatments?

What Does the NBRC Say?

The Entry-Level Examination may ask you a couple of questions related to pediatrics, but this is not the primary proving ground for this area of knowledge. The Registry tests make detailed references to the material in Chapter 43. The Written Registry Matrix contains these items (just a partial list!):

Perinatal data:
- Maternal history
- Perinatal history
- Apgar scores
- Gestational age
- L/S ratio

Recommend procedures:
- Umbilical line
- Transcutaneous monitoring

Inspect the patient:
- Apgar score
- Gestational age
- Retractions
- Nasal flaring

Inspect lateral neck radiograph:
- Epiglottitis
- Subglottic edema
- Foreign bodies

Equipment:
- Oxygen hoods and tents
- Specialized ventilators-oscillators, high frequency

The Clinical Simulation Examination Matrix makes it clear that you will have one pediatric and one neonatal problem. They list these cases as examples:

Neonatal
  Delivery room management, resuscitation, infant apnea, meconium aspiration, respiratory distress syndrome, congenital heart defect.

Pediatric
    Epiglottitis, croup, bronchiolitis, asthma, cystic fibrosis, foreign body aspiration, toxic substance ingestion, bronchopulmonary dysplasia.

While Chapter 43 covers much of this information, you would be wise to consider taking a NALS and PALS course before you take the boards. Here are some sample multiple-choice questions.

135. Which of the following tests would be useful in determining lung maturity?
    A. Sweat chloride
    B. L/S ratio
    C. Fetal hemoglobin
    D. Pneumogram

136. Calculate the Apgar score for a crying infant who has a heart rate of 120, actively moves, sneezes when a catheter is put in the nose, but has blue extremities.
    A. 5
    B. 6
    C. 7
    D. 9

137. A premature infant is experiencing episodes of apnea and cyanosis. The respiratory therapist should recommend which of the following?
    A. Albuterol
    B. Narcan
    C. Exosurf
    D. Aminophylline

138. A 5-year-old child presents in the Emergency Department with complaints of a severe sore throat. The child has inspiratory stridor and muffled phonation. He has a fever of 40 degrees Celsius. His mother states he will not drink anything, so she brought him in. The most likely diagnosis is
    A. Croup
    B. Bronchiolitis
    C. Foreign body aspiration
    D. Epiglottitis

139. A 3-year-old is brought to the emergency department with sudden onset of wheezing. The child has no history of asthma. The mother states the child was playing with her toys when the problem started. Auscultation reveals a coarse wheeze over the right chest only. What is the most likely diagnosis?
    A. Asthma
    B. Croup
    C. Foreign body aspiration
    D. Epiglottitis

140. Which of the following tests is helpful in establishing a diagnosis of cystic fibrosis?
    A. Sweat chloride
    B. L/S ratio
    C. Apgar
    D. Pneumogram

141. An infant born to a woman with a history of heroin use is making weak respiratory efforts after delivery. The respiratory therapist should recommend which of the following?
    A. Albuterol
    B. Narcan
    C. Exosurf
    D. Aminophylline

142. The simplest way to apply CPAP to treat hypoxemia in an infant is to use
    A. Nasal prongs
    B. Nasal mask
    C. Full face mask
    D. An oxygen hood

143. Which of the following is the most appropriate imaging technique to help confirm a diagnosis of croup?
    A. Computerized tomogram
    B. PA chest film
    C. Lateral neck film
    D. Bronchogram

144. A 4-year-old child with LTB presents in the emergency department with moderate stridor and harsh breath sounds. The respiratory therapist should recommend which of the following?
   A. Albuterol
   B. Racemic epinephrine
   C. Immediate intubation
   D. Aminophylline

Food for Thought

If you choose to work in this field it would be a good idea to take the Perinatal/Pediatric Examination to test your knowledge and demonstrate your competence in this specialty area.

Patient Education and Health Promotion

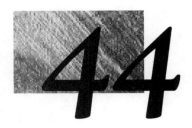

1. Affective domain

—— "Quit worrying about your —— health. It will go away."
Robert Orben

2. Cognitive domain

Teaching can be very satisfying—when learning is taking place! It's equally frustrating to try to learn when teaching is disorganized or the objectives are unclear. Client and community education really go to the far ends of the spectrum. It is tremendously rewarding to help someone quit smoking, learn to be more independent, or to teach a child how to manage his asthma. These are REAL victories in the battle for better health. On the other hand, trying to get your message across to some people can be very frustrating. Chapter 44 provides you with valuable ideas on how to develop, conduct, and measure the outcomes of a health education program. You can use this information in school, with patients, in the community, and in teaching co-workers.

3. Disease prevention

4. Health education

Teacher Talk

I want to make sure you have a good grasp of the key terms in this chapter before you apply them. Write out the definition for each of these terms. You can use the chapter or the glossary.

5. Health promotion

6. Psychomotor domain

Patient Education

Respiratory care practitioners have always been on-the-spot instructors at the bedside, but the role of RCP as formal educator has increased dramatically in the past few years as health care delivery methods and settings have changed.

Overview

7. Describe the first epidemiological revolution—when did it occur, and what happened?

8. What did we learn during the second epidemiological revolution?

9. What are the top five causes of death in the United States?
   A. _____
   B. _____
   C. _____
   D. _____
   E. _____

10. Programs to reduce morbidity and mortality from major illnesses should focus on what aspect of public education?

What's in a Domain?

11. Why should you consider developing written objectives for patient teaching?

12. How can you state an objective in behavioral terms?

13. Give an example of an objective for each of the following learning domains. (Oh, go ahead, take one out of Egan.)

Domain	Objective
A. Cognitive	
B. Affective	
C. Psychomotor	

14. Which of the learning domains (domain is a French word that means realm, estate, or property) should be evaluated before you proceed with patient education?

15. Maslow's hierarchy of needs (which is pretty useful if you apply it) explains why a dyspneic patient will not be very receptive to learning a new skill. How can you assess readiness to learn?

16. What is the key to motivating patients to learn?

17. What is the key to teaching psychomotor skills? How can you confirm that a patient or family member has learned a new skill?

18. Using the text, give an example of how skills a patient uses every day relate to therapy.

F.A.T. T.I.P.S*

Now that you've reviewed some important ideas about teaching, let's take a look at . . .

CRYSTAL CLEAR CLASSROOM COMMANDMENTS

I.   Meet immediate patient needs <u>first</u>.
II. Create an educational setting.
III. Include hearing, seeing, touching, writing, speaking.
IV. Keep sessions short.
V.   Repeat, repeat, repeat!
VI. Allow plenty of time to practice skills.
VII. Spend time preparing for the session.
VIII. Organize your materials and presentation.
IX. Personalize and customize the learning experience.
X.   Be enthusiastic!

If you think about your own learning experiences, you will have no difficulty believing in these powerful ideas for improving your teaching abilities. (Make a copy and mail them to someone!)

Forget Academic Theory, This Is Practical Stuff

Teaching Children

19. How is teaching children different from teaching adults? How is it the same?

20. Where could you find resource materials to help in teaching children with asthma?

21. What suggestions are given for rewarding performance?

Evaluation

22. What process answers the question "Has the patient learned?" When should you begin to develop this process?

23. Describe some of the ways you can tell if a patient has met affective domain objectives.

24. When is it important to go outside the formal teaching mechanisms described above? What does Egan call this situation?

Health Education and Promotion

Naturally, RCPs are expected to be role models who demonstrate healthy behaviors in public. Imagine giving a patient information about nicotine intervention when you smell like cigarettes yourself! However, role models aren't enough to achieve large-scale improvements in public health.

25. What is the primary role of the health educator?

26. State the four central, preventable risk factors for the major causes of death in the United States.
    A. _____
    B. _____
    C. _____
    D. _____

27. Compare the standard medical approach to health in the United States with the public health model.

28. Give goals and examples of each of the following levels of prevention.

Level	Goal	Example
A. Primary		
B. Secondary		
C. Tertiary		

29. Give examples of projects where *RCPs* can participate in organized health promotion activities targeted at primary, secondary, or tertiary goals.
    A. Primary: _____
    B. Secondary: _____
    C. Tertiary: _____

30. Besides the hospital, name four other settings in which RCPs would be likely to function as individual counselors or public health advocates.
    A. _____
    B. _____
    C. _____
    D. _____

Case Studies

Your text has several perfectly good cases in the form of "Mini-Clini's," so let's do something else. Suppose you had to teach your classmates how to use a peak flow meter. Write three objectives for this topic for each domain using behavioral terms.

31. Cognitive domain
    A.

    B.

    C.

32. Affective domain
    A.

    B.

    C.

33. Psychomotor domain
    A.

    B.

    C.

34. How long would your teaching session last?

35. Give examples of how you would involve the following senses in your session.
    A. Hearing

    B. Seeing

    C. Touching

    D. Writing

    E. Speaking

36. Give an example of how you would measure learning for each domain.
    A. Cognitive

    B. Affective

    C. Psychomotor

What Does the NBRC Say?

Not much, except that you should be able to educate a patient. Here's an example.

37. The best way to ensure that a patient learned to properly administer a bronchodilator via MDI is to
    A. Ask the patient to answer questions regarding inhaler use
    B. Give the patient appropriate literature regarding MDI use
    C. Ask the patient to demonstrate how to use the inhaler
    D. Have the patient explain when he is to use the MDI

Food for Thought

38. Why do you think the public should be educated about the risk factors for the top five causes of death? After all, a lot of RCPs are employed taking care of patients who have ignored these risk factors.

39. How is teaching other caregivers different from teaching patients or family members?

Nutritional Aspects of Health and Disease

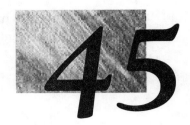

**"To eat is human.
To digest divine."
Mark Twain**

I'm continually surprised at how little attention most of us give to what we eat. Hospitals put a tremendous effort into providing nourishing, specialized diets, with about as much public relations success as the airlines. When was the last time you heard anyone raving about the three-star meal they had after surgery? Dietary habits have far-reaching consequences in terms of overall health, so it should come as no surprise to you that nutrition plays a role in cardiopulmonary function (or that RCPs would get involved).

Eat Your Words

The new terms in Chapter 45 read like a French menu—incomprehensibly. You might need to look up some of these terms before you can match them up with their definitions.

_____ 1. Anergy
_____ 2. Anthropometry
_____ 3. Azotemia
_____ 4. Basal metabolic rate
_____ 5. Gluconeogenesis
_____ 6. Indirect calorimetry
_____ 7. Ketogenesis
_____ 8. Kwashiorkor
_____ 9. Marasmus
_____ 10. Normometabolic
_____ 11. Protein-energy malnutrition
_____ 12. Resting energy expenditure

A. Excess nitrogenous waste in the blood
B. Formation of glycogen from proteins or fatty acids
C. Toxic byproduct of the breakdown of fat
D. Daily resting energy consumption
E. Impaired immune response
F. Science of measuring the human body
G. Hypercatabolic form of malnutrition
H. Hourly resting energy consumption after fasting
I. Energy measurement based on O_2 consumption and CO_2 production
J. Malnutrition associated with starvation
K. Calorimetry REE within 10% of predicted
L. Wasting condition resulting from a deficient diet

Meet the Objectives

13. Describe the food pyramid.

14. What do decks of cards have to do with daily protein requirements?

15. Name the three macronutrients (subgroups for each) that supply your body's energy requirements. State the calorie intake per gram for each main category.

        Macro   *Calories per gram*

A. _____
   1. _____
   2. _____
B. _____
   1. _____
   2. _____
C. _____
   1. _____
   2. _____
   3. _____

16. Write the Harris-Benedict prediction equation for estimating REE. Calculate yours!
   A. Formula: _____
   B. Calculation: _____

17. How many calories will an average adult male who weighs 80 kg need per day to maintain his body weight?

18. Half of the adults in the United States take vitamin supplements. What vitamins and minerals does your text point out as harmful in doses exceeding the RDA?
   A. _____
   B. _____
   C. _____

19. What role do vitamins play in energy metabolism?

20. State two benefits of soluble and insoluble fiber?
   A. Soluble
      1. _____
      2. _____
   B. Insoluble
      1. _____
      2. _____

21. Compare starvation and hypercatabolism malnutrition. Be sure to give at least two clinical examples of each that an RCP would encounter.

22. State the effect of decreases in the following micronutrients through disease or malnutrition (Just a few examples—this is a really huge subject!).
   A. Zinc: _____
   B. Magnesium: _____
   C. Hypophosphatemia: _____

23. What percentage of patients with acute respiratory failure suffer from malnutrition?

24. Give two reasons why malnourished patients are difficult to wean from the ventilator.
    A. _____
    B. _____

25. Why are COPD patients often malnourished?

26. What are the consequences of malnutrition on respiratory muscles and response to hypoxia and hypercapnia?

27. Who normally conducts nutritional assessments in the hospital?

28. State the formula for calculating ideal body weight.
    A. Males: _____
    B. Females: _____
    C. Calculate your own ideal body weight:
    _____

29. Identify one condition that represents each of the following high-risk groups.
    A. Poor intake: _____
    B. Nutrient loss: _____
    C. Hypermetabolism: _____
    D. Drugs: _____

30. List three conditions in which indirect calorimetry may be indicated.
    A. _____
    B. _____
    C. _____

31. What are the contraindications to indirect calorimetry in mechanically ventilated patients?

32. According to the AARC CPG, closed-circuit calorimeters may reduce alveolar volume or increase work of breathing. Explain how these two hazards occur.
    A.

    B.

33. What actions should be taken to prepare a patient for indirect calorimetry?

A. 4 hours before the test

B. 2 hours before the test

C. 1 hour before the test

34. Describe the most significant problem in performing indirect calorimetry on mechanically ventilated patients.

35. Interpret the following RQs and identify the general nutritional strategy.

Value	Interpretation	Strategy
A. >1.0		
1. Interpretation ————————		
2. Strategy ————————		
B. 0.9-1.0		
1. Interpretation ————————		
2. Strategy ————————		
C. 0.7-0.8		
1. Interpretation ————————		
2. Strategy ————————		

36. State the formula for calculating REE using a pulmonary artery catheter.

37. What factors are used to adjust predicted REEs in patients? Give one example.

38. Explain what happens when patients receive too much of the following substrates:

A. Protein

B. Carbohydrates

C. Fat

39. What do the terms *enteral* and *parenteral* mean?
    A. Enteral

    B. Parenteral

40. Explain what is meant by the following tube feeding regimens.
    A. Bolus

    B. Intermittent

    C. Drip

41. How would the RCP confirm suspected aspiration of tube feedings? How is this complication avoided?

42. COPD patients have special dietary needs and problems. Identify four factors that lead to poor nutrition in these patients.
    A. _____
    B. _____
    C. _____
    D. _____

43. What diet is provided to the hypercapnic patient?

44. How and what should COPD patients eat to optimize nutrition?

Chapter Highlights

45. The majority of daily calories should come from _____, fruits, and _____.

46. _____ nutrients supply the body's energy requirements.

47. _____ nutrients play essential roles in normal metabolism and physiology.

48. The _____-_____ equations estimate daily resting energy expenditure.

49. _____ is a state of impaired metabolism in which the intake of nutrients falls short of the body's needs.

50. _____ REEs should be corrected for both stress and activity levels.

51. Nutrients can be supplied _____ or _____, but whenever possible the _____ route should be used.

52. The likelihood of _____ during tube feedings can be minimized by _____ the head of the bed by _____.

Case Studies

Case 1

John Barleycorn, a thin, undernourished COPD patient, tells you that he has difficulty eating because he gets tired and short of breath during meals.

53. What eating pattern should be emphasized to Mr. Barleycorn?

54. Make some suggestions for poor John B. that would increase his nutrient intake.

55. What nutritional supplement was specifically designed for COPD patients?

What Does the NBRC Say?

Sorry folks, while muscle wasting and general appearance do show up in the matrix, and while RCPs are very involved in indirect calorimetry in many institutions, most of this information has not made it to the boards yet. No, this is just practical stuff you can use in patient assessment and patient teaching.

Food for Thought

56. What type of nutritional strategy may help in the weaning of COPD patients from the ventilator?

57. Why is it important to verify tube placement before beginning feeding?

Cardiopulmonary Rehabilitation

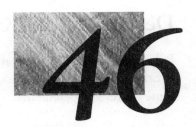

—— "No one is useless in this —— world who lightens the burden of another."
Charles Dickens

Alvan Barach first recommended reconditioning programs for COPD patients over 40 years ago. Unfortunately, it was not until recently that these programs began in earnest around the nation. When I worked in home care in the 1980s, it was often up to the individual therapist to try to provide and encourage these concepts for individual patients. Now there are many well-established inpatient and outpatient programs to meet the physical and psychosocial needs of our patients with chronic lung disease.

While there are many good textbooks and patient teaching aids available, you will find that Chapter 46 provides an excellent overview of the subject. Even if you don't work in rehabilitation, you will be in a position to identify patients who can benefit from these services, and can play a key role in improving the quality of your patient's lives. You may also wish to participate in one of the support groups founded by the American Lung Association, local health care organizations, or affiliations of the American Association for Respiratory Care.

Cerebral Muscle Training

You can build impressive mental muscles by adding these words to your vocabulary. Match the following terms and acronyms to their definitions.

_____ 1. ADL
_____ 2. Borg scale
_____ 3. CORF
_____ 4. Hypoglycemia
_____ 5. METS
_____ 6. OBLA
_____ 7. Reconditioning
_____ 8. Respiratory quotient
_____ 9. Target heart rate

A. Physical activities designed to strengthen muscles and improve oxygen utilization
B. Measure of an individual's ability to perform common tasks
C. Point at which there is insufficient oxygen to meet the demands of energy metabolism
D. Measure of an individual's perception of breathing difficulty
E. Cardiac goal for aerobic conditioning based on 65% of maximum oxygen consumption
F. Ratio of CO_2 production to oxygen consumption
G. Medicare approved facility that provides ambulatory rehab services
H. Low blood sugar levels
I. Indirect measure of physiological work performed during exercise stress testing

Definitions and Goals

Pulmonary rehabilitation is not the same animal as other types of rehab, although it can contain some of the same elements.

10. What is meant by the general term *rehabilitation*?

11. The definition of pulmonary rehabilitation is very long. Please put it into your own words.

12. What are the two specific objectives of pulmonary rehabilitation according to the American Thoracic Society?
    A.

    B.

Scientific Basis for Pulmonary Rehabilitation

Exercise physiology plays an important role in our understanding of the benefits of reconditioning, but physiology alone is not sufficient to achieve desired outcomes in patients with COPD.

13. How do social sciences play a role in establishing ways to improve the patient's quality of life?

14. Why is MVV a useful pulmonary function test in regard to assessing physical activity?

15. How can you estimate MVV using simple spirometry?

16. Identify the three general ways that reconditioning will increase exercise tolerance?
    A. _____
    B. _____
    C. _____

17. Compare the roles of psychosocial and physical methods in terms of outcomes of rehabilitation.

18. Describe the two-way relationship of physical reconditioning and psychosocial support.

Pulmonary Rehabilitation Programs

Program designs may vary, but the desired outcomes and basic components are similar.

19. Why is it so important to have specific objectives for the program goals?

20. State five accepted benefits of exercise reconditioning.
    A. _____
    B. _____
    C. _____
    D. _____
    E. _____

21. Research literature clearly shows that rehabilitation has limits. Name two.
    A. _____
    B. _____

22. List one evaluation tool from each of the three categories shown in Box 46-2 on page 1090 of the text.
    A. _____
    B. _____
    C. _____

23. State three potential hazards of physical reconditioning.
    A. _____
    B. _____
    C. _____

24. What is the first step in patient evaluation for a pulmonary rehabilitation program?

25. Name four tests that should be included with the physical examination.
    A. _____
    B. _____
    C. _____
    D. _____

26. Two tests are usually conducted to assess cardiopulmonary status. State two purposes for these tests.
    A. Exercise evaluation
       1. _____
       2. _____
    B. Pulmonary function testing
       1. _____
       2. _____

27. List two contraindications and two complications of exercise testing.
    A. Contraindications
       1. _____
       2. _____
    B. Complications
       1. _____
       2. _____

28. Identify four physiological parameters that should be monitored during exercise testing.
    A. _____
    B. _____
    C. _____
    D. _____

29. Name two types of patients that are usually excluded from selection for rehabilitation.
    A. _____
    B. _____

30. State the four general groups of patients included in pulmonary rehabilitation programs.
    A. _____
    B. _____
    C. _____
    D. _____

31. What are the benefits of grouping patients together on the basis of severity and overall ability?

32. Give one benefit and one drawback of the open-ended program model.
    A. Benefit: _____
    B. Drawback: _____

33. Give one benefit and one drawback to the traditional closed design.
    A. Benefit: _____
    B. Drawback: _____

34. Describe two ways to set target heart rate for patient exercise.
    A.

    B.

35. Describe a typical walking exercise program.

36. What is the basic concept behind ventilatory muscle training?

37. Briefly discuss the following high-priority program educational components.
    A. Breathing control

    B. Stress management

    C. Medications

    D. Diet

38. What is the ideal class size for a rehabilitation program? What external factor affects this ideal?

39. Give specific examples for each of the following sources of program reimbursement.
    A. Non-governmental health insurance

    B. Federal and state health insurance

    C. Ancillary insurance

    D. Other options

40. What are the most likely causes of lack of measurable improvement within a pulmonary rehabilitation program?

Case Studies

Case 1

Bill Friendly is an alert, 55-year-old man with long-standing asthma and COPD. He is admitted for acute exacerbation of his illness following a "chest cold." This admission is Bill's fourth in the last 3 months. Mr. Friendly tells you that he has had to quit his job and take early retirement because of his lung problems.

41. What concerns does this situation raise?

42. Explain the benefits of entering a rehabilitation program to Mr. Friendly.

Case 2

Jane Deaux is a 57-year-old woman with chronic bronchitis who is enrolled in your pulmonary rehab program. During walking exercises she complains of dyspnea and will not continue with the walk.

43. What assessments would be useful in this situation?

44. Give several possible methods for modifying the exercise program to improve this patient's compliance.

What Does the NBRC Say?

In the case of pulmonary rehabilitation, the Written Registry Examination Matrix is very specific. Up to five questions may be asked. The Matrix states: "Initiate and conduct pulmonary rehabilitation...within the prescription, namely:
• Establish optimal therapeutic goals
• Implement and monitor graded exercise program
• Explain and instruct planned therapeutic goals
• Evaluate patient's progress"

In reality, however, you can expect less than five questions because this area of the matrix also includes home care and assisting in special procedures. Chapter 46 goes into the subject in much greater depth than the boards. The Clinical Simulation Matrix includes identical items but also specifically mentions that you may encounter a case of a patient with COPD who needs pulmonary rehabilitation. This means that rehabilitation is a small but very important part of the advanced practitioner testing. Rehabilitation is not tested on the Entry-Level Examination.

45. A COPD patient has enrolled in a pulmonary rehabilitation program. The patient should be informed that the program will help provide all of the benefits except
A. Increased physical endurance
B. Improved PFT results
C. Increased activity levels
D. Improved cardiovascular function

46. During an exercise test a patient is able to reach a maximum heart rate of 120. His resting heart rate is 70. What target heart rate would you recommend for this patient during aerobic conditioning?
   A. 70 beats per minute
   B. 85 beats per minute
   C. 100 beats per minute
   D. 115 beats per minute

47. Which of the following tests would be useful in assessing ventilatory reserve during exercise testing?
   A. Forced vital capacity
   B. Maximum voluntary ventilation
   C. Body plethysmography
   D. Single breath nitrogen washout

Food for Thought

Chapter 46 (and others) refers to the Borg Scale. This scale is a valuable tool that can be easily used at the bedside or in the rehabilitation setting, but I'm not sure if it is explained in Egan! (So you might have to dig for this one . . .)

48. Describe the Borg Scale.

49. What are the units of measurement on the scale?

50. What is the value of this instrument?

Respiratory Care in Alternative Settings

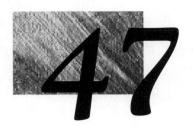

Egan ends with a beginning, and Chapter 47 introduces you to the fastest growing area of respiratory care. As health care is being redefined on many levels, the work setting for our profession is rapidly moving outside the boundaries of the traditional medical center concept. Alternative care settings provide special challenges for the RCP, particularly the new graduate.

Acronyms

No matter what else you got out of this book, you're bound to have a brain full of odd letter combinations. Don't worry, be happy. This is the last of the acronyms for you to write out. (I promise!)

1. AHI

2. DME

3. HCFA

4. NIPPV

5. SAHS

6. SIDS

7. SNF

8. TTOT

Definitions and Goals

9. Name the five areas of subacute or alternate
   care.
   A. _____
   B. _____
   C. _____
   D. _____
   E. _____

10. What is subacute care?

11. In what categories of subacute care are
    RCPs usually involved?

12. What is the most common age-group
    receiving subacute care?

13. What type of agreement is needed for reim-
    bursement of respiratory services under cur-
    rent federal guidelines?

14. State at least three of the benefits of respi-
    ratory home care.
    A. _____
    B. _____
    C. _____

Standards

15. Why does government play a major role in
    setting standards for the regulation of posta-
    cute care?

16. What is the purpose of the Medicare Provider Certification Program?

17. Who is responsible for accreditation of companies that provide home care services?

Traditional Acute Care

18. Why do many RCPs prefer working in the postacute care setting?

19. Compare traditional and alternative settings in terms of the following areas:

Area	Traditional	Alternative
A. Diagnostic tests	_____	_____
B. Equipment	_____	_____
C. Supervision	_____	_____
D. Pt. Assessment	_____	_____
E. Work schedule	_____	_____
F. Time constraints	_____	_____

Discharge Planning

20. Explain the role of the following practitioners in the postacute care team:
A. Utilization and review

B. Social services

C. Physical therapy

D. Physiatrist

E. DME supplier

How can you confirm that a nonprofessional caregiver is able to perform care?

25. Describe the six elements that must be included in a home oxygen prescription.

A.

B.

22. Discuss the equipment requirements necessary in a home environment that must be assessed prior to discharge.

C.

D.

Oxygen Therapy

23. Why do so many people use home oxygen in the United States?

E.

F.

24. State three of the documented benefits of home oxygen therapy.

A. _____

B. _____

C. _____

26. What is the purpose of the Certificate of Medical Necessity?

27. What are the two primary uses of compressed oxygen cylinders in the alternative setting?
   A. E cylinder

   B. H cylinder

28. How do flowmeters used in alternative settings differ from those used in the hospital?

29. Let's compare the advantages and disadvantages of the oxygen supply systems available for use in alternative settings.

System	Advantage	Disadvantage
A. Cylinders		
1. _____	_____
2. _____	_____
B. Liquid		
1. _____	_____
2. _____	_____
C. Concentrator		
1. _____	_____
2. _____	_____

30. Liquid oxygen is weighed to determine the amount available. If a patient was using 3 L/min with an 80 lb system that was 1/4 full, how many hours would the gas last?
   A. Formula: _____
   B. Calculations: _____
   C. Answer: _____

31. Explain how an oxygen concentrator works.

32. What is the typical range of oxygen percentage a concentrator will supply at 2 L/min? At 4 L/min?
   A. 2 L/min: _____
   B. 4 L/min: _____

33. What effect will the concentrator have on a patient's electrical bill?

34. Describe some of the methods for avoiding communication problems with patients receiving home oxygen therapy.

35. In addition to providing a backup supply, what other precautions should be taken in terms of concentrator power supply?

36. List at least four areas that should be evaluated when checking a home patient's oxygen concentrator.
    A. _____
    B. _____
    C. _____
    D. _____

37. When a patient is placed on an oxygen-conserving device, how would you determine the correct liter flow to use?

38. What actions should a patient who is wearing transtracheal oxygen take if they believe the catheter isn't working properly?

39. In theory, how would a demand-flow oxygen-conserving system benefit the patient?

40. What are the two main drawbacks to demand-flow systems?

41. In what situations should a patient or caregiver be instructed to alter the prescribed flow setting?

42. State the three main problems associated with insertion of the transtracheal catheter.
    A. _____
    B. _____
    C. _____

43. Describe the basic methods for avoiding complications of transtracheal catheters.

Ventilatory Support

44. Give examples for each of the three main groups of patients who are placed on ventilators in the alternative care setting.
    A. Nocturnal ventilation
       1. _____
       2. _____
       3. _____
    B. Continuous mechanical ventilation
       1. _____
       2. _____
       3. _____
    C. Terminally ill
       1. _____
       2. _____

45. Identify the three common settings where ventilatory support is delivered outside the hospital.
    A. _____
    B. _____
    C. _____

46. Invasive long-term ventilation is always provided via what type of airway?

47. Describe the emergency situations a family must be able to deal with in caring for a home ventilator patient.

48. Describe three reasons why noninvasive ventilation may be preferable to invasive ventilation in the alternative setting.
    A.

    B.

    C.

49. Identify at least 3 situations where NIPPV is partly contraindicated.
    A. _____
    B. _____
    C. _____

50. Identify at least three situations where NIPPV is absolutely contraindicated.
    A. _____
    B. _____
    C. _____

51. What options exist for patients who do not want invasive ventilation and cannot use NIPPV?

52. What options are available on invasive positive pressure ventilator systems during power failures, or if a patient wishes to be mobile?

53. What is the biggest challenge associated with NIPPV?

54. Identify the three basic types of negative pressure ventilators.
   A. _____
   B. _____
   C. _____

Other Modes of Postacute Respiratory Care

55. What is the primary use of bland aerosols in the postacute setting?

56. What is the major problem with delivery of bland aerosols?

57. What are the two limits on Medicare reimbursement for compressor-driven SVNs in the alternate setting?
   A. _____
   B. _____

58. Identify the three requirements for approval of reimbursement for compressor-driven nebulizers?
   A. _____
   B. _____
   C. _____

59. How can you prevent bacterial growth on suction catheters that are used repeatedly?

60. State three common problems associated with SAHS.
   A. _____
   B. _____
   C. _____

61. What is the primary treatment for this condition?

62. When should nasal masks be replaced?

63. Discuss solutions to the common complaint of nasal dryness.

64. What infant condition suggests the use of apnea monitoring?

Patient Assessment and Documentation

65. Describe the main areas you would check during initial screening of a patient following admission to a postacute care facility.

66. What areas would be important to assess *besides* the usual vital signs and evaluation of the respiratory system?

67. Once the initial assessment is done a treatment plan is initiated. When is formal reassessment performed?

68. How often should a member of the home care team perform a follow-up evaluation for patients receiving respiratory care treatments? What factors should be considered in determining the frequency of visits?

Equipment Disinfection and Maintenance

69. Describe the process for cleaning a home nebulizer (for example).

   A.

   B.

   C.

   D.

70. Describe the ARCF guidelines for using water in humidifiers and nebulizers.

71. What is the most important principle of infection control in the home setting?

Case Studies

Case 1

Jim Billings is a 70-year-old man with COPD who is discharged with an order for home oxygen. The patient's room air blood gas prior to discharge is

pH	7.47
$PaCO_2$	33 mm Hg
PaO_2	62 mm Hg
SaO_2	92%

Medicare returns the CMN as disapproved on the basis that this patient does not meet the criteria for saturation of pO_2 for home oxygen.

72. Make an argument for keeping the patient on oxygen based on your knowledge of respiratory physiology. (This is a real case and we did get reimbursement!)

Case 2

Steve Bete is a home care patient you are seeing who uses an oxygen concentrator. Mr. Bete calls you (late at night, of course) to say that he doesn't think he is getting an adequate amount of flow from his cannula.

73. What are some possible causes of this problem?

74. What would you suggest Steve should do at this time?

Case 3

Cathy Chow, an active 49-year-old with alpha$_1$-antitrypsin deficiency, is to be discharged with home oxygen. The prescription is for 2 L/min of continuous oxygen.

75. What system would you recommend for Ms. Chow to use at home?

76. What about a portable system?

What Does the NBRC Say?

A small but important section of the Advanced Practitioner examinations is devoted to home care. Since most RCPs are working in acute or subacute care, it is easy to overlook this information. It is reasonable to expect that the newly revised tests will include some information on subacute care, but that hasn't happened yet. The matrix includes:

- Monitor and maintain home care equipment
- Assure safety and infection control
- Modify procedures for use in the home
- Evaluate patient's progress
- Maintain apnea monitors

The Clinical Simulation Matrix adds that you may encounter a COPD patient in a home care setting.

77. A patient with a tracheostomy is to receive humidification via a nebulizer in his home. With regard to water for the nebulizer, which of the following would be the most appropriate choice for the home setting?
   A. Sterile distilled water should be obtained from the DME provider
   B. Tap water is sufficient for the home setting if the nebulizer is cleaned properly
   C. Bottled water can be used as long as it is distilled
   D. Tap water that is boiled may be used for up to 24 hours

78. Which of the following actions would an RCP perform during the monthly check of a home oxygen concentrator system?
   I. Replacement of the silica pellets in the sieve bed
   II. Analysis of the FIO_2 delivered by the concentrator
   III. Filter replacement
   IV. Evaluation of the concentrator's electrical system
   A. I, II only
   B. II, III only
   C. II, IV only
   D. II, III, IV only

79. A patient who is wearing a transtracheal oxygen catheter suddenly becomes dyspneic. The first action the patient should take would be to
   A. Call the physician
   B. Clean the catheter
   C. Increase the oxygen flow to the catheter
   D. Remove the catheter and proceed to the emergency room

80. A patient who is using oxygen at home occasionally needs to go out for health care appointments. What type of portable system would you recommend for this patient?
   A. E cylinder with standard flowmeter
   B. E cylinder with conserving device
   C. Small liquid oxygen reservoir
   D. Patients can go out for short periods without supplemental oxygen

81. A respiratory care practitioner determines that a cuirass-type negative pressure ventilator is now reading a pressure of -20 cm H_2O, when it should be cycling at -35 cm H_{20}. The patient is in no distress, but the measured tidal volume is 200 ml lower than the desired volume. The practitioner should
   A. Begin manual ventilation of the patient
   B. Check for leaks in the system
   C. Increase the vacuum setting
   D. Increase the amount of air in the cuff

Food for Thought

82. Where could you find the local regulations that apply to providers in your state?

Your textbook indicates that there is some controversy over the best way to disinfect reusable equipment and supplies in the home setting.

83. State three types of solutions that can be used.
   A. _____
   B. _____
   C. _____

84. What are the advantages of using acetic acid (white vinegar, not red wine!) as a disinfectant?

85. What are the disadvantages?

Answer Key

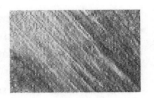

Chapter 1

Word Wizard

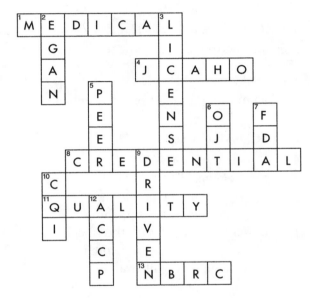

Meet the Objectives

1. Page 4
   A. Personnel
   B. Equipment
   C. Method or manner in which care is provided

2. Page 12
   A. Institutional monitoring (care plan audits, case study exercises)
   B. Centralized government monitoring (JCAHO)

3. Pages 4-5

Protocols improve the allocation of respiratory resources by reducing misallocations such as over-ordering. Studies (Table 1-1) show reductions of 28%-72% in oxygen for patients who had adequate oxygenation. Protocols also reduce costs. (Table 1-4, page 16)

Chapter Highlights (pages 16-17)

4. Medical

5. Misallocation

6. Protocols

7. Registered

8. National Board for Respiratory Care (NBRC).

9. Patient-focused

10. Continuous Quality Improvement.

11. Licensure and voluntary credentialing.

Case Studies (pages 8-10)

12. A. SOB
    B. Tachycardia
    C. Diaphoresis
    D. Confusion

13. The pulse oximeter shows good saturation. The patient has no clinical signs of hypoxemia and no history that suggests heart or lung disease. Respiratory rate and heart rate are normal. Oxygen therapy is not indicated.

14. Place the patient on room air and recheck the saturation. The history of abdominal surgery suggests starting the patient on incentive spirometry.

15. Mr. Day has a history of smoking and lung disease and has had surgery. His radiograph shows atelectasis. Pulse oximetry is acceptable. He should be started on hyperinflation therapy such as incentive spirometry (q1 hour) and a bronchodilator such as Albuterol (qid).

Board Exam Business

16. A. Oxygen therapy (page 8)

17. D. Aerosolized bronchodilator therapy (page 7)

18. A. Increase the liter flow to the cannula (page 8)

19. B. Postoperative patients (page 10)

Food for Thought

20. Successful protocol programs involve many elements, including collaboration with physicians and nurses, trained therapists, committed medical direction, and active quality monitoring. Failure to take all of these actions could result in poor outcomes. Protocols themselves must be well designed. (page 6, Fig 1-2). Quality assurance efforts are also complex. (page 12, Box 1-6, page 13, Box 1-7). Timely audits must be conducted and follow-up actions to resolve problem areas must be taken.

21. The basic design of a quality improvement program would be similar in any setting. (See benchmarks on page 13, Box 1-8). Policies and procedures have to be adapted to alternate care settings (page 12, Box 1-5). Alternate care settings may have different patient populations (aged) that have different issues. Caregivers in alternate settings may not be as familiar with respiratory modalities.

Chapter 2

Word Power (page 19)

You'll Get a Charge Out of This
ground, macroshock, microshock, fibrillation

Burn, Baby, Burn
nonflammable   combustible   cigarettes

Keep it Moving! (pages 20-21)

4   Dangle the patient.
3   Sit them up.
5   Assist to a standing position.
6   Encourage slow, easy breathing.
1   Lower the bed and lock the wheels.
2   Move the IV pole close to the patient.
7   Provide support while walking.

Meet the Objectives

1. Page 20
   A. Patient movement and ambulation
   B. Electrical hazards
   C. Fire hazards

2. A. Good body mechanics (page 20)
   B. Ground equipment not the patient (page 23)
   C. Remove flammable materials used near oxygen, keep ignition sources such as smoking, away from patients using oxygen. (page 26)

3. Minimizes the likelihood of injuries. (page 20)

4. Level of consciousness, color, breathing, strength, complaints. (page 22)

5. A. Attitude
   B. Culture
   C. Self-concepts
   D. Feelings
   E. Prior experiences (pages 27-8)

6. Page 29
   A. Share information instead of telling
   B. Relate to people instead of controlling
   C. Value disagreement as much as agreement
   D. Eliminate threatening behavior
   E. Use effective nonverbal communication

7. A. Poor communication: supervisor not willing to accept different points of view for dealing with a difficult patient. (page 31)
   B. Structural problems: conflict increases in larger organizations. (page 31)
   C. Personal behavior: personalities, attitudes, behavior traits. (page 32)
   D. Role conflict: clinical supervisor trying to manage staff and students at the same time. (page 32)

8. A. Written picture of occurrences and situations pertaining to a patient throughout his or her stay in a healthcare institution. (page 33)
   B. Medical records are the property of the institution.
   C. Only those individuals directly caring for the patient.

9. A. Legal: no documentation means that no care was given. (page 33)
   B. Practical: brief, accurate, clear charting using standard terms. (page 35)

10. A. SOAP = subjective, objective, assessment, plan. (page 36)
    B. Examples (page 37, Box 2-4)
       1. S: "My chest hurts when I breathe"
       2. O: Awake, alert, and oriented. HR 98, RR 25, BP 118/80
          Bronchial breath sounds in right lower lobe
       3. A: Pneumonia continues
       4. P: Postural drainage and percussion every 4 hours

Chapter Highlights (page 38)

11. Ambulation
12. Microshock
13. Grounding
14. Oxygen
15. Communication
16. Conflict
17. Legal
18. Document

Case Studies

19. Portable oxygen source: E cylinder or liquid.

20. Color, breathing (rate, pattern, use of accessory muscles), strength, patient complaints (shortness of breath). A pulse oximeter might be useful in evaluating adequacy of oxygenation. (page 22)

21. Take time to unplug the power cords from the wall. Cords plugged into the wall but disconnected from the IV pump or pulse oximeter represent a significant electrocution hazard.

22. Status and perception of the problem may result in conflict. The doctor and the nurse are concerned with transporting a critically ill patient as quickly as possible. Physicians and nurses may perceive their "rank" as higher than other practitioners. (page 31.) Some form of collaboration or compromise, or avoidance strategy, is indicated. For example, you could ask someone else to bag the patient, or you could keep bagging and ask someone else to take care of the cords as you leave (page 32).

Board Exam Blues

23. C. I and III only (page 35, Box 2-3)

24. D. I, II, III The new order must be noted in the chart for legal and reimbursement purposes. You should communicate with the RN regarding the patient's care plan. The supervisor will need to know about the change in order to plan workload scheduling.

Food for Thought

25. Back injuries are the most common injuries in almost all work settings.

26. Night shift. There are less workers overall, workers are less likely to be alert for various reasons, and patients who are sleepy or medicated are more likely to fall.

Chapter 3

Slam the Door on Infections

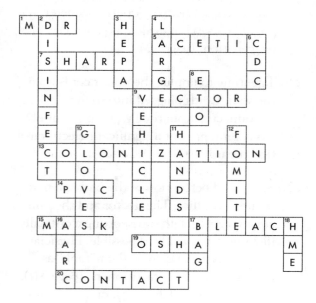

Meet the Objectives

1. Cleaning, usually by washing, is the first step in processing. (page 43)

2. Pasteurization is the application of moist heat at temperatures below the boiling point of water. It does not kill spores. (page 44)

3. Glutaraldehydes, hydrogen peroxide, peracetic acid, and sodium hypochlorite are all high-level disinfectants. Glutaraldehyde is commonly used in respiratory care. Bronchoscopes and spirometry tubing are examples. (page 45)

4. Page 46

Method	Equipment
A. Incineration	Disposables
B. Dry heat	Glassware, metal instruments
C. Boiling	Metals, some plastics
D. Autoclave	Metal instruments, linens
E. Ionizing radiation	Food, supplies
F. Ethylene oxide	Heat sensitive items

5. Page 59

Indicator	Example
A. Chemical indicators	Packaging tape
B. Biologic indicators	Bacterial spores

6. A. Handwashing—the single best way! (page 53)
   B. Protective wear—mask, gown, gloves
   C. Patient placement and transport procedures

Chapter Highlights (page 60)

7. 10% and 40%, surfaces

8. Glutaraldehyde

9. Large-volume nebulizers

10. Sterile

11. Wash your hands

12. All

13. Masks and goggles

14. Contaminated

15. "Sharps"

Case Studies

16. Surgical incision, pain, anesthesia, intubation, and narcotics all impair host defenses. (page 40)

17. Skin of visitors and health professionals (contact transmission) (page 42)

18. A. Rigorous handwashing
    B. Use of gloves
    C. Isolate the infected patients (page 42)

19. Gloves protect caregivers from contamination when contacting patients' blood and body fluids. Gloves also protect patients from bacteria that colonizes the caregivers' hands. You still have to wash your hands because gloves may have very small defects, and you may contaminate your hands when removing the gloves. (page 53)

20. Obviously this situation is a source of conflict; it involves both communication and ethical issues. The student will have difficulty telling the caregiver they are wrong, and may be uncomfortable in telling someone what the caregiver is doing.

21. Airborne (page 56)

22. Patients should be wearing masks, preferrably specialized masks for use with TB. (page 56)

23. These patients should be placed in special isolation rooms. If these rooms are not available, they should be cohorted, or placed in rooms together. (page 56)

24. 1. Only perform these procedures if essential.
    2. Perform the procedures in special rooms or enclosures designed to meet ventilation requirements for airborne isolation.
    3. Patients should be instructed to cover their mouth and nose with tissue when coughing.
    4. Specialized nebulizers may be used. See Box 3-13 on page 57 for a complete discussion.

25. Since these are prisoners, there are additional concerns regarding practitioner safety and maintenance of security.

What Does the NBRC Say?

26. D. Sterile distilled water (Box 3-3, page 48)

27. B. I, II, and IV only (Box 3-3, page 48)

28. B. Wash your hands after every patient contact (page 53)

Food for Thought

29. This situation presents another opportunity for discussion of ethics and for review of your program's clinical policies.

30. Some programs or colleges offer low-cost vaccinations. The risk of hepatitis B far outweighs the risk of the vaccine.

Chapter 4

Word Power

Answers on pages 67-72. Also found in the glossary of key terms.

criminal, civil, plaintiff, defendants, tort, negligence, assault, battery, or slander, libel, confidential

Case Studies

1. Confidentiality is both a legal and an ethical issue. Discussion of cases or patients should not be held in the cafeteria, elevators, and other public places. (pages 67, 72)

2. The student could be reprimanded or even asked to leave the program for violation of confidentiality. While this situation has relatively low risk of harm, the ultimate consequence of breach of confidentiality is possible litigation by the family over breach of confidentiality. (pages 67-68)

3. This case, like the Mini-Clini on page 68, provides opportunity for discussion of how to deal with confidentiality issues. One simple response would be to remind the classmate about talking about patients in the cafeteria. See the "AARC Code of Ethics" on page 65.

4. The American Hospital Association Patient's Bill of Rights reaffirms the patient's right to refuse a treatment. Forcing or threatening could be illegal in some cases. (page 66)

5. It would be important to adopt a non-threatening approach in explaining the importance of the therapy and the consequences of not taking a treatment. (page 66)

6. Refusal to take a treatment must be documented in the medical record.

   It might be important to discuss this with the nurse and/or physician, and pass the information on to your instructor or supervisor. (page 66)

7. This patient is clearly hypoxic, a condition that can affect mental status and ability to make rational decisions. Failure to recognize and treat the hypoxia could meet the criteria for negligence (page 71), or breach of contract (page 73).

8. Continue to attempt to place the oxygen back on the patient after explaining. Seek help from the nursing staff. It is necessary to inform the physician of the situation.

9. With proper documentation and a physician order, restraints are an acceptable method of preventing a patient from harming themselves or others. Unauthorized contact may be considered battery, but implied consent exists in this situation as well. Oxygen is not an unusual or experimental procedure. (page 72)

What About Ethics?

See page 65 for the AARC Code of Ethics.

Case Studies

10. In actions of benevolent deception the truth is withheld. It is rarely practiced in the United States outside of pediatrics or in cases of potential suicide. (page 66)

11. Opportunity for discussion. A Harris poll showed 94% of Americans surveyed would want to know everything about their case, even bad news. (page 66)

12. The appropriate action is to instruct Mr. Miller to discuss this with his physician. It is important to make sure that the physician is notified of the patient's concerns. (page 66)

13. Informing the patient when he has indicated he will kill himself if he has HIV.

14. Patient, nurse, doctor, RCP, family

15. Confidentiality, beneficence, autonomy, veracity

16. The primary physician

17. Medically, the goal is to provide adequate oxygenation to ensure normal mentation. Also, the RCP should observe the patient and report suicidal ideations. In terms of the health care team, the RCP should participate in the discussion. Regardless of the decision, the RCP should provide emotional support.

18. Short term consequences of informing the patient could include depression, despair, suicide. Not informing the patient would seem to have little short-term effect. In fact, the patient could be equally despairing over not knowing what is wrong when he suspects. Long term consequences of not telling the patient include loss of trust in the health care system/practitioners. This could result in the patient not getting life-sustaining medical treatment.

19. It's your call—you make the decision.

20. Precautions to prevent suicide. Appropriate counseling and psychological support. Informing the patient of available treatment and outcomes.

21. Staffing is an immediate issue. Breakdown of the chain of command.

22. Refusing to care for a patient is generally considered unethical (see AARC statement on page 65). Exceptions are possible when the caregiver could suffer harm, such as a pregnant RCP caring for a patient with measles. Refusing to care for a patient could be considered abandonment, which is usually illegal (see Mini-Clini on page 64).

23. First, I would privately discuss the situation with the RCP. If that was not successful, it might be necessary to take administrative action after you determine the legal rights involved in each specific situation. The supervisor might need to contact the Human Relations Department and the Technical Director. In some situations it would be appropriate to have another practitioner deliver the therapy while the situation was being resolved. Ultimately, the RCP might be terminated.

Chapter Highlights (Answers on page 75)

24. <u>dilemmas</u>

25. <u>ideal</u>

26. <u>formalism</u> and <u>consequentalism</u>

27. <u>Public</u>

28. <u>malpractice</u> <u>harm</u>

29. <u>Defending</u>, <u>legal</u>

Food for Thought

30. Consider whether to keep this material private or use as a tool for a confidential classroom discussion of ethics.

Chapter 5

Unlock Your Brain

Yes, but it's a dry heat
<u>absolute</u>, <u>relative</u>, <u>body</u>, <u>deficit</u>, <u>evaporation</u>

Some like it hot
<u>evaporation</u>, <u>conduction</u>, <u>radiates</u>, <u>convection</u>

Obey the Laws

1. The volume of gas will expand. (page 97)

2. Charles' Law

3. Pressure will increase in the cylinder. (page 97)

4. Guy-Lussac's Law

5. Decreases

6. Boyle's Law (page 97)

Try It, You'll Like It!

7. The balloon inflates or expands.

8. Charles' Law (page 97)

9. The paper rises, or lifts up.

10. Bernoulli Principle/Effect (page 102)

11. They move inward toward each other.

12. The biggest straw

13. Water is the easiest

14. Poiseuille's Law (page 101)

Case Studies

15. P_B 226 Torr (Mini-Clini on page 96)
    P_I 0.21 × 226 = 47 Torr

16. 0.70 × 226 = 158 Torr (Mini-Clini on page 96)

17. Dalton's Law (pages 94-95)

18. Increased temperature increases the partial pressure. (page 96)

19. $PaCO_2$ increases about 5% per degree C, so we would expect a 15% increase, or 6 mm Hg. The new value = 46 mm Hg. (page 96)

20. Metabolism and cardiovascular changes also occur with body temperature changes. These are difficult to measure and may make temperature conversions invalid clinically. (page 96)

Mathemagic

21. Formula: Degrees K = degrees C + 273 (page 81)
    Solution: 30 + 273
    Answer: 303°K

22. Formula: Degrees C = 5/9 (F-32) (page 81)
    Solution: C = 5/9 (68-32) ... 5/9 (36) ... 180/9
    Answer: 20°C

23. Formula: Degrees F = (9/5 C) + 32 (page 81)
    Solution: F = (360/5) + 32 ... 72 + 32
    Answer: 104°F

24. Formula: Relative Humidity = Content/Capacity 100 (page 90)
    Solution: RH = 22 mg/L 43.8 mg/L × 100
    Answer: RH = 50%

25. Formula: Humidity deficit = content−capacity (37°C) (page 91)
    Solution: Humidity deficit = 43.8 mg/L−22 mg/L
    Answer: Humidity deficit = 21.8 mg/L

26. Formula: cm H_2O = mm Hg × 1.36
    Solution: cm H_2O = 10 mm Hg × 1.36
    Answer: 13.6 cm H_2O

27. Formula: kPa = cm H_2O d 10 (precisely 10.2) (page 94)
    Solution: kPa = 10 cm H_2O ÷ 10
    Answer: 1 kPa

28. Formula: PIO_2 = Pb × FIO_2 (page 95)
    Solution: PIO_2 = 760 mm Hg × 0.21 (0.209 more precisely)
    Answer: 160 mm Hg (or 159.6 or 159)

29. Formula: PIO_2 = Pb x FIO_2 (page 95)
    Solution: PIO_2 = 500 mm Hg × .21
    Answer: PIO_2 = 105 mm Hg

Chapter 6

Keys to the Highway

Computereze
hardware (page 110), software (page 113), disks (page 111), CD-ROMs (page 111)

Talk to me!
Internet, (page 117), modem (page 117)

Computers in Health Care

1. Page 118, 119
   A. Laboratory information management
   B. Nursing care documentation
   C. Resource scheduling
   D. Billing systems
   E. Patient data/medical records
   F. Direct interface to diagnostic equipment

2. Page 121
   A. Monitoring—ventilation, hemodynam-
      ics, ECG
   B. Diagnostic—ABG analyzers, PFTs

3. Page 124
   Monitoring systems can collect data and suggest actions or provide information (open-
   loop), or take actions automatically (closed-
   loop). The servo-controlled humidifier is the
   simplest example of a closed loop system.

4. Page 125
   A. Pulmonary function test interpretation
   B. Arterial blood gas interpretation
   C. Hemodynamic assessment
   D. ECG interpretation
   E. Fitness profiles

5. Pages 134, 135
   A. Confidentiality—Computers may allow
      access to sensitive information. Pass-
      words and other protection systems may
      help prevent this problem.
   B. Technical skills—"Black box mentality"
      and lack of technical understanding
      may result in practitioners who cannot
      detect failures in computerized systems.
      Computerized equipment adds the need
      for additional computer skills.
   C. Software errors/Patient harm—Just as
      software may fail or have incompatabili-
      ties in home computers, the same prob-
      lem occurs in health care with more
      serious consequences. The FDA now has
      quality guidelines for medical software.
   D. Lay access to medical information—
      There are two sides to this issue. Inter-
      net access has increased consumer
      knowledge. It also produces misinforma-
      tion. The Health on the Net Founda-
      tion (HON) established a code of con-
      duct for sites that provide health care
      information.

Case Studies (pages 115-130)

6. Database

7. Spreadsheet

8. Word processing

9. This question provides an opportunity for
   discussion/demonstration of the use and
   limitations of the word processing programs
   you use.

10. URL means Universal Resource Locator.
    (page 130)

11. A. Protocol
    B. Domain name
    C. Document location

12. A. HTTP protocol: http://—Web page
       transfer
    B. Domain name: www.aarc.org—Server's
       name
    C. Document location:
       /cpgs/cpg_index.html—Path on the
       server to the document you want to
       view

13. Use a bookmark (Netscape) or Favorite
    (Explorer)

Practice Makes Perfect!

Chapter 7

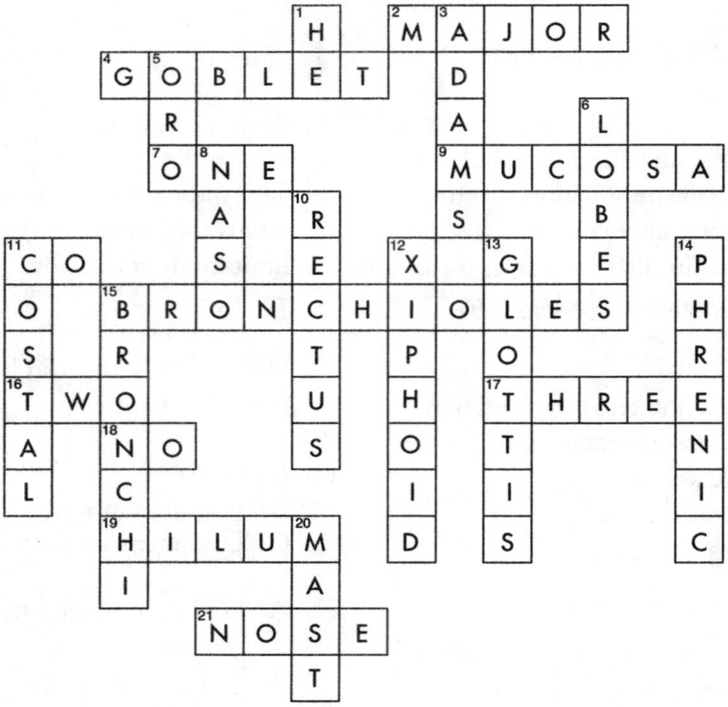
H M A J O R
G O B L E T D
R A L
O N E M U C O S A
A R S B
C O S E X G E P
O B R O N C H I O L E S H
S R T P O R
T W O U H T H R E E
A N O S O T N
L C I I I
H I L U M D S C
I A
N O S E
T

A Picture is worth a thousand . . .

1. (Figure 7-1, page 141)
   A. Apex (R)
   B. Right upper lobe
   C. Left upper lobe
   D. Right middle lobe
   E. Right lower lobe
   F. Left lower lobe

2. (Figure 7-2, page 141)
   A. Right midclavicular line
   B. Left midclavicular line
   C. Midsternal line

3. (Figure 7-3, page 142)
   A. Anterior axillary line
   B. Midaxillary line

4. (Figure 7-14, page 150)
   A. Scalenus anterior
   B. Sternomastoid
   C. Pectoralis major
   D. Internal intercostal
   E. Diaphragm
   F. Rectus abdominus

5. (Figure 7-19, page 158)
   A. Nasopharynx
   B. Oropharynx
   C. Hypopharynx
   D. Tongue
   E. Epiglottis
   F. Thyroid cartilage
   G. Cricothyroid membrane
   H. Cricoid cartilage

6. (Figure 7-24, page 162)
   A. Epiglottis
   B. Thyroid cartilage
   C. Cricothyroid ligament
   D. Cricoid cartilage
   E. Trachea

7. (Figure 7-30, page 167)
   A. Respiratory cilia
   B. Gel layer
   C. Sol layer

8. (Figure 7-34, page 171)
   A. Alveolar macrophage
   B. Pore of Kohn
   C. Capillary
   D. Alveolar type II cell
   E. Red blood cell
   F. Alveolar type I cell

Lobes and Segments (Table 7-3, page 165)

Right Lung	Left Lung
Right upper lobe	*Left upper lobe*
	Upper portion
1. Apical	1 and 2. Apical posterior
2. Posterior	
3. Anterior	3. Anterior
Right middle lobe	*Lower portion (lingula)*
4. Lateral	4. Superior
5. Medial	5. Inferior
Right lower lobe	*Left lower lobe*
6. Superior	6. Superior
7. Medial basal	7 and 8. Anteromedial
8. Anterior basal	
9. Lateral basal	9. Lateral basal
10. Posterior basal	10. Posterior basal

Meet the Objectives

9. Page 153
   A. Diaphragm: Phrenic nerve, C3-5; injury results in paralysis of diaphragms.
   B. Intercostal: Intercostal nerves, T2-T11; injury results in decreased respiratory muscle function, both inspiratory and expiratory.
   C. Larynx: Recurrent laryngeal nerves, branches of vagus nerves, injury results in vocal cord paralysis, hoarseness, loss of voice, ineffective cough.

10. Page 157

Division	Function
A. Nasal cavity	Conduct gas, warm, filter, humidify
B. Oral cavity	Digestion, speech, accessory respiratory passage
C. Pharynx	Conduct gas, protective functions during swallowing
D. Larynx	Conduct gas, protective functions during swallowing, phonation

11. Table 7-4, page 166
    Air passes through the conducting airways: trachea, mainstem bronchi, lobar bronchi, segmental bronchi, subsegmental bronchi, bronchi, and terminal bronchi. Next it enters the smaller airways: bronchioles and terminal bronchioles. Gas exchange occurs: respiratory bronchioles, terminal respiratory bronchioles, alveolar ducts, and finally the alveoli.

Chapter Highlights (page 174)

12. Thorax
13. Diaphragm
14. Heats and humidifies, foreign
15. Conducts, zones
16. Lobes, segments
17. Alveoli, surface

Case Studies (pages 145-160)

18. The lung would collapse.
19. Air would enter the pleural space.
20. Pneumothorax
21. Insertion of a chest tube.
22. Narrowing of the oropharynx and hypopharynx. Relaxation of the tongue and other muscles. Obesity contributes to the problem.

23. OSA is a condition in which the upper airway closes during sleep even though respiratory efforts continue. Treatment includes CPAP, medications, weight loss, and surgery.

24. Both of these groups have upper airway obstruction, partial or complete.

25. A head-tilt maneuver (extension) would be appropriate in many cases.

More on this subject in Chapter 30.

Food for Thought

26. Airways narrow due to smooth muscle contraction, mucosal edema, and increased secretions. The alveoli are not directly affected by asthma (initially).

27. Emphysema results in destructive changes to the small airways and alveoli. Loss of elastic tissue occurs. Loss of alveolar surface area for gas exchange occurs.

Chapter 8

Language of the Heart
1. Afterload   <u>F</u>

2. Automaticity   <u>H</u>

3. Baroreceptors   <u>D</u>

4. Cardiac output   <u>B</u>

5. Chemoreceptors   <u>G</u>

6. Pericardium   <u>A</u>

7. Preload   <u>C</u>

8. Stenosis   <u>E</u>

Meet the Objectives
9. Page 177
   Pulmonary edema and decreased compliance.

10. Page 180
    Special properties of heart muscle tissue include conductivity and inherent rhythmicity (automaticity). Nodal tissues, bundle branches, and Purkinje fibers coordinate conduction. Nodal tissues conduct impulses slowly (5cm/sec), which allows time for the ventricles to fill. Purkinje fibers conduct impulses at 400 cm/sec, which results in coordinated ventricular muscle fiber contraction.

11. Page 184
    Local control involves smooth muscle tone in vessels. It is affected by perfusion pressures and metabolic substances such as oxygen, lactic acid, and carbon dioxide. This is mostly occurring in the capillary beds. Central control mainly involves the sympathetic division of the autonomic nervous system. Adrenergic beta-receptors respond to norepinephrine. Central control is primarily precapillary in nature.

12. Page 184
    In exercise, the vascular beds dilate to prevent increased pressure in the face of increased blood flow. When blood loss occurs, the vessels constrict to try to increase pressure back to normal.

13. Page 191-192

Electrical Event	Mechanical Event
A. P wave	Atrial depolarization
B. QRS complex	Ventricular depolarization
C. T wave	Ventricular repolarization

Chapter Highlights (page 192)
14. cardiovascular, homeostasis

15. output, afterload, heart rate

16. sympathetic, autonomic

17. metabolic

18. arterioles (Page 181)

19. Purkinje

Case Studies (Pages 177, 187)

20. Narrowing of the mitral valve

21. Increased resistance to blood flow raises the pressure in the left atrium. Pressure in the pulmonary vascular bed also increases. Increased hydrostatic pressure results in fluid being forced into the pulmonary interstitial spaces.

22. Hypoxemia should be treated with oxygen administration.

23. A. Sympathetic stimulation increases rate, contractility or both
    B. Parasympathetic stimulation decreases heart rate.

24. A. Sympathomimetic—Mimics the effect of sympathetic stimulation to cause smooth muscle relaxation in the airway.
    B. Parasympatholytic—Blocks the smooth muscle constriction caused by parasympathetic stimulation.

25. Increased stimulation of the heart may accompany airway muscle relaxation due to receptor stimulation. Heart rate should increase no more than 20 during a treatment.

Food for Thought

26. Page 182
    A. Sympathetic venous tone
    B. Skeletal muscle pumping (milking) of vessels (plus valves)
    C. Cardiac suction
    D. Thoracic pressure differences caused by ventilation

27. The thoracic pump describes the effect of inspiration on venous return to the chest. As intrathoracic pressure drops, blood flow is enhanced from the abdominal vessels and the head. Positive pressure ventilation like IPPB, impedes venous return by increasing intrathoracic pressure.

Just for Fun . . . ?

L	N	A	V	C	H	O	R	D	A	E	E	Y	Y
A	A	Y	O	E	R	L	V	T	J	N	B	R	O
R	Y	R	T	R	I	G	O	H	D	A	E	U	T
T	R	H	T	I	T	N	J	O	R	T	T	T	R
E	A	G	Z	I	C	A	T	O	R	P	A	P	I
R	L	A	U	T	M	I	R	A	U	R	K	N	C
I	L	Y	F	K	O	E	T	T	C	G	W	K	U
O	I	U	O	W	C	C	D	A	V	A	H	I	S
L	P	E	O	E	A	C	M	I	M	A	Z	D	P
E	A	D	P	R	H	C	T	N	T	O	L	I	I
S	C	T	D	E	E	E	H	B	T	O	T	V	D
P	O	I	M	D	A	O	L	E	R	P	R	U	E
R	A	O	D	A	O	L	R	E	T	F	A	A	A
C	F	M	U	I	D	R	A	C	I	R	E	P	C

AFTERLOAD   CHORDAE
AORTA   ENDO
ARTERIOLES   MITRAL
ARTERY   OUTPUT
AUTOMATICITY   PERICARDIUM
BARORECEPTOR   PRELOAD
CAPILLARY   TRICUSPID
CARDIAC   VALVE
CAROTID   VEIN
CHEMO

Chapter 9

(Figure 9-1, page 197)

First Things First

<u>Ventilation</u>, <u>acidemia</u>, <u>spirometer</u>, <u>plethysmograph</u>, <u>pneumotachometer</u>, <u>work</u>, <u>respiration</u>, <u>ascites</u>, <u>kyphoscoliosis</u>, <u>ankylosing spondylitis</u>, <u>distensible</u>

Picture this . . .

1. (Figure 9-1, page 197)
   A. Transrespiratory pressure
   B. Transpulmonary pressure
   C. Transthoracic pressure

Can I have another . . . ?

2. (Figure 9-14, page 209)
   A. Apex: -10 cm H_2O
   B. Base: -2.5 cm H_2O

3. The base of the lung

Work of Breathing

4. PEEP or CPAP therapy

5. Pursed-lip breathing, slow deep breaths (page 206)

6. Smooth muscle spasm (bronchospasm), mucosal edema, increased secretions

7. Bronchodilators, cromolyn sodium, nedocromil, inhaled steroids (See Chapter 28)

8. Active exhalation is a sign of respiratory distress. You have to look for the cause of the distress and try to eliminate it.

9. Patients who cannot use their abdominal muscles frequently have difficulty coughing. Assisted cough techniques may be needed.

10. Slow deep breaths and exhalation against pursed lips (page 206)

11. Work of breathing is a complex subject. This is a good time to review and see your instructor if you have not gained a basic understanding of the factors that affect WOB.

Deadspace

12. A. Anatomic deadspace (VD anatomic)
    B. Physiologic deadspace (VD physiologic)
    C. Alveolar deadspace (VD alveolar)

13. One ml per pound of ideal body weight (2.2 ml/kg) or 150 ml (pages 211-212)

14. The patient will try to increase minute ventilation by increasing rate and/or volume. (Page 213)

15. Hyperventilation is excessive ventilation that results in a lower $PaCO_2$. Hyperpnea is increased ventilation that occurs when metabolic rate is increased, such as in exercise. (Page 214)

Mathemagic

16. Page 211
    Formula: Minute ventilation = tidal volume × frequency
    Calculation: 800 ml × 8 breaths per minute = 6400 ml
    Answer: Minute ventilation = 6.4 L/min.

17. Page 211
    Formula: Anatomic deadspace = 1 ml per pound of body weight.
    Calculation: 180 lbs × 1 ml
    Answer: Anatomic deadspace = 180 ml

18. Page 211
    Formula: Alveolar ventilation = frequency (Tidal volume − deadspace)
    Calculation: Alveolar ventilation = 8 (800 − 180)
    Answer: Alveolar ventilation = 4.96 L/min

19. D. 7200 ml (Page 211)

20. A. 3200 ml (Page 211)

21. A. 10   600 (Page 213)

Chapter 10

All Aboard

oxyhemoglobin, Bohr, carbaminohemoglobin, Haldane, carboxyhemoglobin, (page 210)

I think we're in Kansas

Kansas, Ranier, methemoglobin, sickle cell

Mathemagic

1. Page 216
   Formula: $PAO_2 = (PB - PH_2) FIO_2 - PaCO_2 \div 0.8$
   Solution: $PAO_2 = 713 \times 0.21 - 40 \div 0.8$ or 149.73-50
   Answer: $PAO_2 = 99.73$ mm Hg (100)

2. Page 217
   Formula: A-a gradient = $PAO_2 - PaO_2$
   Solution: A-a gradient = 100 − 90
   Answer: A-a gradient = 10 mm Hg

3. Page 217
   Formula: $PAO_2 = (PB - PH_2O) FIO_2 - PaCO_2$ ...(FIO_2 is ≥ 0.6)
   Solution: $PAO_2 = 713 \times 0.6 - 40$ or 428 − 40
   Answer: 388 mm Hg

4. Formula: A-a gradient = $PAO_2 - PaO_2$
   Solution: A-a gradient = 388 − 90
   Answer: A-a gradient = 298 mm Hg

Kodak Moment

5. A. Red blood cells
   B. Capillary membrane
   C. Interstitial fluid
   D. Alveolar membrane
   E. Pulmonary surfactant

Mathemagic

6. Page 223
   Formula: Oxygen content = $1.34 \times Hb \times SaO_2 + PaO_2 \times 0.003$
   Solution: $1.34 \times 15 \times 0.97 + 100 \times 0.003$ or 19.50 + 0.3
   Answer: 19.53 volume percent or 19.53 ml/dl

7. Page 223
   Formula: Oxygen content = $1.34 \times Hb \times SaO_2 + PaO_2 \times 0.003$
   Solution: $1.34 \times 15 \times 0.80 + 50 \times 0.003$ or 16.08 + 0.150
   Answer: 16.32 volume percent or 16.53 ml/dl

8. Page 223
   Formula: Oxygen content = $1.34 \times Hb \times SaO_2 + PaO_2 \times 0.003$
   Solution: $1.34 \times 10 \times 0.97 + 100 \times 0.003$ or 12.998 (13) + 0.3
   Answer: 13.3 volume percent or 13.3 ml/dl

Throw me a curve

For questions 9-12: (Please note that the numbers in Egan are slightly different than other texts.)

	PaO_2	SaO_2
9.	40 mm Hg	70%
10.	50 mm Hg	80%
11.	60 mm Hg	90%
12.	100 mm Hg	97%

For questions 13-18

	Factor	Shift
13.	Acidosis	Right
14.	Hypothermia	Left
15.	High 2,3 DPG	Left
16.	Fever	Right
17.	Hypercapnia	Right
18.	Carboxyhemoglobin	Left

Bad Gas Exchange

19. Hypoxia (page 232)

20. Hypoxemia (page 232)

21. Shunt (page 232)

22. Perfusion (page 232)

23. Diffusion (page 233)

24. Shock (page 232)

25. Ischemia (page 236)

26. Dead (page 237)

27. Minute or alveolar (page 233)

28. Perfusion (page 237)

Bohr-ed Exams

29. B. Acute hyperventilation

30. B. 12.97 ml O_2/dl (page 223)

31. A. 97 mm Hg (page 217)

Case in Point

32. Pulse oximeters are unreliable when abnormal hemoglobins are present.

33. Carbon monoxide poisoning

34. Give oxygen. Consider hyperbaric chamber. (page 229)

35. Hypoxia

36. Loss of 2,3-DPG (page 228)

37. Lots of possibilities-Blood reaction, pain, small pneumothorax, surgical complications

38. Arterial blood gas, consider co-oximetry

39. The CO_2 level is low, indicating hyperventilation. The oxygen level indicates mild hypoxemia. Hyperventilation raises the level of oxygen, which would be lower with normal ventilation.

40. Hemoglobin (page 223)

41. Absolute anemia is simply a low level of hemoglobin in the blood. It results in a low oxygen content. Blood transfusion is the immediate treatment. (pages 233, 235)

42. Drug overdose results in decreased alveolar ventilation, which results in an increased CO_2 level. (page 233)

43. Decreased alveolar ventilation may result in a lowered P_{AO_2} simply because the CO_2 is elevated. (page 233)

Food for Thought

44. Cyanide poisoning (page 236)

45. (Septic shock, ARDS) When oxygen demand exceeds oxygen delivery. (page 236)

46. When oxygen is inadequate for cellular metabolism, lactic acid is formed. (page 236)

Chapter 11

Drowning in Words

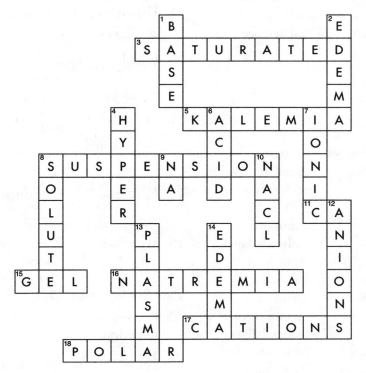

Water, water everywhere . . .

1. Page 249.

   <u>3</u>   Males
   <u>5</u>   Newborns
   <u>4</u>   Children
   <u>2</u>   Females
   <u>1</u>   Obese individuals

2. Page 249 (Answers given for an adult male as percent of total body weight.)

Compartment	%H_2O
A. Intracellular	45 (also listed as ⅔ of total body H_2O)
B. Extracellular	15-20 (also ⅓ of total body H_2O)
1. Interstitial	11-15 (also as 15% of body weight)
2. Intravascular	4.5 (also 5% of body weight)

Where has all the water gone, long time passing. . . .

	Source	Amount
3.	Sensible	1,200-1,400 ml/day
	A. Urine	1,000-1,200 ml
	B. Intestinal	200 ml
	C. Sweat	0 ml (up to 2,000 per hour max)
4.	Insensible	900 ml/day
	A. Skin	700 ml
	B. Lung	200 ml

5. 1,000 ml of fluid is lost for each degree of temperature above 99° F that persists for 24 hours or more. (page 250)

6. Table 11-4 (page 250)

Source	Amount
A. Ingestion	2,000-2,600 ml/day
1. Fluids	1,500-2,000 ml
2. Solids	500-600 ml
B. Body metabolism	250 ml average

Electrifying Information

7. Pages 253-255

Electrolyte	Symbol	Purpose
A. Sodium	Na	Regulates total body water
B. Chloride	Cl	Anion that maintains electrolyte balance
C. Bicarbonate	HCO_3	Acid-base balance
D. Potassium	K	Cation that maintains electrolyte balance
E. Calcium	Ca	Neuromuscular, cellular enzyme function
F. Magnesium	Mg	Muscle function, neural conduction
G. Phosphorus	HPO_4	Energy metabolism

8. B Bicarbonate   A. 140 mEq/L

9. D Calcium   B. 24 mEq/L

10. E Chloride   C. 4.0 mEq/L

11. G Magnesium   D. 5.0 mEq/L

12. F Phosphorus   E. 100 mEq/L

13. C Potassium   F. 1.2 mEq/L

14. A Sodium   G. 1.3 mEq/L

Answers in Table 11-5, page 253

For questions 15-19.

	Imbalance	Cause	Symptom
15.	Hyponatremia	Sweating	Weakness, apathy
16.	Hypokalemia	Diuretics, steroids	Muscle weakness, paralysis
17.	Hypo-phospatemia	Starvation	Diaphragmatic weakness
18.	Hypercalcemia	Hyperthyroidism	Fatigue, depression
19.	Hyperkalemia	Chronic renal disease	ECG changes

Case Studies (page 252)

20. A low-sodium diet helps to prevent water retention.

21. Potassium is replaced intravenously in the hospital, with supplements in the home.

22. Pulse oximetry or arterial blood gases to assess oxygenation and ventilation. Oxygen is likely to be the initial treatment to treat hypoxemia and reduce work of the heart.

23. Pulmonary edema resulting from fluid backing up in the lung secondary to ventricular failure.

24. Albumin. Mr. Wilson is malnourished. (pages 250-251)

25. When blood protein levels are low, hydrostatic pressure in the capillaries forces fluid out into the lungs resulting in interstitial edema. (page 252)

26. Pulse oximetry or arterial blood gases to assess oxygenation and ventilation. Oxygen is likely to be the initial treatment.

Mathemagic

27. Page 246
    Formula: W/V solutions = grams of solute per 100 ml solution
    Solution: A 5% solution = 5 grams of solute per 100 ml
    Answer: 5

28. Page 246
    Formula: Mg = ml x percent
    Solution: 1 ml $\times$ 5
    Answer: 5 mg

29. Page 246
    Formula: C1 $\times$ V1 = C2 $\times$ V2
    Solution: 5% $\times$ 1 ml = ? $\times$ 3 ml or
    0.05 $\times$ 1 $\div$ 3
    Answer: 0.0166% (or 0.017%)

What About Those Board Exams?

30. D. ECG rhythm (page 253)

31. C. I and III only (pages 253-254)

32. D. Increased hematocrit.

33. C. 0.90% (pages 243-244)

Food for Thought

34. Draws water out of cells. (page 243)

35. Cells absorb the water. (page 243)

36. Osmosis (page 243)

Chapter 12

Interpret What?

1. **J** Acidemia

2. **A** Volatile acid

3. **H** Anion gap

4. **C** Hyperventilation

5. **K** Metabolic acidosis

6. **B** Alkalemia

7. **F** Kussmaul's breathing

8. **O** Hypoventilation

9. **E** Fixed acid

10. **I** Respiratory alkalosis

11. **G** Metabolic alkalosis

12. **M** Standard bicarbonate

13. **N** Base excess

14. **D** Respiratory acidosis

15. **L** Buffer

Where has all the acid gone?

16. Page 258
    Ventilation
    $$CO_2 + H_2O \leftarrow H_2CO_3 \leftarrow HCO_3^- + H^+$$
    $$\uparrow$$
    $$HHb \rightarrow H^\ddagger Hb^-$$

17. Increased ventilation eliminates CO_2, which "pulls" the hydration reaction to the left, which compensates for increased fixed acids. (page 258)

18. Buffers are a mixture of acid and base components. (page 259)

19. Bicarbonate reacts to form the weaker carbonic acid and a neutral salt (NaCl). (page 259)

20. Bicarbonate buffers (open system)— carbonic acid+bicarbonate ions (page 259) Nonbicarbonate buffers (closed system)— phosphates and proteins (Hb)

21. Ventilation actually removes CO_2. It is the bicarbonate that combines with the Hydrogen ions. (page 259)

22. The kidney is responsible for the removal of fixed acids. This action is necessary in addition to lung removal of CO_2 to maintain normal balance. (page 262) Kidneys also affect HCO_3 levels. (page 263)

Balancing Act

23. Page 267

	Low Normal	to High Normal
A. pH	7.35	7.45
B. $PaCO_2$	35 mm Hg	45 mm Hg
C. HCO_3^-	22 mEq/L	26 mEq/L

24. Page 260
$$pH = \frac{6.1 + \log[HCO_3]}{(PCO_2 \times 0.03)}$$

25. Table 12-4, page 268

Disorder	Primary defect	Compensation
A. Respiratory acidosis	Increased $PaCO_2$	Increased HCO_3
B. Respiratory alkalosis	Decreased $PaCO_2$	Decreased HCO_3
C. Metabolic acidosis	Decreased HCO_3	Decreased $PaCO_2$
D. Metabolic alkalosis	Increased HCO_3	Increased $PaCO_2$

26. The plasma HCO_3 rises by 1 mEq/L for every 10 mm Hg increase in $PaCO_2$ above 40 mm Hg. (page 268)

27. Plasma bicarbonate rises by approximately 5 mEq/L for each 10 mm Hg increase in $PaCO_2$. (page 272)

Try it, You'll Like it!

28. pH 7.34
$PaCO_2$ 60 mm Hg
HCO_3^- 331 mEq/L (page 271)

Partially compensated respiratory acidosis. The pH shows acidosis. The $PaCO_2$ shows acidosis.

The bicarbonate is elevated higher than the expected change for acute respiratory acidosis (We would expect 28).

29. pH 7.38
$PaCO_2$ 60 mm Hg
$HCOO_3^-$ 34 mEq/L

Compensated respiratory acidosis. The pH is within the normal range, but on the acid side of 7.40. The bicarbonate is significantly elevated, suggesting a chronic problem.

Welcome to the Gap!

30. Box 12-4, page 275
    A. Lactic acidosis
    B. Ketoacidosis
    C. Renal failure

31. Dyspnea and hyperpnea. Kussmaul's breathing may be present. (page 275)

32. Neurologic symptoms range from lethargy to coma. (page 275)

Bicarb Blues

33. Page 268
    Formula: Predicted HCO_3 = 24 + (Measured $PaCO_2$ − 40) ÷ 10
    Solution: Predicted HCO_3 = 24 + (50 − 40) ÷ 10
    Answer: Predicted HCO_3 = 25

34. Page 268
    Formula: Predicted HCO_3 = 24 + (Measured $PaCO_2$ − 40) ÷ 10
    Solution: Predicted HCO_3 = 24 + (70 − 40) ÷ 10
    Answer: Predicted HCO_3 = 27

35. Page 272
    Formula: Predicted HCO_3 = 24 + (Measured $PaCO_2$ − 40) ÷ 2
    Solution: Predicted HCO_3 = 24 + (70 − 40) ÷ 2
    Answer: Predicted HCO_3 = 39

Hassle?

36. Page 260

    Formula: $pH = 6.1 + \log(HCO_3) \div [PaCO_2 \times 0.03]$

    Solution: $pH = 6.1 + \log(30) \div [40 \times 0.03)$

    Answer: $pH = 6.1 + \log 30 \div 1.2$ or $6.1 + \log 25$ or $6.1 + 1.4 = 7.5$

37. Formula: $pH = 6.1 + \log(HCO_3) \div [PaCO_2 \times 0.03]$

    Solution: $pH = 6.1 + \log(24) \div [40 \times 0.03)$

    Answer: $pH = 6.1 + \log 24 \div 1.2$ or $6.1 + \log 16.7$ or $6.1 + 1.22 = 7.32$

38. Formula: $pH = 6.1 + \log(HCO_3) \div [PaCO_2 \times 0.03]$

    Solution: $pH = 6.1 + \log(24) \div [60 \times 0.03)$

    Answer: $pH = 6.1 + \log 24 \div 1.8$ or $6.1 + \log 13.33$ or $6.1 + 1.12 = 7.22$

Gap?

39. Formula: $Anion\ gap = Na - (Cl + HCO_3)$

    Solution: $Anion\ gap = 140 - (105 + 24)$

    Answer: $Anion\ gap = 11$. This is a normal gap. Normal gaps accompanying acidosis are the result of lots of bicarbonate. The most common cause is diarrhea.

40. Formula: $Anion\ gap = Na - (Cl + HCO_3)$

    Solution: $Anion\ gap = 140 - (105 + 12)$

    Answer: $Anion\ gap = 23$. Elevated gaps accompanying metabolic acidosis are the result of lactic acidosis, keto acid, renal failure, or acid ingestion.

Case Studies

42. Acute respiratory acidosis. The elevation of the bicarbonate is secondary to the acutely increased CO_2. (p. 268)

43. Hypoventilation secondary to CNS depression from the drug overdose

44. Acute respiratory alkalosis (page 272)

45. Hyperventilation secondary to anxiety. (page 272)

46. Acute metabolic alkalosis. (page 275)

47. Loss of hydrogen ions from vomiting. (page 275)

48. Acute metabolic acidosis (page 274)

49. Ketoacidosis secondary to diabetes. (page 274)

50. Compensated respiratory acidosis (page 271)

51. Retention of bicarbonate by the kidney (page 271)

52. Compensated metabolic acidosis (page 275)

53. Hyperventilation to achieve respiratory alkalosis (page 275)

54. Partially compensated metabolic alkalosis (page 276)

55. Hypokalemia is a possible cause of metabolic alkalosis (see Box 12-5, page 276). Other possibilities are loss of chloride, bicarb ingestion, and hypovolemia.

What About Those Board Exams?

56. D. I and III only (page 276)

57. D. Normal ABG (pages 262-263)

58. A. Increase the rate of ventilation (page 270)

59. C. Uncompensated hyperventilation (page 272)

60. C. Kussmaul's breathing (page 275)

Food for Thought

61. Acute respiratory alkalosis superimposed on chronic respiratory acidosis (page 273)

62. Grandpa is hypoxemic and is hyperventilating to try to bring up his PO_2.

Chapter 13

Reading, Writing, and Regulating

```
            ¹V
²R E C E ³P T O R S   ⁴M   A
        O       ⁵H E R I N G
    ⁶A P N E A   D       A
    P   S       U       L
    N           L
    ⁹P E R I P H E R A L   ⁸C
    U       N   A       H
    S       T           E
¹⁰B I O T S   ¹¹I R R I T A N T
    I       A           E
    ¹²C S F   L
```

Where's the Action (Fig. 13-1, p. 284)

1. A. Pons
   B. Medulla oblongata
   C. Spinal cord
   D. Pneumotaxic center
   E. Apneustic center
   F. Dorsal respiratory groups
   G. Ventral respiratory groups

2. Dorsal groups send impulses to the motor nerves of the diaphragm and external intercostals. They receive impulses from the vagus and glossopharyngeal nerves and others. Ventral groups send impulses to the laryngeal and pharyngeal muscles, and to the internal intercostals and abdominal muscles. (page 284)

3. The apneustic center is an ill-defined area. If the nerves to it are cut, a breathing pattern of prolonged inspiratory gasps is initiated. The pneumotaxic center controls inspiratory time. The exact relationship of the apneustic and pneumotaxic centers is poorly understood. Together they appear to control depth of inspiration. (page 285)

4. Head trauma, cerebral hypoxia, narcotics, decreased cerebral blood flow, alkalosis, and COPD or other conditions with increased CO_2. (pages 290-291)

Automatic Pilot (pages 285-286)

For questions 5-10.

	Reflex	Stimulus	Response	Location
5.	Hering Breuer	Inflation	Inhibition via vagus	Airway muscle
6.	Deflation	Collapse	Strong insp. effort	?
7.	Head	Inflation	Increased effort	?
8.	Vago-vagal	Physical irritation	Cough, sneeze, tachypnea, bronchospasm	Epithelium in airways
9.	C fiber	Alveolar inflammation	Rapid shallow breaths, dypsnea	Near the capillaries
10.	Proprioceptor	Movement, pain	Stimulate ventilation	Muscle, tendon

Central Chemoreceptors

11. CO_2 diffuses from the blood into the CSF. There it reacts to water and forms hydrogen ions and bicarbonate. The hydrogen ions stimulate the chemoreceptors. (page 287)

12. Increases of only 2 mm Hg cause an almost instantaneous increase in ventilation. This response declines over 1-2 days as compensation from bicarbonate occurs. (page 287)

Peripheral Chemoreceptors

13. Peripheral receptors respond to decreased PaO_2 levels in arterial blood by stimulating ventilation. (page 288)

14. Drive to breathe is increased as PaO_2 drops below 60 mm Hg. This increases until the PaO_2 falls to 30 mm Hg. PO_2 below 30 mm Hg exhibits a depressant effect. (page 288)

15. Increased ventilation at altitude results in alkalemia, which decreases the central drive to breathe. As compensation occurs, the drive to breathe increases again at about 24 hours to its maximum level. (page 288)

16. Peripheral receptors account for about 20%-30% of the ventilatory response to hypercapnia. This response is by hypoxemia. Peripheral receptors respond more rapidly than central receptors because they are directly exposed to arterial blood. (page 288)

No One Understands Me!

17. Low concentrations: 24%-28% (page 290)

18. Arterial blood gases allow you to monitor oxygen, carbon dioxide, and blood pH. (page 290)

19. COPD patients usually do not have shunting. Also, their blood oxygen levels are usually on the steep part of the Hb-O_2 dissociation curve, so small increases in PaO_2 lead to large increases in saturation. (page 290)

Ouch!

20. Respiratory rate and tidal volume gradually increase, then decrease, followed by a period of apnea. Then the cycle repeats. CHF, low cardiac output, and brain injuries may cause Cheyne-Stokes. (page 290)

21. Biot's breathing is caused by increased ICP. It is similar to Cheyne-Stokes, except that the tidal volumes are constant. (page 290)

22. Apneustic breathing indicates damage to the pons. (page 290) It is a gasping pattern with poorly defined expirations. (page 285)

23. The two patterns are central neurogenic hyperventilation and hypoventilation. Head trauma, severe brain hypoxia, and decreased cerebral blood flow are possible causes. (pages 290-291)

Case Studies

24. Deliberate hyperventilation to achieve CO_2 levels of 25-30 mm Hg to reduce intracranial pressure by cerebral vasoconstriction. (page 291)

25. As compensation occurs, the vasoconstrictive effect diminishes. (page 291)

26. Reduce the inspired oxygen. This will reduce the PaO_2 and increase stimulus to breathe. You can also stimulate Grandpa to take deep breaths and blow off some of that CO_2 and improve his V/Q. (pages 289-290)

27. A PaO_2 of about 60% will produce adequate oxygenation and maintain drive. (pages 289-290)

What About Those Board Exams?

28. A. 28% Venturi mask (page 290)

29. B. Administer oxygen via 24% Venturi mask (page 290)

30. C. Change the oxygen to 2 L/min via nasal cannula (page 290)

31. C. Increase rate and volume of ventilation with a resuscitation bag (page 291)

Experiment

32 Breath-holding time should increase with moderate hyperventilation.

33. Pulse oximeter readings shouldn't vary too much.

34. Hyperventilation reduces arterial CO_2. Since this is what stimulates you to breathe, breath-holding time should increase. Free-divers use this technique to increase time under water. The pulse oximeter readings don't change because the length of time is not sufficient to significantly reduce the level of oxygen in the blood.

35. The new breath holding time should be even longer than the previous ones.

36. 20 minutes is the theoretical maximum. This is limited by a person's response to drive induced by CO_2. The response varies.

Students who are interested in this subject will find some research papers available in the literature.

Food for Thought

37. Since respiratory rate is under conscious control, an individual may alter their rate when they are being observed. (page 284)

38. Pain, fear, anxiety. Pain may further modify breathing, depending on its location.

Chapter 14

Word Power

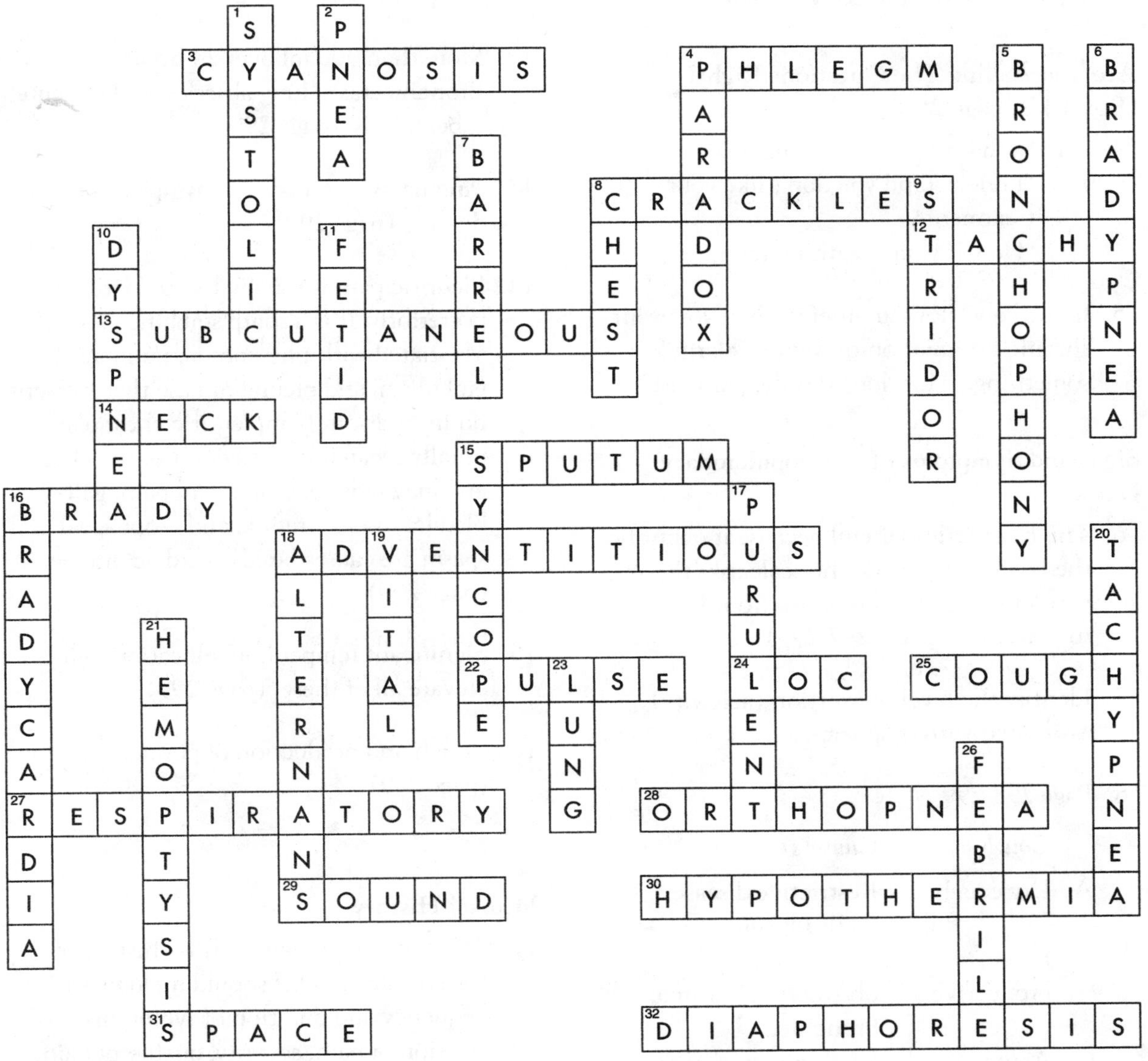

1 SYSTOLIC
2 PNEA
3 CYANOSIS
4 PHLEGM
4 PARADOX
5 BRONCHOPHONY
6 BRADYPNEA
7 BARREL
8 CRACKLES
8 CHEST
9 STRIDOR
10 DYSPNEA
11 FETID
12 TACHY
13 SUBCUTANEOUS
14 NECK
15 SPUTUM
15 SYNCOPE
16 BRADY
16 BRADYCARDIA
17 PURULENT
18 ADVENTITIOUS
18 ALTERNAN
19 VITAL
20 TACHYPNEA
21 HEMOPTYSIS
22 PULSE
23 LUNG
24 LOC
25 COUGH
26 FEBRILE
27 RESPIRATORY
28 ORTHOPNEA
29 SOUND
30 HYPOTHERMIA
31 SPACE
32 DIAPHORESIS

Start at the very beginning . . .

1. Read the patient's medical record to determine history of present illness, chief complaint, past medical history, family/environmental history, and the systems review. (page 300)
2. Give a brief introduction of who you are and the purpose for the visit. Stay in the social space, about 4-12 feet away. Provide privacy if the room is not private by drawing the curtain. Move closer to the personal space and try to place yourself at eye level. (page 296)

3. Box 14-1, page 297
   A2. "Good morning Mr. Johnson."
   B2. Sit in a chair at the bedside
   C2. Keep your clipboard on your lap
   D1. "Do you need anything right now?"
   E1. "I'll be back to see you in one hour"

Are You Asking The Questions Right? (Box 14-2, page 298)

4. A1. "What are you coughing up?"
   B1. "I understand you don't like your treatments.
   C1. "How is your breathing today?"

5. Closed questions are useful when you want specific information or want to clarify something. "How long did the pain last?"

Signs and Symptoms of Cardiopulmonary Disease

6. The Borg scale is useful because it quantifies the level of dyspnea. The scale asks the patient to rate their dyspnea from 1, least, to 10, worst. (pages 297-298)

7. Identify the level of exertion (acitivity) associated with dyspnea.

8. Page 298-299

Cough	Cause(s)
A. Dry cough	Restrictive disease: CHF, fibrosis
B. Loose, productive	Inflammation, obstruction: asthma, bronchitis
C. Acute, self-limiting	Viral infection of the upper airway
D. Chronic	Asthma, postnasal drip, reflux, chronic bronchitis

9. Mucus is normally produced by healthy airways. When the amount of mucus is increased and expectorated it is called sputum. (page 299)

10. Color, viscosity, and quantity should be charted. (page 299)

11. Small amounts of blood associated with infection, lung cancer, tuberculosis, trauma, and pulmonary embolism. (page 299)

12. More than 300 ml over 24 hours. Bronchiectasis, lung abscess, aold or acute tuberculosis. (page 299)

13. Angina, which may be a symptom of heart disease. (page 299)

14. Pleuritic pain is usually located laterally or posteriorly. It is a sharp stabbing pain associated with pneumonia, pulmonary embolism, and pleural disease that worsens on inspiration. Nonpleuritic chest pain is usually located in the center of the chest and may radiate. Chest wall pain, gall-bladder disease, reflux, and esophageal spasm are causes besides cardiac disease. (page 299)

15. Significant temperature elevations will elevate all of these. (page 299)

16. Cough and production of purulent sputum. (page 299)

Medical History

17. CC—chief complaint. HPI—history of present illness. HPI should include: Onset, frequency and duration of symptoms, location of pain, severity, quality of pain, aggravating and alleviating factors, associated manifestations. (Box 14-3, page 301)

18. PMH means past medical history and should include childhood diseases, hospitalizations (injuries, major illness), allergies, drugs and medications. (pages 300-301)

19. Page 300-301

	Finding	Significance
A.	Weak, emaciated	General ill health and diaphoretic malnutrition Fever, stress, acute anxiety
B.	Appears anxious	Severity of problem; level of cooperation
C.	Sitting up, leaning with arms on table	Typical position for patients with obstructive lung diseases such as emphysema

Is anyone home?

20. An alert, well-oriented person knows who they are, where they are, and the time or day. (page 302)

21. Lethargic refers to a sleepy patient that is easily aroused and responds appropriately when aroused. Obtunded patients are difficult to arouse, but still respond appropriately once aroused. (Box 14-5, page 302)

22. Stuporous patients don't wake up completely. They do respond to pain, and may respond slowly to verbal stimulus. Comatose patients are unconscious, and have loss of reflexes and other response to stimuli. They usually don't move voluntarily. (Box 14-5, page 302)

23. The RCP should assess oxygenation. (page 302)

Vital Information

24. Pages 302-305

	Sign	Avg. Normal	Low	High
A.	Temperature	98.6 (37° C)	Hypothermia	Hyperthermia
B.	Pulse rate	72/ minute	Bradycardia <60	Tachycardia >100
C.	Respiratory rate	12-18	Bradypnea	Tachypnea
D.	Systolic BP	120 mm Hg	90 mm Hg	140 mm Hg
E.	Diastolic BP	80 mm Hg	90 mm Hg	60 mm Hg

25. Page 303

	Site	Disadvantage
A.	Oral	Can't be used with all patients. Affected by food, etc.
B.	Axilla	Underestimates core temperature.
C.	Rectum	No fun! (But accurate)
D.	Ear	Requires special device.

26. Page 303-304
    A. % Tachycardia
    B. # Bruits
    C. @ Amplitude
    D. ! Paradoxical pulse
    E. * Pulsus alternans
    F. $ Bradycardia

27. A. % Tachypnea
    B. ! Eupnea
    C. # Orthopnea
    D. * Trepopnea
    E. $ Hyperpnea
    F. @ Bradypnea

28. Count their respiratory rate immediately after the pulse, while keeping your fingers on the wrist. (page 304)

29. Page 304
    A. Postural hypotension
    B. Move them slowly from supine to upright
    C. Administer fluid or vasoactive drugs

30. Page 305. Paradoxical pulse is present. Caused by decrease in intrathoracic pressure during inspiration. Usually caused by hyperinflation such as asthma, or cardiac restriction from tamponade. (page 304)

Examining the Chest and Lungs: The Big Four

31. Page 307

Bad Chests	Description
A. Barrel	Increased A-P diameter, horizontal slope of ribs
B. Kyphosis	Abnormal anteroposterior curvature of the spine
C. Kyphoscoliosis	Combination of kyphosis and scoliosis
D. Pectus carinatum	Abnormal protrusion of the sternum
E. Pectus excavatum	Abnormal depression of the sternum
F. Scoliosis	Abnormal lateral curvature of the spine

32. Page 308, and Table 14-1, page 308

Condition	Pattern of Breathing
A. Asthma	Prolonged exhalation, possible retractions
B. Atelectasis	Tachypnea—Rapid, shallow breathing
C. Chest trauma	Paradoxical chest wall movement
D. Epiglottitis	Prolonged inspiratory phase
E. Increased ICP	Biot's respirations—Irregular with periods of apnea
F. Metabolic acidosis	Kussmaul—Deep and fast

33. Outward excursion of the abdomen on inspiration is one sign.

34. Excessive motion of the neck, upper chest muscles.

35. Older individuals are more likely to have kyphotic and emphysematous changes.

36. Depends on where you live!

37. Vocal—Vibration produced by speech; Tactile—When you feel the vibration. (pages 308-309)

Rhonchial—Vibration produced by mucus.

38. Emphysema causes decreased fremitus because of hyperinflation. Pneumonia usually increases the intensity of fremitus because of consolidation. (page 309)

39. Subcutaneous air forms when air leaks from the lung and gets under the tissue layers of the skin. The crackling sensation is called crepitus. (pages 309-310)

Questions 40-42 require lab completion and instructor supervision.

40. Describe the temperature of your partner's skin.

41. Were there any areas of abnormal fremitus? Why (why not?)?

42. Estimate the amount of chest expansion in centimeters. What is normal adult expansion?

43. Page 310 Terms in parentheses are common but not used in the chapter.

Condition	Percussion Note
A. Emphysema	Increased resonance (Hyperresonant)
B. Atelectasis	Decreased resonance (Dull or flat)
C. Pleural effusion	Decreased resonance (Dull or flat)
D. Pneumothorax	Increased resonance (Hyperresonant or tympanic)
E. Pneumonia	Decreased resonance (Dull or flat)

44. Abnormalities that are small or deep can't be easily detected. (page 310)

45. Resonance should increase slightly with a deep breath, decrease with forced exhalation.

46. Table 14-2, page 313

Breath Sound	Pitch	Intensity	Where is it heard?
A. Vesicular	Low	Soft	Peripheral lung
B. Bronchial	High	Loud	Over trachea
C. Bronchovesicular	Moderate	Moderate	Upper chest, between scapulae

47. Coarse, low-pitched crackles are often caused by secretions being moved by air in the airways. Fine, end-inspiratory crackles are probably caused by sudden opening of peripheral airways and are associated with restrictive disorders like fibrosis, atelectasis, and pulmonary edema. (page 314)

48. Monophonic wheezes indicate a single obstructed airway. The wheezing may be heard on inspiration or expiration. Mucus or a foreign object might be the cause. Polyphonic wheezes suggest multiple obstructed airways and are heard on exhalation. They are most likely to be caused by bronchospasm or CHF. (page 314)

49. Rhonchi are low-pitched continuous sounds usually heard on exhalation. Crackles are discontinuous sounds that usually appear on inspiration, although they may be heard on exhalation (coarse). (Table 14-3, page 313)

Extremity Exam

50. Normal refill time is less than 3 seconds. It is assessed by pressing briefly on the fingernail. (page 318)

51. Usually the feet and legs are checked. Fluid settles there due to gravity. (page 318)

52. Page 318 Peripheral cyanosis may be caused by poor blood flow in the extremity. There are many causes. Central cyanosis is a sign of significant desaturation of hemoglobin. (page 306)

Case Studies

53. Obstructive lung disease—possibly emphysema. (page 307)

54. Sponginess of the nail. (page 317)

55. Lung cancer is a possible cause. (page 317)

56. Shock (low BP), causing poor cerebral perfusion. (page 304)

57. There is evidence of hypoxia. Pulse oximetry to assess oxygenation. (page 302)

58. Blood pressure. (page 304)

59. Ausculation and percussion may help reveal a pneumothorax.

60. While a chest tube is treatment for a pneumothorax, oxygen should be administered immediately.

61. A chest radiograph would help rule out a pneumothorax. An ECG would help rule out an MI, althought the history and nature of the pain do not suggest MI.

62. An air leak from the lungs.

63. Page 299 The history, crackles, and dry cough suggest an acute restrictive disease such as atelectasis or CHF. (page 298)

64. Chest radiograph.

65. Since Mr. Garcia has dyspnea, cough, tachypnea, and tachycardia, he may have hypoxia. Oxygen is indicated. If the chest radiograph shows atelectasis, a lung inflation procedure such as IS may be indicated. (page 298)

What About Those Board Exams?

66. B. The patient should be suctioned (page 308)

67. D. Difficulty breathing when lying down (page 297)

68. B. Stridor (page 312)

69. D. Lethargic (page 302)

70. A. Wheezes (page 313)

71. D. Bradypnea (page 304)

72. D. I, II, III (page 302)

73. A. A bacterial infection of the lung (page 299)

74. C. Pectus excavatum (page 307)

75. B. Stridor (page 312)

76. A. Presence of cyanosis (page 306)

Chapter 15

A Picture is worth . . . (Fig. 15-2, p. 323)

1. Superior vena cava

2. Right atrium

3. Tricuspid valve

4. Right ventricle

5. Interatrial septum

6. Interventricular septum

7. Left atrium

8. Mitral valve

9. Left ventricle

10. Sinoatrial node (SA)

11. Interatrial conduction tract (Bachmann's bundle)

12. Internodal-atrial conduction tracts

13. Atrioventricular node (AV)

14. Bundle of His

15. Left bundle branch

16. Right bundle branch

17. Purkinje fibers

More Pictures? (Figure 15-3, page 324)

For questions 18-21

Wave	Represents
18. P wave	Atrial depolarization
19. QRS complex	Ventricular depolarization
20. T wave	Ventricular repolarization
21. U wave	Not usually seen. Possible electrolyte abnormalities.

22. Obscured by the QRS complex. (page 324)

23. No longer than 0.20 seconds. Longer intervals indicate a block. (page 324)

24. Myocardial infarction is one cause of ST segment abnormality. (page 324)

Making Measurements

25. 25 mm/second (page 325)

26. 0.04 seconds, 0.20 seconds. (page 325)

27. 10 small boxes, 2 large boxes. (page 325)

Start at the very beginning . . .

28. 7, 70. (page 325)

29. 4, 75. (page 325)

30. Sinus bradycardia (page 326)

31. Sinus tachycardia (page 326)

Try it, You'll Like it!

32. 0.28

33. First degree heart block

Try it, You'll Like it!

34. 0.08 seconds

35. Upright

Try it, You'll Like it!

36. Depressed

37. Regular

Labba Dabba Doo!

38. Page 331
    A. Infection
    B. Patient's immune system is generating a significant response

39. Page 331
    A. Lymphoma
    B. Chemotherapy or radiation therapy
    C. Elderly patients with overwhelming infection

40. Table 15-2, page 332
    A. Bacterial—neutrophils
    B. Viral—lymphocytes

41. Page 332
    A. Anemia
    B. Blood transfusion is a treatment for severe life-threatening anemia

42. Page 332
    A. 12-16 g/dl
    B. Hemoglobin is important to maintain oxygenation

43. Secondary polycythemia (page 332)

44. Platelets and prothrombin time (page 333)

Lytes, Camera, Action

45. 3.5-4.8 mEq/L (page 333)

46. Hyperkalemia and hypokalemia can result in muscle weakness and arrythmias. Failure to correct abnormalities could render the patient unable to maintain adequate ventilation during weaning. (page 334)

47. Carbon dioxide (page 333)

48. Arterial blood gases to assess acid-base status. (page 334)

49. BUN and creatinine (page 334)

Enzymes

50. Page 335

	Old	New
A.	SGOT	AST
B.	SGPT	ALT

51. CK2-MB (creatine kinase) (page 335)

Sputum is our Bread and Butter!

52. Few (< 25per low-power field) pus cells and many epithelial cells. (page 335)

53. Culture aids in identification and determination of antibiotic sensivity. (page 336)

Case Studies

54. Stop suctioning. Atropine is a possible drug treatment if the rhythm does not improve. (pages 617-618)

55. Vagal stimulation.

56. Stop suctioning. Give the patient oxygen.

57. Hypoxemia. (page 326)

58. Jeff should call for help. He should then ventilate the patient.

59. The initial treatment calls for rapid defibrillation. CPR, oxygen, and antiarrythmic drugs are also indicated. (page 331)

What About Those Board Exams?

60. D. Bronchitis (pages 335-336)

61. B. Electrolyte analysis (page 334)

62. C. Defibrillation (page 331)

Food for Thought

63. Cancer and cancer treatments are a possibility. The most likely cancer is lymphoma or leukemia. AIDS is an important possibility to consider as well. (page 331)

64. Trained athletes may have heart rates below 60 without symptoms or need of treatment.

Chapter 16

Life's a Gas

Meet the Objectives

1. Oxygen molecules cross a membrane and enter an electrolyte solution. A chemical reaction causes current to flow between two electrodes. The amount of current reflects the amount of oxygen molecules present. (page 338)

2. Page 338
   A. Galvanic
   B. Polarographic

3. Galvanic analyzers use a gold anode and a lead cathode. Current flow across these poles is generated by a chemical reaction.

Polarographic analyzers use a silver anode and a platinum cathode. Current flow is generated by a polarizing voltage applied to these poles. The flow of electrons reduces the oxygen molecules and increases the current. Polarographic analyzers have a faster response time. (page 338)

4. Step 1 is to expose the electrode to 100% O_2 and calibrate the reading to 100%. Step 2 is to expose the electrode to 21% O_2 and calibrate the electrode. (page 339)

5. The arterial blood gas. This means ABGs are the standard against which other methods of analysis are measured. (page 339)

6. Page 339
   A. It is near the surface and easy to palpate.
   B. Collateral circulation is provided by the ulnar artery.
   C. The radial artery is not near any large veins.
   D. This site may be less painful.

7. Page 340 and Figure 16-3, page 342
   A. You occlude the radial and ulnar arteries and have the patient make a fist. Then release the ulnar artery.
   B. Flushing of the hand within 10 seconds is a positive result demonstrating collateral circulation.

8. Page 339
   A. Brachial
   B. Femoral
   C. Dorsalis pedis
   D. Temporal (infants)

9. Page 341
   A. Healthy, breathing spontaneously—at least 5 minutes
   B. COPD (or critically ill)—20 to 30 minutes

10. Administration of a local anesthetic (lidocaine) prior to the arterial puncture. (page 344)

11. Page 343
    A. Anticoagulants
       1. Heparin
       2. Coumadin (warfarin)
    B. Thrombolytics
       1. Streptokinase
       2. Tissue plasminogen activator (TPA)

12. Page 344
    A. Anaerobic sample
    B. Anticoagulated sample
    C. Immediate expulsion of air bubbles
    D. Analyze within 15 minutes

13. Apply standard or universal precautions such as wearing gloves. (pages 349-50; also Chapter 3). With blood gases you should avoid recapping and dispose of sharps properly. (page 341)

14. Page 348
    A. pH
    B. PCO_2
    C. PO_2

15. A hemoximeter (cooximeter) (page 348)

16. $+/- 3\%-5\%$ (page 360)

17. Page 361
    A. Assess perfusion at the monitoring site
    B. Agreement between the pulse oximeter heart rate and actual rate
    C. Confirm the adequacy of the output signal

18. Make a direct measurement of SaO_2 with an ABG or hemoximeter. (page 362)

19. Pages 350-351
    A. Gas electrodes are calibrated with precision mixtures of oxygen and carbon dioxide. The pH electrode is calibrated with standard pH buffer solutions. Calibration is a two-point process using high and low values. The analyzer automatically adjusts the response so the low output equals the low input, and so on.
    B. Once the machine is calibrated, control chemicals that mimic real blood samples are analyzed. At least two levels are tested every 8 hours, and three levels every 24 hours. Analyzed results are compared with expected values.
    C. Five unknown samples are analyzed at least three times per year. Results are reported. If the values are not acceptable, remediation must be performed and documented or reimbursement may be suspended.

20. Infants and small children. (page 346)

21. Failure to properly warm the skin and squeezing the puncture site. (page 348)

22. pH and PCO_2 give rough estimates compared to arterial blood. PO_2 is not valuable from a capillary sample. (page 346)

23. Pages 353-335
    A. Advantages
        1. Noninvasive
        2. Continuous
    B. Disadvantages
        1. Poor correlation of values in some cases, such as older patients
        2. Not useful during short procedures or emergencies
        3. Labor intensive and complex

24. During a short procedure, or during an emergency when results are needed immediately. (page 355)

25. Infants where hyperoxia is a concern. Saturation measured by the pulse oximeter is not specific enough to monitor PO_2. (page 354)

26. Between the patient and the wye connector. (page 364)

27. Normal end-tidal CO_2 is approximately 35-43 mm Hg (5%-6%), or about 1-5 mm Hg less than arterial values. (page 364)

28. Page 365
    A. Cardiac arrest
    B. Esophageal intubation

Could also indicate a leak or a disconnection.

29. An elevated baseline indicates rebreathing. (page 366)

30. Figure 16-21, page 367
    A. COPD/airway obstruction
    B. Left ventricular failure/shock

Chapter Highlights

31. A. Low battery
    B. Sensor depletion
    C. Electronic failure

32. A. Ventilation
    B. Acid-base balance
    C. Oxygenation

33. 15 minutes

34. A. Benefits
        1. Ready access for blood sampling
        2. Continuous pressure monitoring
    B. Hazards
        1. Increased risk of infection
        2. Increased risk of thrombosis

35. Point of care testing allows for measurement of blood gas and other values at the bedside. This reduces turnaround time, may improve care and may lower cost. It may also decrease the need for personnel and complex lab equipment. (page 352)

36. Capnometry is the measurement of CO_2 in respiratory gases. A capnometer is the actual measuring device. Capnography is the graphic display of CO_2 levels during breathing.

Case Studies

37. Tachycardia, tachypnea, abnormal breath sounds, labored breathing.

38. The pulse oximeter will give falsely high %Hb O_2 in the presence of carbon monoxide (HbCO) poisoning. (Table 16-7, page 361)

39. Elevated levels of carbon monoxide in the blood. Consider the carbonaceous sputum, history, breath sounds, and soot on Biff's face.

40. An ABG should be drawn and part of the sample analyzed with a co-oximeter (hemoximeter). (page 359)

41. PaO_2 levels of 100-600 are capable of giving pulse oximeter readings of 100%. (page 363)

42. Transcutaneous monitoring will provide a noninvasive way to assess oxygenation in terms of keeping a minimally acceptable PaO_2 and avoiding hyperoxia. (page 354)

43. Pulse oximetry is a useful way to monitor the adequacy of arterial oxygenation. It is simple, quick, and noninvasive. (page 362)

44. It's important to check acid-base and ventilatory status of long-term COPD patients on admission to establish baseline values, and to establish agreement between the SaO_2 and the SpO_2. (page 362)

45. Capnometry is continuous and noninvasive —since you will be relying on maintaining a low $PaCO_2$ for this patient. (AARC CPG—Indications for Capnometry page 365)

46. Between the endotracheal tube and the wye connector of the circuit. (page 364)

47. Rebreathing. (page 366)

48. Manually ventilate or increase the ventilation provided by the ventilator to reduce the CO_2. The capnometer will be useful in assessing this change.

49. CO_2 is vasoactive. Increased levels cause vasodilation. As the blood vessels dilate, they take up more space in the head. Since the skull doesn't expand, the pressure goes up.

What About Those Board Exams?

50. C. Performing an Allen test on the patient (page 340)

While pulse oximeters can be used to perform an Allen test, the test itself is used prior to radial artery puncture.

51. B. I, II only (page 341)

52. C. Co-oximetry (page 359)

53. A. Replace the battery (page 339)

54. B. Room air contamination of the transcutaneous electrode (page 356)

55. C. Capnometer (page 366)

56. D. End-tidal CO_2 monitoring (page 365)

57. A. Pulmonary embolus (page 343)

58. B. The electrode membrane has water condensation on its surface.

59. D. II, III, IV only (page 361)

60. B. An air bubble has contaminated the sample. (Table 16-1, page 344)

61. D. Endotracheal tube connector (Figure 16-19, page 364)

62. A. $TcPO_2$ should be checked with arterial blood samples. (page 355)

Food for Thought

63. Apply pressure to the site longer. Check carefully for post-puncture bleeding. The text recommends checking after 20 minutes.

64. Some analyzers (point of care for example) require immediate analysis of unchilled blood. Accurate potassium analysis requires this also. Thirty minutes of icing in a plastic syringe may erroneously increase PaO_2. Glass syringes are recommended for long delays in analysis. (page 344)

65. Shock or burns to the patient (page 363)

66. Capnometers are indicated to assess adequate blood flow generated during CPR since pulmonary blood flow is required generate exhaled CO_2. Pulse oximeters rely on perfusion at a peripheral site, which may not be available during CPR. (Pulse oximeter, page 361; capnometer pages 365, 368)

Chapter 17

Initially . . .

1. E   DL

2. P   ERV

3. A   VT

4. J   IRV

5. K   RV

6. C   TLC

7. F   VC

8. I   IC

9. L   FRC

10. B   MVV

11. M   FVC

12. D   PEFR

13. H $FEF_{200\text{-}1200}$

14. O   FEV1

15. N $FEF_{25\%\text{-}75\%}$

16. G FEV_1/FVC

First things first (Figure 17-1, page 375)

Volume/Capacity	Value
A. TLC	6000 ml
B. VC	4800 ml
C. IC	3600 ml
D. FRC	2400 ml
E. IRV	3100 ml
F. VT	500 ml
G. ERV	1200 ml
H. RV	1200 ml

Meet the Objectives

18. Residual volume (page 374)

19. Functional residual capacity, total lung capacity (page 374)

20. Page 376
    A. Helium dilution
    B. Nitrogen washout
    C. Body plethysmography

21. All the gas in the thorax including the lungs, trapped air, and air in the pleural space. Measured by the plethysmograph. (page 376)

22. They may be larger in disease states. (page 379)

23. A leak will alter the values by increasing them, giving the appearance of hyperinflation. (page 380)

24. Page 392
    A. Height
    B. Age
    C. Gender
    D. Ethnicity

25. Page 382-383
    A. Duration—At least 6 seconds
    B. Variance of two best FVCs—Not more than 5% or 200 ml
    C. Satisfactory start—Abruptly and without hesitation, extrapolated volume less than 5% or 150 ml
    D. Minimum number—3 acceptable tests

26. Page 383
    A. FVC—The largest FVC from an acceptable test
    B. FEV1—The largest FEV1, even if not from the largest FVC

27. PEFR (page 384)

28. PEFR, FEV_1, $FEF_{200\text{-}1200}$ (page 394)

29. $FEF_{25-75\%}$ (page 394)

30. Within 3%. For example, a 3-liter syringe is used. The values must be within 2.91-3.09 L. (page 385)

31. A calibrated, large-volume syringe, or super syringe. (page 385)

32. The patient breathes as deeply and rapidly as possible for 12-15 seconds. (page 386)

Normal is 160 L/min. (page 391)

33. Low concentrations of CO_2. (page 386)

34. Helium is used as a tracer gas and to allow measurement of TLC by a single breath helium dilution. (page 388-389)

35. Hemoglobin and hematocrit. (page 388-389)

36. Figure 17-3, page 390

Anatomy	Phase	Patho	Measure
A. Obstructive			
Airways	Expiration	Increased Raw	Flow rates
B. Restrictive			
Parenchyma/ pump	Inspiration	Decreased CL	Volume/ capacity

37. Table 17-4, page 391

Degree of Impairment	% Predicted
A. Normal	80-120%
B. Mild	65-79%
C. Moderate	50-64%
D. Severe	35-49%

38. Non-white normals reduced by 12%-15% (page 394)

39. Page 394
    A. Normal—70% or greater
    B. Obstructed—Less than 70%
    C. Restricted—Absolute values reduced, but ratio will be 70% or greater

Case Studies

40. Obstructive lung disease

41. Pre- and post-bronchodilator spirometry to assess reversibility.

42. Within normal limits—At the bottom of normal

43. First of all, Jim's ethnicity. Second, smoking history. Third, family history, childhood illness. Fourth, occupational history before entering school.

44. Probable restrictive lung disease.

45. Nitrogen washout or other determination of lung volumes. Chest radiograph. Consider DLCO.

46. Smoking history. What did he do at the shipyard?

47. Mixed restrictive and obstructive disease.

48. Specific information on the dyspnea—How long, how severe, etc. Smoking and family history. Employment history or other exposure.

49. TLC suggests hyperinflation. FEV_1/FVC shows obstruction. The DLCO is reduced indicating alveolar capillary membrane pathology.

50. Emphysema

51. The large residual volume

What About Those Board Exams?

52. B. FEF_{25-75} (page 398)

53. D. Spirometry with flow-volume loops (page 397)

54. A. The results are within normal limits (page 385) (also page 374, ATS standards)

55. B. I, IV (page 377)

56. C. Functional residual capacity (page 391)

57. D. Obstructive lung disease

58. C. 15% (page 398)

59. B. tidal volume (page 374-375)

60. A. Emphysema (page 397)

Food for Thought

61. It makes the results invalid (or less valid) since the test measures diffusion of CO_2 into the blood. Environmental exposure can also have the same effect. (page 388)

62. Inspiratory capacity (page 392)

63. I think it's a good idea to review this in class prior to performing spirometry on each other. I find a lot of errors when these calculations are performed by hand.

Chapter 18

Word Wizard

radiograph, radiolucent, radiopaque, hydrothorax, infiltrates, pneumothorax

Step-by-Step

1. Compare the position of the ends of the clavicles (anterior structure) to that of the spinous processes (posterior structure). (page 404)

2. Overexposed lung fields lose the blood vessels in the periphery show an overly darkened parenchyma. (page 404)

3. Lack of visualization of the vertebral bodies through the heart shadow. (page 404)

4. The lungs appear whiter and may be misinterpreted as congestion or infiltrates. (page 404)

5. Page 405
   A. Chest wall and pleura
   B. Lung parenchyma
   C. Mediastinum

6. Page 405
   A. Fluid in the pleural space (hydrothorax)
   B. Air in the pleural space (pneumothorax)

7. Fractures (page 405)

8. 80%-90% of the lung tissue has bone overlying it. (page 405)

9. One half the diameter of the chest. (page 405)

10. The diaphragm. (page 406)

Identifying Abnormalities

11. The angle between the diaphragm and the chest wall. (page 406)

12. The pleural meniscus sign. (page 406 and Figure 18-3, page 407)

13. The decubitus view. The patient is positioned so they are lying on the side with the suspected effusion. (page 406)

14. Identifying exudative pleural effusions. Sonography can also be used to guide pleural drainage procedures. (page 407)

15. Computerized tomography. (page 407)

16. Page 409
    A. Rupture of a bleb
    B. Biopsy
    C. Barotrauma

17. Upright chest film obtained during exhalation. (page 409)

18. Page 410
    A. Inferiorly displaced hemidiaphragm
    B. Mediastinum shifted away from the affected side

19. Immediate decompression with a chest tube. (page 410)

20. Page 410
    A. Alveoli
    B. Interstitium (supporting structures of the lung)

21. Patchy areas of increased density (page 410)

22. They appear the same. (page 410)

23. Air bronchograms occur when their is an alveolar infiltrate surrounding the airway. (page 411)

24. Interstitial lung disease. (page 412, 413)

25. Refers to ability to visualize the heart border along with a lung density. The right heart border is visible in a right lower lobe infiltrate, obscured with a right middle lobe infiltrate. (page 411)

26. Page 413
    A. Pulmonary opacification
    B. Elevation of the diaphragm
    C. Shift of trachea and mediastinal structures
    D. Narrowing of the space between the ribs.

27. Page 414

Lung Volume	Anterior Ribs
A. Poor inspiration	Less than 6
B. Good effort	6-7
C. Hyperinflation	More than 7

28. Page 414
    A. Primary
       1. Loss of pulmonary vascular markings
       2. Appearance of bullae
    B. Secondary
       1. Increased A-P diameter
       2. Retrosternal and retrocardiac air spaces
       3. Flattening of the diaphragms

29. The standard chest radiograph is relatively insensitive. CT may show evidence of emphysema even when PFTs are normal. This is because CT can be used to measure lung density. (page 415)

30. The radiopaque line can be seen on the film. The film may also demonstrate if placement has caused any complications. (page 416)

31. 5 cm above the carina in an adult. (page 416)

32. The right mainstem bronchus. (page 416)

33. Pneumothorax or hydrothorax (page 416)

34. Pulmonary infarction (page 419)

35. Between the lungs (page 419)

36. Computed tomography (page 419)

Case Studies

37. The right lower lobe, since the right heart border is visible (page 411)

38. Pulmonary infiltrates such as pneumonia (page 411)

39. Auscultation, diagnostic percussion, palpation of chest wall motion

40. About 5 cm above the carina (page 416)

41. Pull the tube out at least 2 cm.

42. Suggests hyperinflation (page 414)

What About Those Board Exams?

43. C. A chest radiograph (page 409)

44. C. A dark area without lung markings
    (page 409)

45. D. Right-sided atelectasis (page 413)

46. B. 2 cm above the carina (5 cm is the rec-
    ommended level in the text, however,
    since the tube can move about 2 cm in
    either direction with head movement,
    2 cm is the minimum. (page 416)

46. B. Decubitus radiographic projection
    (page 406)

Food for Thought

48. Extension results in an upward movement.
    Flexion moves the tube down. The two
    positions may move the tip as much as
    4 cm. (page 416)

Chapter 19

Classification and Pathogenesis

1. Therapy based on the most likely cause of
   the infection when the specific organism is
   still unknown. (page 426)

2. Lower respiratory tract infection that develops in hospitalized patients > 48 hours after
   admission (excluding incubating community acquired infections) (page 426)

3. Second-most frequent nosocomial infection
   in the United States 15%-18% of all nosocomial infections. 250,000 cases per year.
   (page 426)

4. Page 426 70% mortality
   A. ICU patients
   B. Bone marrow transplant recipients

5. Table 19-2, page 427
   A. TB
   B. Histoplasmosis
   C. Cryptococcus
   D. Coccidioidomycosis (Also Q fever,
      legionellosis)

6. Page 427
   A. Narcotic use
   B. Alcohol intoxication
   C. Prior stroke
   D. Seizure disorders (also cardiac arrest,
      syncope)

7. Intubated patients (page 427)

8. The suction catheter passes through the oro-
   or nasopharynx picking up bacteria which
   then inoculate the trachea. (page 427)

9. *P. carinii* pneumonia in immunocompromised or HIV patients. Cytomegalovirus is
   another example. (page 427)

Microbiology

10. Knowledge of organisms associated with
    pneumonia helps with differential diagnosis
    and selection of empirical antimicrobial
    therapy. (page 427)

11. *Streptococcus pneumoniae* or pneumococcus
    accounts for 20%-75%. (page 428)

12. Page 428
    A. *Legionella* species
    B. *Chlamydia pneumoniae* (also *Mycoplasma
       pneumoniae*)

13. Inability of patient to produce sputum fail-
    ure to check, viruses and anaerobic bacteria
    not cultured, new types of pathogens are
    not recognized. (page 428)

14. Page 428
    A. Virus
       1. Influenza
       2. RSV (respiratory syncytial virus)
    B. Winter months

Clinical Manifestations

15. Page 428
    A. Cough
    B. Sputum production
    C. Pleuritic chest pain (also dyspnea)

16. Page 428
    A. Acute bronchitis
    B. Chronic bronchitis (could also be TB)

17. High fever, shaking, chills, productive cough (page 429)

18. Page 429
    A. New onset of fever
    B. Purulent secretions suctioned from ET tube
    C. New pulmonary infiltrate on chest radiograph

19. Lobar consolidation, patchy infiltrates (bronchopneumonia), pleural effusion (bacterial) (page 429)

20. Bronchitis and pneumonia have similar appearance. Preexisting conditions such as CHF and ARDS may mask the signs. (page 429)

Risk Factors

21. Page 430; Table 19-1, page 431

Factor	Description
A. Age	> 50 years of age
B. Gender	Male
C. Vital signs	BP <90, HR > 125, RR > 30, T > 40 C
D. Arterial pH	< 7.35
E. High-risk causes	Gram-negative, *aureus*, aspiration
F. Comorbid illness	Cancer, liver/kidney disease, CVA, CHF

22. Page 431
    A. Diabetes mellitus
    B. Malignancy
    C. Chronic heart disease
    D. Chronic lung disease
    E. Renal failure

23. Page 431
    A. ET or nasogastric tube
    B. Contaminated H_2O or ventilator equipment
    C. Prior antibiotic therapy
    D. Neutralization of gastric pH

Diagnostic Studies

24. High predictive value for selection of appropriate antibiotic therapy and identification of resistant organisms. (page 432)

25. Rinse mouth, deep cough, prompt transport to lab. (page 432)

26. > 25 leukocytes, < 10 squamous epithelial cells per high power field (page 432)

27. Page 433

	Test	Organism
A.	Acid-fast stain	*Mycoplasma* (M. *tuberculosis*)
B.	Direct fluorescent stain	*Legionella*
C.	Toluidine blue	*P. carinii*
D.	Potassium hydroxide	Fungi—histo, blasto, cocci

28. Patient between ages 15-54 who has *H. influenzae* or pneumococcal pneumonia, especially if the patient has behaviors that put them at risk for HIV. (page 434)

29. Severe cases, immunocompromised individuals who may have opportunistic infections, or if HIV or *P. carinii* is suspected. (page 434)

30. Box 19-3, page 435
    A. Clinical diagnosis
    B. Fiberoptic bronchoscopy: PBB, BAL, direct visualization
    C. Therapist-directed mini-BAL
    D. Transthoracic fine-needle aspiration

Therapy

31. Antibiotics (page 435)

32. Page 436; Table 19-9, page 437

Organism	Agent of Choice
A. Pneumococcal infection	Vancomycin (or penicillin)
B. *Mycoplasma*	Erythromycin (macrolides)
C. *P. carinii*	Trimethoprim-sulfamethoxazole/pentamidine
D. *Legionella*	Erythromycin (may add rifampin, doxy-cycline)

33. 10-14 days for community-acquired (page 436); 14 days minimum for nosocomial. (page 437)

34. Page 437
    A. Young—1 month (90% of individuals under 50)
    B. Older—> 1 month (70% of cases) or those with underlying illness

Prevention

35. Page 438
    A. Influenza
    B. *S. pneumoniae*

36. Page 438
    A. Individuals > 60 years
    B. Health care workers (including RCPs)
    C. Individuals with chronic heart or lung disease

37. Table 19-10, page 438
    A. Handwashing
    B. Isolation of patients with resistant organisms
    C. Infection control/surveillance techniques

38. Semi-erect (not recumbent) (page 438)

39. Sucralfate (Carafate) (page 438)

Case Studies

40. Community-acquired pneumonia. Probably pneumococcal. Patient has fever, chills, pleuritic pain, purulent rust-colored sputum. Page 428, 429

41. Oxygen

42. Box 19-1, page 431
    A. Male over 50 years
    B. HR 125
    C. RR 30
    D. Temp 104° F
    E. pH < 7.35

    He also is likely to have comorbity such as COPD, liver disease, heart disease.

43. Endotracheal tubes promote exposure of the lung to microorganisms. (page 431)

44. Sputum culture and sensitivity. If not successful, bronchoscopic exam. (Pages 432, 434, 435)

Food for Thought

45. RCPs should know the at risk populations and benefits since they come in contact with elderly and COPD patients. (page 438)

46. That depends on the season. Immunization is recommended for healthcare workers to reduce risk of spreading influenza to patients. (page 438)

Chapter 20

Sputum Power

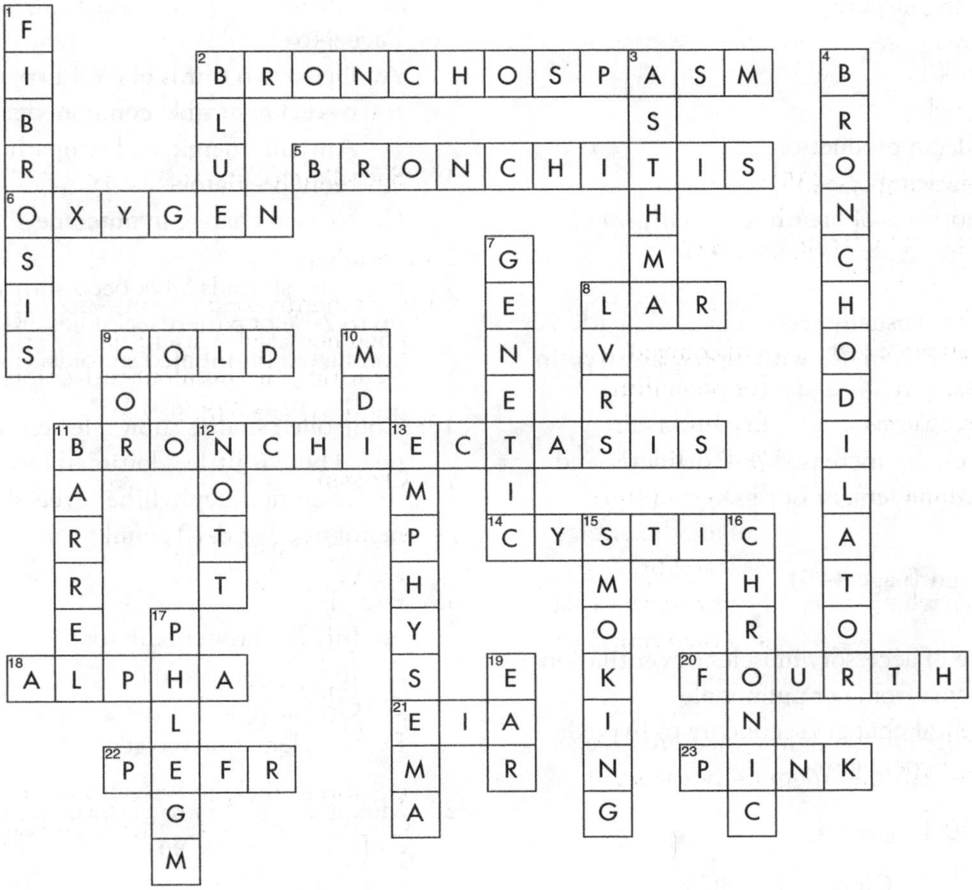

Across and down answers (crossword grid):

- 1 Down: FIBROSIS
- 2 Across: BRONCHOSPASM
- 3 Down: ASTHMA
- 4 Down: BRONCHODILATATOR
- 5 Across: BRONCHITIS
- 6 Across: OXYGEN
- 8 Across: LAR
- 9 Across: COLD
- 11 Across: BRONCHIECTASIS
- 14 Across: CYSTIC
- 18 Across: ALPHA
- 20 Across: FOURTH
- 21 Across: EIA
- 22 Across: PEFR
- 23 Across: PINK

Chronic Obstructive Pulmonary Disease

1. Page 442
   A. Gastroesophageal reflux
   B. Asthma
   C. Post-nasal drip

2. Chronic bronchitis—14 million, Emphysema—2 million (page 442)

3. COPD is fourth leading cause of death, so heart attack and stroke are more common. But death rate from COPD is rising, and that of heart disease is not. (page 442)

4. 24 billion dollars per year in United States (page 442)

5. Page 443
   A. Alpha$_1$ antitrypsin deficiency
   B. Intravenous ritalin abuse (also HIV, Marfan's syndrome, Ehler-Danlos disease)

6. About 15% of all smokers experience a more rapid decline of lung function than non-smokers. (page 443)

7. Elastin is protected by the protein alpha$_1$-antitrypsin from neutrophil elastase, which is attracted to the lung by inflammation or infection. Decreased levels of alpha$_1$-antitrypsin result in digestion of elastase. Cigarettes create inflammation and inhibit lung defenses. (pages 443, 444)

8. Page 444
   A. Inflammation and obstruction of small airways
   B. Loss of elasticity
   C. Bronchospasm

9. Page 444
   A. Cough
   B. Phlegm production
   C. Wheezing
   D. Shortness of breath, especially on exertion

10. Dyspnea is usually seen in late 60s, early 70s with COPD, in 40s with alpha$_1$-antitrypsin deficiency. (page 444)

11. Barrel chest (increased A-P diameter and outward movement of ribs).

Hoover's sign (page 445)

12. Page 445
    A. Use of accessory muscles of ventilation
    B. Edema from cor pulmonale
    C. Mental changes secondary to hypoxia and hypercapnia

13. Table 20-1, page 445

	Features	Chronic Bronchitis	Emphysema	Alpha$_1$
A.	Age of onset	60-70	60-70	40-50
B.	Family history	Not necessarily	Not necessarily	Common
				Common
C.	Smoker	Often heavy	Often heavy	Not necessarily
D.	Lung volume	Normal	Increase	Increase
E.	DLco	Normal	Decrease	Decrease
F.	FEV$_1$/ FVC	Decrease	Decrease	Decrease
G.	Radiograph	"Dirty lungs"	Hyperinflation, especially at apex	Hyperinflation, especially at base

14. Treatment is different. (page 446)

15. 12% and a 200 ml rise in FEV$_1$. (page 446) Note that this differs from the 15% value found elsewhere in the text. This represents the more recent standard.

16. Page 446
    A. Up to two thirds of COPD patients have a reversible component
    B. Anticholinergic and sympathomimetic bronchodilators
    C. No real change in outcome

17. Systemic steroids have been shown to help up to 29% of patients. Studies are being conducted on inhaled steroids. (page 446)

18. Controlled studies show a lessening of dyspnea. There is little additional bronchodilation. Serum theophylline levels should be maintained at 8-10 µg/ml.

19. Page 447
    A. Inhaled bronchodilators
    B. Intravenous steroids
    C. Oral antibiotics
    D. Supplemental oxygen

20. Maximized ability to perform activities of daily living. (page 447)

21. Rehab improves exercise capacity, but has no effect on lung function or long-term survival. (page 448)

22. Page 448
    A. Instruction
    B. Group counseling
    C. Nicotine replacement therapy

23. Oxygen therapy. (page 448)

24. Aggressive bronchodilator therapy will help up to one third of patients enough to avoid long-term supplemental oxygen. (page 448)

25. Page 448
    A. Influenza—Annual
    B. Pneumonia (pneumococcal)

26. Pages 448, 449
    A. Lung transplantation—COPD is the most common current indication. Patients must be < 65 years old and have FEV_1's level of $< 20\%$ of predicted. Single-lung transplant is usually performed with a 40% survival rate at 5 years. The surgery is associated with significantly improved quality of life.
    B. Lung volume reduction surgery—Removes a portion of the diseased hyperinflated lung. FEV_1, walking endurance, and oxygen are improved. Currently, studies are being conducted to clarify the indications and expected outcomes.

Asthma

27. Older definitions emphasized airway reactivity and reversible obstruction. Current emphasis is placed on the inflammatory aspects of the disease. (page 450)

28. A little over 5% of the population. (page 450)

29. Asthma mortality is rising. Death rates have increased by 31% from 1980-1987. (page 450)

30. Page 450
    A. Airway inflammation
    B. Bronchial hyperreactivity

31. The antigen cross-links to specific IgE molecules on the surface of mast cells in the bronchial mucosa. Degranulation occurs, and multiple mediators are released, resulting in airway inflammation and bronchospasm. (pages 450, 451)

32. Page 451
    A. EAR—Immediate hypersensitivity reaction that usually lasts about 30-60 minutes.
    B. LAR—Response that occurs in about 50% of asthmatics and lasts 3-8 hours. Characterized by increasing influx and activation of inflammatory cells such as eosinophils, mast cells, and lymphocytes.

33. History (page 451)

34. Page 451
    A. Episodic wheezing
    B. Shortness of breath
    C. Chest tightness
    D. Cough

35. Page 451
    A. Tumors
    B. Laryngospasm
    C. Aspiration of a foreign object
    D. Tracheal stenosis
    E. Vocal cord dysfunction

36. Pre- and post-bronchodilator measurement of FVC and FEV_1. A 12% increase (at least 200 ml) or 15% increase of self-recorded peak flow rates. (page 451)

37. Page 452
    A. Drug—methacholine (cold air, exercise, hypertonic saline also used)
    B. Response—20% decrease in FEV_1

38. ABGs are used in staging of an asthma attack. They may be normal between attacks, and have no real diagnostic value. Mild asthma shows a normal PO_2 with decreased CO_2 and increased pH. PO_2 declines in a moderate attack. In severe attacks, the PO_2 is low, CO_2 is normal or high, and pH is normal or decreased. (See Mini-Clini, page 452)

39. Table 20-2, page 453

Severity	Symptoms	Long-term meds
A. 1–Intermittent	$< 1x$ per week	None
B. 2–Mild persistent	$> 1x$ per week, $<$ daily	Steroids–MDI, cromolyn, long-acting dilator for noc.
C. 3–Moderate persistent	Daily symptoms	Steroids–MDI, long-acting dilator for noc. Steroids–MDI, long-acting dilator for noc.
D. 4–Severe persistent	Continuous	Same as above. Consider adding oral steroids.

40. Page 453
    A. Symptoms—Minimal to no symptoms
    B. Beta$_2$ agonists—Infrequent to no need
    C. Exercise—No exercise or activity limitations
    D. PEFR—> 80% predicted, less than 20% diurnal variation

41. Table 20-2, page 453

Zone	PEFR % predicted	Treatment/ Action
A. Green	≥ 80%	Inhaled beta/$_2$ agonist PRN
B. Yellow	> 60 < 80 %	Inhaled beta/$_2$ agonist 3-4 x day
C. Red	≤ 60%	Inhaled beta/$_2$ agonist prn for symptoms

42. Inhaled corticosteroids are the most effective medication for treatment of the inflammatory response. They act locally on the airway to suppress the primary disease process. Bronchodilators are used to relieve the symptoms of airway spasm. (page 454)

43. Page 454
    A. Candidiasis
    B. Dysphonia
    C. Control/reduce—Use spacer, rinse mouth after treatment

44. Page 454
    A. Indications
       1. Adults—Prevent cough-variant and exercise-induced asthma
       2. Children—Prevent atopic (allergic) asthma
    B. Acute attacks—Not useful

45. Similar to cromolyn but more potent. Used as an alternative to cromolyn.

46. Beta agonists. (page 456)

47. Primary use is for treatment of nocturnal asthma. The role in chronic management is still evolving. (page 456)

48. Sustained-release theophylline is useful for nocturnal asthma. IV or oral theophylline may be used in hospitalized patients. (page 456)

49. Daily use has not been established. May be helpful for cough-variant asthma. Can also be used when first-line bronchodilators are ineffective. (page 456)

50. Page 456
    A. Symptoms
    B. PEFR
    C. ABGs

51. A. PaO$_2$—PaO$_2$ > 60 mm Hg
    B. PEFR—Patient's best or > 70% of predicted
    C. Symptoms—No nocturnal symptoms, return to preadmission state
    D. Discharge meds—12-24 hour stability on discharge meds

52. Immunotherapy is one potential method. Avoidance and standard pharmacotherapy are the usual recommended method. (page 457)

53. Page 457
    A. Outdoor
       1. Ragweed
       2. Grass
       3. Pollen (and molds)
    B. Indoor
       1. Pets
       2. House-dust mites
       3. Molds

54. Page 457
    A. EIA—Asthma triggered by exercise, especially in cold air. The causes are poorly understood.
    B. Prophylaxis
       1. Beta$_2$-agonist drugs
       2. Cromolyn
       3. Leukotriene inhibitors

55. Asthma caused by exposure to a specific sensitizing agent in the workplace. It is the most common form of occupational lung disease in industrialized nations. Toluene diisocyonate used in the plastics industry is the most common cause. (page 458)

56. Total cessation of exposure. (page 458)

57. Ipratroprium (page 458)

58. Page 458
    A. Sustained-release theophylline
    B. Salmeterol
    C. Antacids

59. Use acetaminophen and avoid aspirin and NSAIDs. (page 458)

60. One third get better control, one third worsen, one third stay the same. Poor control of asthma increases perinatal mortality, prematurity, and low birth weight. (page 458)

61. Theophylline, beta$_2$ agonists, inhaled steroids, and cromolyn are safe. (pages 458, 459)

Bronchiectasis

62. Chronic production of large amounts of purulent sputum. (page 459)

63. "Fine-cut" CT scanning (page 459)

64. Page 459
    A. Local
       1. Foreign body
       2. Benign tumors
    B. Diffuse
       1. Cystic fibrosis
       2. Ciliary dyskinesia
       3. Serious lung infections (also rheumatoid arthritis, alpha$_1$-antitrypsin deficiency, aspergillosis, and hypogammaglobulinemia)

65. Page 459
    A. Antibiotics
    B. Bronchopulmonary hygiene techniques

66. Surgical resection. (page 459)

Cystic Fibrosis

67. Page 459-460
    A. Airflow obstruction
    B. Exocrine pancreatic insufficiency (malabsorption)
    C. Abnormally high sweat electrolytes

68. Viscid mucus (with stasis and obstruction) (page 460)

69. In 1969 the median survival age was only 14. Current median survival age is 29. By the year 2000, nearly one half of all patients with CF will be adults. (page 460)

70. Sodium or chloride concentrations in sweat greater than 60 mEq/L. (page 460)

71. Page 460
    A. Chest physical therapy and postural drainage
    B. Mucolytics
    C. Bronchodilators
    D. Antibiotics (Late-oxygen, lung transplant)

72. Page 460
    A. *Staphylococcus aureus*
    B. *Pseudomonas* species

Case Studies

73. Emphysema (page 455)

74. 100 pack-years (see workbook introduction)

75. Smoking cessation. (page 448)

76. Chronic bronchitis. (page 455)

77. Collect a sample for gram stain, culture and sensitivity.

78. Oxygen therapy. (page 447)

79. Inhaled bronchodilators—both beta agonist and ipratropium. Consider steroids. (Figure 20-5, page 447)

Alpha$_1$-antitrypsin deficiency. He is young, a nonsmoker, and has a familial history. He shows signs of emphysema: barrel chest, decreased breath sounds. The chest radiograph shows basilar hyperinflation. (page 445)

81. Lung transplant therapy, administration of purified alpha$_1$-antitrypsin. (page 449)

82. EIA (page 457)

83. Methacholine or other type of challenge. (page 452)

What Does the NBRC Say?

84. B. Expiratory wheezing (page 451)

85. A. Acute respiratory alkalosis (see Chapter 12)

86. C. Nasal cannula at 2 L. The hypoxemia is mild and cannulas are well tolerated by asthmatics. You could make an equally valid claim for the entrainment mask based on the abnormal breathing pattern, but a 50% produces a relatively low total flowrate. (see Chapter 34)

87. B. 0.5 ml Proventil (albuterol) via SVN (page 456)

88. C. Oxygenation

89. D. Intubation and mechanical ventilation (page 453). The patient is now having a severe attack bordering on respiratory failure. Of course, there are other strategies that could be attempted to avoid intubation.

90. C. II, III

91. B. Air-entrainment mask at 28% (see Chapter 34)

92. D. Bronchiectasis (page 459-460)

93. A. Emphysema (page 455)

94. B. II only (page 451)

Food for Thought

95. There is also an increased risk of lung cancer and cardiovascular disease. Second-hand smoke represents another hazard. (see Chapter 25)

96. Purified alpha$_1$-antitrypsin is available from donated human blood. The therapy must be taken weekly, and may improve PFTs, improve survival, and slow the decline of lung function. It costs $25,000-50,000 per year and poses risks of bloodborne pathogens. (page 449)

97. These drugs block or prevent the release of leukotrienes which play an important role in the pathogenesis of inflammatory asthma. They are new drugs. (page 454)

Chapter 21

Game, Set, and Match!

1. F Asbestosis

2. H Corticosteroids

3. D Cytotoxic agents

4. I Eosinophilic granuloma

5. C Hypersensitivity pneumonitis

6. A Idiopathic pulmonary fibrosis

7. B Interstitial lung disease

8. J Lupus erythematosus (systemic)

9. E Occupational lung disease

10. K Pneumoconiosis

11. M Rheumatoid arthritis

12. G Sarcoidosis

13. L Silicosis

Clinical Signs and Symptoms of ILD

14. Page 465
    A. Exertional dyspnea
    B. Nonproductive cough

15. Bilateral inspiratory "Velcro" rales in the bases.

16. Page 465
    A. Sarcoidosis may involve the airways
    B. Localized wheezing may represent focal narrowing from inflammation or scarring.

17. Page 465
    A. Digital clubbing
    B. Signs of pulmonary hypertension such as extremity edema, JVD

18. Page 466
    A. Joint inflammation
    B. Joint deformity
    C. Muscle weakness
    D. Skin rash

19. Bilateral reticulonodular infiltrates. Also volume loss in the bases. Late-honeycombing. (pages 466, 467)

20. Page 467

Variable	Effect of ILD
A. FEV_1	Decreased
B. FVC	Decreased
C. FEV_1/FVC	Normal or supranormal
D. DLCO	Decreased
E. Lung volumes	Decreased
F. PaO_2	Decreased as disease progresses
G. Compliance	Stiff poorly compliant lungs

Specific Types of ILD

21. Page 468
    A. Asbestosis
    B. Silicosis
    C. Pneumoconiosis of coal workers

22. Impairment usually occurs late in the disease after long-term exposure. Pulmonary function findings are similar. (pages 468, 469)

23. Box 21-2, page 465

Category	Example
A. Antibiotic	Nitrofurantoin, Sulfasalazine
B. Antiinflammatory	Aspirin, Methotrexate, Gold
C. Cardiovascular	Amiodarone, Tocainide
D. Chemotherapeutic	Bleomycin, Busulfan, Azathioprine
E. Illegal drugs	Heroin, Methadone, Propoxyphene
F. Miscellaneous agents	O_2, Radiation, Hydrochlorothiazide

24. The patients are usually inactive due to pain and joint problems so dyspnea on exertion is not detected. (page 469)

25. P. 469
    A. Rheumatoid arthritis
    B. Scleroderma (also polymyositis/dermatomyositis)
    C. Systemic lupus erythematosus (SLE)

26. Chronic hypersensitivity pneumonitis (page 470)

27. Careful environmental history. (page 470)

28. Unknown origin. (page 470)

29. Pages 470,471

	IPF	Sarcoidosis
A. Age	50-70 years old	Young adults
B. Symptoms	DOE, NPC	Cough, dyspnea, wheezing
C. Treatment	Prednisone, azothioprine	None (or corticosteroids)
D. Prognosis	Poor—death in 5 years	Varies—Often benign

Treatment

30. Avoiding exposure to the antigen or toxic substance. (page 471)

31. Corticosteroid (page 471)

32. Cytotoxic agents (page 471)

33. Idiopathic pulmonary fibrosis (page 472)

34. Lung transplantation (page 472)

Case Studies

35. Hypersensitivity pneumonitis (page 470)

36. Moldy hay—*Aspergillus* or *Micropolyspora* organisms. Could also be be caused by animal proteins or chemicals used in farming. (Table 21-1, page 466)

37. Asbestosis or asbestos-related pulmonary disease. (page 468)

38. Finding out what Mr. Kealoha did at the shipyard.

39. Restrictive lung disease. (page 467)

Food for Thought

40. Restrictive (see Chapter 17)

41. Partial list in Box 21-1, page 464; also see Table 21-1, page 466
    A. Talc pneumoconiosis (talc workers)
    B. Hard metal fibrosis (such as grinders)
    C. Sugar cane workers
    D. Tombstone cutters (and other granite/stone workers)
    E. Working with animals, especially birds

Chapter 22

Hey Buddy, Got a Match?
(Answers in glossary)

1. B

2. D

3. F

4. A

5. G

6. C

7. H

8. E

9. K

10. L

11. I

12. M

13. N

14. J

15. P

16. O

17. Q

The Pleural Space

18. The pleural spaces of the buffalo are connected. Humans are separate. For the buffalo this meant that puncture of either lung resulted in collapse of both lungs. Humans are put in this situation following lung volume reduction surgery and bilateral lung transplantation surgery. (page 476)

19. The space is about 10-20 microns in width and is filled with a small amount of pleural fluid. (page 476)

20. Normal pressure is negative relative to atmospheric pressure and results in a net movement of fluid into the pleural space when it is in communication with adjacent sites. (page 476)

21. The weight of the lung and gravity are pulling the lung down so that the visceral pleura at the top is pulled away from the parietal pleura, thus increasing negative pressure. The opposite effect occurs at the base. (page 476)

Pleural Effusions

22. Pages 477, 478

Condition	Mechanism
A. CHF	Elevated pulmonary venous pressure forces fluid into the interstitium and reduces removal of fluid via intercostal veins.
B. Hypoalbuminemia	Low protein levels allow fluid to leak out of vessels into the interstitial space.
C. Liver disease	Ascites force fluids into the the pleural space via small holes in the diaphragm.
D. Lymph obstruction	Normal drainage is slowed by blocked lymphatics.
E. CVP line	Accidental placement into the pleura.

23. CHF. (page 477)

24. Inflammation in the lung or pleura. (page 479)

25. Pages 479-480

Effusion	Cause
A. Parapneumonic	Increased lung H_2O and pleural fluid from inflammation. Complicated effusions have fibrin clots.
B. Malignant	Cancer metastasized into the pleura.
C. Chylothorax	Rupture or blockage of the thoracic duct.
D. Hemothorax	Bleeding into the space—usually after trauma.

26. Restriction, especially decrease in FVC. (page 481)

27. The costophrenic angles. (page 481)

28. In the lateral decubitus film the patient lies on the affected side. (page 481)

29. Ultrasound is good but CT is the most sensitive (with contrast) (page 481)

30. Page 482
    A. Intercostal artery laceration
    B. Infection
    C. Pneumothorax

31. Figure 22-3, page 482
    A. Fluid collection chamber—Keeps fluid out of the water seal
    B. Water seal—Prevents air leak back into the lung
    C. Suction chamber—Standardizes pressure applied to the chest

Pneumothorax

32. Page 483
    A. Sharp chest pain (nearly every patient)
    B. Dyspnea (two thirds of all cases)

33. Iatrogenic pneumothorax. Often not treated. Common causes include needle aspiration lung biopsy, thoracentesis, and CVP catheter placement. (page 484)

34. Penetrating chest trauma (non-iatrogenic) is usually caused by knife or gunshot wounds. Blunt trauma can fracture ribs, which tear the lung, or may rupture the alveoli. Treatment for penetrating trauma is usually a chest tube, unless uncontrolled bleeding occurs. Blunt trauma may or may not require a chest tube. (page 484)

35. Transillumination. (page 484)

36. Primary spontaneous pneumothorax occurs without lung disease. Probably rupture of a small bleb. Usually occurs in tall, slender, young males. 90% are smokers. Secondary spontaneous pneumothorax occurs in COPD patients who have emphysema, or in hyperinflated asthmatics or cystic fibrosis patients. Some pulmonary fibrosis patients may experience spontaneous pneumothorax. (pages 484, 485)

37. Page 485
    A. Air in the pleural space at greater than atmospheric pressure.
    B. Mediastinal shift away from the affected side, diaphragm depression, and rib expansion.
    C. Hypotension, hypoxemia, tachycardia, decreased breath sounds, and hyperresonance to percussion
    D. Needle decompression, then a chest tube.

38. Mortality rate is low (7%) with early recognition. Delay by as little as 30 minutes raised mortality to over 30%. (page 485)

39. Most of the gas in a pneumothorax is nitrogen. Oxygen replaces the nitrogen and is absorbed, since this increases the pressure gradient for nitrogen from the pleural space into the tissues. (page 486)

40. Large prolonged air leak. Positive pressure ventilation adds air to the pleural space. Lowering tidal volumes, lowering PEEP, positioning, double-lumen tube ventilation, and adding PEEP to chest tubes may help (among others). (page 489)

Case Studies
41. Right-sided pleural effusion because
    1. Hypoxemia (page 481)
    2. Chest radiograph shows opacification on the right (page 481)
    3. Dull percussion note (page 310)
    4. Shift of structures to the left
    5. CHF commonly causes effusions (page 477)

42. Administer oxygen.

43. Thoracentesis to drain the effusion may be necessary, but it is more important to treat the underlying CHF. (page 477)

44. A. Pneumothorax because
    1. Chest radiograph—dark area without lung markings (Chapter 18)
    2. Increased resonance to percussion (page 310)
    3. Pain on inspiration (page 483)
    4. History of tall, thin, young male (page 484)
    5. Breath sounds (Chapter 14)

45. All patients with pneumothorax should be placed on oxygen. O_2 helps resolve the pneumothorax as well as the respiratory distress and mild hypoxemia. (page 486)

46. If the pneumothorax is small, it may resolve without treatment. Otherwise, simple aspiration may be successful (page 486), or insertion of a chest tube. (page 487)

What Does the NBRC Say?
47. B. Chest radiograph (pages 484, 485)

48. A. A water seal (page 482)

49. D. Pneumothorax (page 484)

50. B. Lateral decubitus chest film (page 481)

51. A. Pulmonary edema in the right lung (page 485)

52. D. Lung compliance measurement.

53. B. Initiate oxygen therapy

54. C. Recommend a chest radiograph.

Food for Thought

55. Ascites is fluid accumulated in the abdomen. It restricts downward movement of the diaphragm. (page 477)

56. No more than 1,000 ml should be removed at one time. (page 485)

57. Subcutaneous emphysema is the presence of air in the soft tissues, and under the skin. It means that alveolar disruption has occurred, probably from barotrauma. It may or may not occur with a pneumothorax. (page 483)

Chapter 23

Word Power

hypertension, embolism, infarction, pulmonale

Meet the Objectives

1. 300,000-650,000 (page 492)

2. 50,000-100,000 (page 492)

3. Deep veins of the lower extremities or pelvis (page 492)

4. The lung has two blood supplies—pulmonary arterial circulation and bronchial circulation. At the capillary level there are extensive connections between the two systems. (page 493)

5. PE increases the number of ventilated but unperfused alveoli. (page 493)

6. Hypoxemia develops because of circulatory shock, $\dot{V}/\dot{Q}$ mismatch, and shunt. (page 493)

7. Increased resistance to blood flow through the lung. The final result is increased right ventricular work. (page 493)

8. Page 494
   A. Dyspnea (73%)
   B. Pleuritic pain (66%)

9. Page 494
   A. Tachypnea
   B. Crackles
   C. Tachycardia

10. 13%-20% (page 494)

11. Only 13%. But the abnormalities are nonspecific in 70%-75% of the cases. (page 494)

12. Page 494
    A. Tachycardia
    B. ST segment depression

13. It rules out other abnormalities such as pneumothorax. A normal chest radiograph in a dyspneic patient may be a clue to the presence of PE. (page 494)

14. ABGs are not helpful in ruling out PE. ABGs are useful in documenting hypoxemia, and in patients with poor cardiopulmonary reserve they document the CO_2 levels. (page 495)

15. Page 495
    A. Venography
    B. Compression ultrasonography
    C. Impedance plethysmography

16. Venography (page 495)

17. Compression ultrasonography. It is not a good screening tool for high-risk asymptomatic patients. (page 495)

18. Page 495
    A. Ventilation/perfusion lung scans
    B. Pulmonary angiography

19. A large segmental perfusion defect without a corresponding ventilation defect is highly suggestive of PE. A perfusion defect with a corresponding ventilation defect has a lower probability of PE. Multiple matched defects indicates a low probability. (Box 32-2, page 496)

20. Page 497
    A. Spiral computed tomography
    B. MRI

21. Page 499
    A. Pharmacologic prophylaxis
       1. Low-dose subcutaneous heparin
       2. Warfarin
       3. Low-molecular weight heparin (also heparinoids, dextran)
    B. Mechanical prophylaxis
       1. Early ambulation
       2. Elastic stockings
       3. Pneumatic calf compression devices (and electrical calf muscle stimulation)

22. Pages 499-500
    A. Drug—Heparin
    B. Action—Inhibits the coagulation system
    C. Risks—Bleeding, thrombocytopenia

23. Thrombolytics lyse existing clots. Anticoagulants prevent new clots. The two drugs should not be administered together. (page 500)

24. Page 500
    A. Streptokinase
    B. Urokinase
    C. TPA

25. Pulmonary embolectomy, catheter tip embolectomy, and catheter tip fragmentation. (page 501)

26. Usually when DVT is present and the patient has poor cardiopulmonary reserve. Filters can also be used with multiple trauma, chronically immobilized patients, and when anticoagulants are contraindicated. (page 501)

27. Primary pulmonary hypertension is defined as mean PA pressure > 25 mm Hg at rest, or > 30 mm Hg during exercise along with increased pulmonary vascular resistance, normal left heart function, and absence of secondary causes of pulmonary hypertension. (page 501)

28. Page 501
    A. Age—Can occur at any age but 30-40 is most common
    B. Gender—More common in females than males
    C. Genetics—About 7% of the cases are familial
    D. Symptoms—Dyspnea, angina, and syncope are the most common.
    E. Mortality—Often fatal. Only 33% live for 5 years after diagnosis.

29. Basically by ruling out all other possible causes. This means having ECG, echocardiography, $\dot{V}/\dot{Q}$ scan, CT, chest radiograph, and PFTs. (page 501)

30. Page 502
    A. Supplemental oxygen
    B. Anticoagulation with coumarin
    C. Vasodilators

31. Lung transplantation (page 502)

32. 50% (page 503)

33. Alveolar hypoxemia causes potent pulmonary vasoconstriction which increases pulmonary artery pressure and vascular resistance. This results in increased right ventricular work and eventual failure. (page 503)

34. Loss of vascular bed caused by destruction, compression of vessels from hyperinflation, and polycythemia. (page 503)

35. Oxygen therapy (page 503)

Chapter Highlights (pages 503-504)

36. Thromboembolism, mortality

37. Embolism, one

38. Lower, pelvis, 86%

39. Non-specific

40. Prophylactic

41. Heparin, warfarin

42. Young

43. Coumadin, calcium

Case Studies

44. Orthopedic surgery in an older patient. (page 492)

45. Chest radiograph and ECG. (page 494)

46. Oxygen therapy. He has increased work of breathing and heart, and an SpO_2 at the low end of normal. (page 500)

47. Anticoagulants such as IV heparin. (page 500)

What Does the NBRC Say?

48. C. Pulmonary embolism (page 493)

49. B. Pulmonary angiography (page 496)

50. B. Acute pulmonary embolus (page 496)

Food for Thought

51. Schistosomiasis. (page 502)

52. A $\dot{V}/\dot{Q}$ scan may help confirm the diagnosis. The accuracy of clinical diagnosis is less than 50%. (page 492) However, critically ill patients have a higher risk of PE, and moving a critically ill patient has the potential for disaster! There are also potential technical difficulties in performing the test on a ventilator patient.

Chapter 24

Acronym Soup

1. ALI—acute lung injury

2. APRV—airway pressure release ventilation

3. ARDS—acute respiratory distress syndrome

4. CHF—congestive heart failure

5. ECMO—extracorporeal membrane oxygenation

6. $ECCO_2R$—extracorporeal carbon dioxide removal

7. GIT—gastrointestinal tract (page 512)

8. HFV—high frequency ventilation

9. MODS—multiple organ dysfunction syndrome

10. PMNs—neutrophils (page 511) (polymorphs)

11. PEEP—positive end expiratory pressure

Meet the Objectives

12. Table 24-4, page 512

Category	Conditions
A. Cardiac	Left ventricular failure Cardiac valvular disease
B. Vascular	Systemic hypertension Pulmonary embolism
C. Volume overload	Excessive fluid administration Renal failure

13. Table 24-2, page 509
    A. Primary
       1. Pneumonia
       2. Gastric aspiration
       3. Toxic inhalation
       4. Near drowning (also lung contusion)
    B. Secondary
       1. Sepsis
       2. Burn injuries
       3. Prolonged systemic hypotension (shock)
       4. Multiple trauma (and others: pancreatitis, OB-Gyn, drugs, and so on)

15. Table 24-3, page 512

	CHF	ARDS
A. Chest radiograph		
1. Heart	Cardiomegaly	Normal (can be enlarged)
2. Effusions	Present	Present or not
3. Infiltrates	Diffuse alveolar and interstitial in both	
B. PCWP	> 18 mm Hg	< 18 mm Hg
C. BALF	Nonproteinaceous	Proteinaceous

16. Increased pulmonary venous pressures force fluid into the lungs. (pages 508, 511)

17. Systemic inflammatory response leads to microvascular injury that results in leaky capillaries. (page 511)

18. (Box 24-1, page 514)
    A. Avoid oxygen toxicity
    B. Prevent aspiration
    C. Prevent barotrauma/volutrauma
    D. Identify and treat infections
    E. Early extubation

19. Box 24-1, page 514
    A. Minimize demand by reducing metabolic rate-control fever, anxiety and pain.
    B. Support cardiovascular system with fluids and pressors to maintain adequate BP, reverse lactic acidosis, and maintain urine output.

20. Optimum PEEP is the PEEP that improves oxygenation but preserves cardiac output and lung compliance. This may be lower than the PEEP that results in the highest PaO_2. (See Mini Clini, page 515; and Figure 24-4)

21. 8-15 cm H_2O (page 515)

22. Provide adequate oxygenation, ensure adequate tissue oxygenation, maintain alveolar patency during ventilation, avoid barotrauma. (page 517)

23. Maintain a PaO_2 of at least 60 mm Hg with an FIO_2 below 60%. (page 517)

24. Conventional tidal volumes are usually 10-15 ml/kg. In ARDS, tidal volumes of 5-7 ml/kg are optimal. (page 516)

25. Permissive hypercapnia allows $PaCO_2$ to rise above normal. CO_2s of 60-80 mm Hg with pH as low as 7.25 is acceptable to avoid volutrauma. This strategy should be accomplished over time and may require sedation or paralysis. (pages 517-518)

26. Page 518
    A. Elevated intracranial pressure: increased $PaCO_2$ may increase ICP resulting in brain injury.
    B. Unstable hemodynamic status: decreased pH may affect cardiac function.

27. A ventilator technique that uses high rates (up to 300) and low volumes (3 ml/kg). The technique has been successful with neonates, but is not proven in adults. (page 518)

28. In conventional ventilation, I:E ratios are maintained at 1:2 or greater. In IRV, exhalation is allowed to last longer than inspiration.

29. No study has shown a significant survival benefit. Routine use is not advocated at this time. (pages 518-519)

30. Page 519
    A. Heavy sedation
    B. Paralysis

31. Page 519
    A. Recruits collapsed alveoli
    B. Minimizes ventilator-induced barotrauma

32. APRV appears to be better tolerated by patients. One study showed much lower peak airway pressures and alveolar recruitment. (page 519)

33. Prone positioning has dramatically improved oxygenation in some patients. It is difficult to accomplish with critically ill adults. (page 520)

34. Blood is diverted into an artificial lung. (page 520)

35. They are restricted to controlled clinical trials and are not recommended for routine use. (page 520)

36. Lungs are partially filled with a perfluorocarbon solution, then the patient is ventilated with a conventional ventilator. (page 521)

37. Perfluorocarbon compounds can hold large quantities of dissolved oxygen—2.5 times as much as air. (page 521)

38. Alveofact, or surfactant similar to human surfactant, is instilled into the lung. Aerosolization did not work. (page 520)

39. Nitric oxide is a potent vasodilator that preferentially enters well ventilated portions of the lung and causes local vasodilation. (page 521)

40. Patients with high pulmonary vascular resistance. (page 521)

41. Methemoglobin. (page 521)

42. Severe pulmonary vasoconstriction. (page 521)

43. High dose corticosteroids have been used to treat uncomplicated pulmonary fibrosis following ARDS. (page 521)

Chapter Highlights

44. Respiratory, clinical

45. Hydrostatic, vasculature

46. Inflammatory

47. Bronchoscopy, pulmonary artery catheterization

48. Gas exchange, organ

49. Induced, injury, PEEP, tidal, oxygen

Case Studies

50. ARDS secondary to sepsis (pages 508-509)

51. Increase the PEEP (and try to reduce the FIO_2) (page 517)

52. Reduce the volume to 325-450 ml (5-7 cc/kg) (page 516)

53. PIP no higher than 35 cm H_2O (page 516), and mean airway pressure no higher than 35 cm H_2O (page 517)

53. Cardiogenic (hydrostatic) pulmonary edema caused by congestive heart failure. (page 512)

54. This patient is at the borderline of the minimally acceptable values. You would probably need to improve cardiac function with drugs prior to increasing the PEEP. (pages 515, 517) Treating the underlying CHF and improving blood pressure will improve tissue oxygenation. (page 514)

What Does the NBRC Say?

55. B. Initiating PEEP (page 515)

56. B. 10 cm H_2O 60 mm Hg 4.3 L/min (pages 515, 519)

57. B. Inspiratory crackles (see Chapter 14)

58. C. Change to inverse ratio ventilation (page 581)

59. D. Pulmonary artery catheter (pages 514, 517)

60. D. I, II, III only (page 510)

61. C. I, II, III only (pages 518-519)

Food for Thought

62. It's not recommended.

63. Heterogeneous. Gattinoni suggests 3 distinct zones in ARDS lungs. The overall state is one of reduced overall lung volume, but the aerated portions of the lung are basically normal. Ventilation techniques will affect each area of the lung differently. (page 516)

Chapter 25

New Words

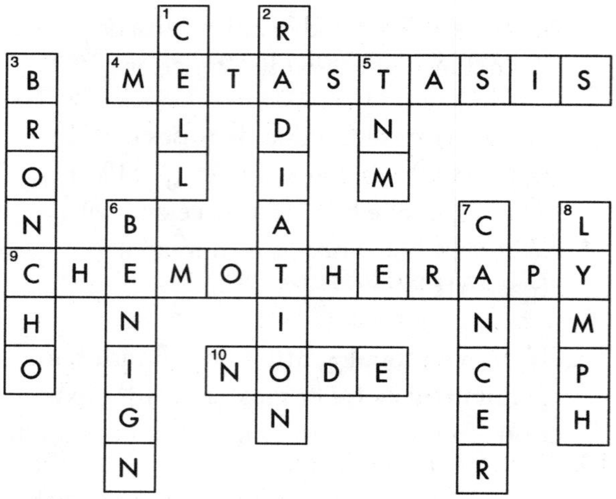

1 CELL
2 RADIATION
3 BRONCHO
4 METASTASIS
5 TNM
6 BENIGN
7 CANCER
8 LYMPH
9 CHEMOTHERAPY
10 NODE

Meet the Objectives

1. Page 526
   A. 178,100 in United States
   B. 2 million new cases worldwide

2. Page 526
   A. 28% of cancer deaths
   B. 6% of all deaths

3. The peak incidence of lung cancer in white and black men occurred in the mid 1980s. The rate for women of all races continues to increase. (page 526)

4. Smokers in general have a ten to twenty-five fold increase in lung cancer compared with non-smokers. (page 526)

5. Page 526
   A. Number of cigarettes smoked
   B. Duration in years of smoking
   C. Early age at the initiation of smoking
   D. Depth of inhalation
   E. Tar and nicotine content of cigarettes

6. Page 526
   A. United States smokers—46 million adults
   B. Percentage of population: 26%
   C. Men: 24 million
   D. Women: 22 million

7. Second-hand smoke. (page 527)

8. Passive exposure increases the risk of bronchogenic cancer. The average risk for a spouse of a smoker is increased by 30%. Spouses of long-term heavy smokers have an 80% excess risk. Second-hand smoke results in about 3,000-5,000 deaths each year. (page 527)

9. Page 527
   A. Atmospheric pollution
   B. Occupational factors
   C. Dietary factors
   D. Genetic factors

10. Exposure to smoke and a synergistic factor increases the overall risk more than either factor alone. Exposure to radon is an example. (page 527)

11. Page 527-529

Type of Cancer	Percent	Description
A. Adenocarcinoma	30-35	Forms glandular structures (4 types)
B. Squamous cell	30-32	Flat epithelial cells.
C. Large cell	15-20	Large, aggressive peripheral lesions, mets
D. Small cell	20-25	Centrally located in bronchi, metastasizes

12. Page 529
    A. CNS
    B. Cervical lymph nodes

13. 15% (page 529)

14. Page 529
    A. Cough
    B. Wheezing
    C. Hemoptysis
    D. Dyspnea
    E. Hoarseness (also dysphagia, chest pain)

15. Page 529
    A. Chest pain
    B. Dyspnea
    C. Cough

16. Page 529
    A. Excessive production of bronchial secretions
    B. Indicates extensive lung involvement

17. Extrathoracic manifestations caused by nonmetastatic complications. (page 529)

18. Page 530
    A. Hypercalcemia
    B. Inappropriate antidiuresis
    C. Cushing's syndrome
    D. Neurologic syndromes (also clubbing, weight loss, fever, malaise)

19. Page 532
    A. Sputum cytology
    B. Fiberoptic bronchoscopy
    C. Transthoracic needle aspiration
    D. Thoracotomy

20. Tumor staging is the most important prognostic variable in bronchogenic carcinoma. (page 532)

21. Page 533
    A. T = Tumor
    B. N = Nodes
    C. M = Metastases

22. There are only two: limited and extensive. Limited means the cancer is confined to one side of the chest and suggests that radiation will be a possible treatment. (page 532)

23. Resection offers the best chance of long-term survival. (page 535)

24. Stage IIIB (locally advanced) and Stage IV (metastatic) are not surgical candidates. (page 535)

25. RCPs might perform pulmonary function testing, usually spirometry. (page 535)

26. A preoperative FEV_1 of at least 2 liters, or 70% of predicted indicate adequate lung reserves. If the FEV_1 is less than 70%, then a postoperative prediction should be made. If the predicted postop FEV_1 is less than 40% of predicted, DLCO (predicted postop) is less than 40%, and the patient has significant dyspnea, postoperative mortality is likely. In any case, a pre-op FEV_1 of less than 35% of predicted is a contraindication to surgery. (page 535)

27. Page 535
   A. Endobronchial laser therapy
   B. Endobronchial radiation

28. Treatment is usually nonsurgical, and chemotherapy is the choice. Cis-platinum and etoposide are commonly used. (page 536)

29. 1-3% (page 536)

Chapter Highlights (page 536)

30. Bronchogenic

31. 85%

32. Adenocarcinoma

33. TNM, survival

34. Small cell

35. Radiation, chemotherapy

36. Smoking

Case Studies

37. Pancoast tumors may affect cervical sympathetic nerves. While drooping of the eyelids may also show up in neuromuscular diseases such as myasthenia gravis, the cancer patients will also have constricted pupils and lack of sweating on the affected side. (Mini Clini, page 530)

38. Stroke. But these symptoms can also show up in paraneoplastic syndromes. (page 530)

39. Many of these patients have underlying COPD. They may benefit from bronchial hygiene and bronchodilator therapy. (page 535)

40. Bronchoscopy. (page 530)

Food for Thought

41. COPD, cardiovascular disease, and others (such as eye disorders, diabetes)

42. Screenings of patients with high risk for lung cancer have been done using chest radiographs and sputum cytology, but they made no improvement in overall survival. There is no current consensus that high-risk patients should have annual tests. (page 535)

43. Endobronchial radiation. Radioactive material is placed into the airway. (page 535)

Chapter 26

Power Words

1. B

2. D

3. F

4. G

5. I

6. A

7. C

8. E

9. H

Meet the Objectives

10. Page 540
    A. Upper airway
    B. Chest wall
    C. Diaphragm (and some add abdominals)

11. Page 540
    A. Atelectasis
    B. Hypoxemia
    C. Ventilatory insufficiency

12. Page 540
    A. Exertional dyspnea
    B. Fatigue
    C. Orthopnea

13. Box 26-1, page 540

Location	Diseases
A. Cortex, upper motor	Stroke, traumatic brain injury
B. Spinal cord	Trauma, transverse myelitis, multiple sclerosis
C. Lower motor neurons	ALS, poliomyelitis, spinal muscular atrophy
D. Peripheral nerves	Guillain-Barré, Lyme disease
E. Neuromuscular junction	Myasthenia gravis, Lambert-Eaton, botulism
F. Muscle tissue	Duchenne's muscular dystrophy, polymyositis
G. Interstitial lung tissue	Polymyositis, dermatomyositis, neurofibromatosis

14. Restrictive (page 541)

15. Page 541
    A. Vital capacity
    B. Inspiratory pressures
    C. Arterial blood gases

16. It doesn't. Respiratory muscle weakness is not uniform. (page 541)

17. Cor pulmonale, daytime somnolence, and sleep disturbances. (page 542)

18. Page 542
    A. Primary muscle disease that decreases ability to generate effective contraction.
    B. Duchenne's muscular dystrophy— muscle wasting
    C. Myotonic dystrophy (also polymyositis)

19. Nocturnal ventilation (usually PPV) is used effectively in muscular dystrophy and Duchenne's muscular dystrophy. It is usually instituted in response to desaturation. PPV improves daytime muscle function as well, but prophylactic use early in the disease has not shown to be beneficial. (pages 542-543)

20. Production of antibodies (anti-ACh-r) against the ACh receptors which inactivates the receptors and ultimately destroys them. (pages 543-544)

21. Anticholinesterase inhibitors (page 543)

22. Thymectomy (page 543)

23. (Box 26-4, page 545)
    A. Viral infections
    B. Pregnancy
    C. Hodgkin's lymphoma
    D. General surgery

24. One third. (page 545)

25. High cervical cord injury. (page 545)

26. Cardiac surgery. (page 545)

27. The paralyzed diaphragm is still curved but is displaced upward on a standard xray view. (page 545)

28. Under flouroscopy, when the patient is asked to sniff, the diaphragm on the affected side moves upward. (page 546)

29. Page 547
    A. 10,000 new cases/year
    B. 5%-10%

30. Page 547
    A. High: C1-C2
    B. Middle/Low: C3-C8

31. Pages 547-548

Level	Muscle Groups
A. C1-C2	Complete respiratory muscle paralysis
B. C3-C5	Diaphragm
C. C4-C8	Shoulder girdle
D. T1-T12	Intercostals
E. T7-L1	Abdominals

32. Abdominal paradox—Inward movement of the abdomen while the thorax expands on inspiration. (page 548)

33. 80% (page 548)

34. Acute interruption of blood flow to the brain. (page 548)

35. Page 548
    A. Thrombotic/embolic
    B. Hemorrhagic

36. (Table 26-1, page 549)

Location	Effect on Respiration
A. Cerebral cortex	Impaired speech, mild hyperventilation, sleep apnea
B. Bilateral hemispheric infarct	Cheyne-Stokes breathing
C. Lateral medulla	Apnea (rare condition)
D. Midpons	Loss of conscious control of breathing (also rare)

37. Page 549
    A. Neurogenic pulmonary edema
    B. Hypersecretion of mucus

In addition, apnea may occur from head injuries severe enough to result in loss of consciousness.

38. Page 549
    A. Kyphosis—Posterior angulation of the thoracic cage
    B. Scoliosis—Lateral curvature of the spine

39. Page 550
    A. Ventilation—Hypoventilation and hypercapnia (eventually pulmonary hypertension)
    B. Pulmonary function—Restrictive defect with decreased compliance, decreased TLC and VC.

40. Surgical stabilization. (page 550)

41. Nocturnal ventilation is effective. Both positive and negative pressure devices are used. (page 550)

42. The destabilized segment of the chest moves outward with exhalation and collapses inward during inspiration (with spontaneous breaths). (page 550)

43. Page 550
    A. Pulmonary contusion
    B. Hemothorax
    C. Pneumothorax

44. Page 550
    A. Positive pressure ventilation
    B. Surgical stabilization of the ribs if needed
    C. Adequate analgesia

Chapter Highlights (pages 550-551)

45. Brain, neuromuscular, muscles

46. Ventilatory

47. Hyperventilation, apnea, atelectasis

48. Dyspnea, cough

49. Total, vital, maximal

Case Studies

50. Myasthenia gravis. (page 543). Naturally there are other possible causes, but Martha fits the classic MG profile: young woman, weakness after exertion, difficulty swallowing, descending weakness.

51. A rapid-acting anticholinesterase inhibitor such as Tensilon would be appropriate. (page 543)

52. Measurement of maximal inspiratory pressure (or expiratory) is a more sensitive test than vital capacity. (page 544)

53. Guillain-Barré Syndrome. (page 546)

54. Presence of protein in the CSF is typical in GBS at the height of the disorder. Few WBCs will be present (albuminocytologic dissociation).

55. A. Intravenous immunoglobulin infusion
    B. Plasmapheresis

What Does the NBRC Say?

56. D. Initiate mechanical ventilation

57. C. Intubation and mechanical ventilation (page 546)

58. C. 15 ml/Kg (page 546)

59. B. Neostigmine (page 543), unless the patient is in cholinergic crisis.

60. A. Flail chest (page 550)

Food for Thought

61. What is the long-term prognosis for the following conditions?
    A. Myasthenia gravis: Lifelong illness in most cases, controlled by drugs.
    B. Guillain-Barré syndrome: 20% have disability one year after the episode. It can recur. Mortality is about 3%-6%. (page 545)
    C. Duchennne's muscular dystrophy: Wheelchair by age 12, death by age 20 in most cases. (page 542)

Chapter 27

Acronym-o-philia

1. BiPAP—Bilevel positive airway pressure

2. CSA—Central sleep apnea

3. CPAP—Continuous positive airway pressure

4. EDS—Excessive daytime sleepiness (page 554)

5. EEG—Electroencephalogram (page 555)

6. EPAP—Expiratory positive airway pressure

7. IPAP—Inspiratory positive airway pressure

8. OSA—Obstructive sleep apnea

9. PSG—Polysomnogram (page 557)

10. UVPPP—Uvulopalatopharyngoplasty (page 565)

11. UARS—Upper airway resistance syndrome

Meet the Objectives

12. Repeated episodes of complete cessation of airflow for longer than 10 seconds. (page 554)

13. Obstructive apnea is due to upper airway closure. Central apnea is caused by lack of ventilatory effort. (page 554)

14. 2%-4%, or roughly equivalent to that of asthma or diabetes in the adult population. (page 554)

15. When you sleep the upper airway dilator muscles are less active and the airway narrows or closes. (page 554)

16. Box 27-1, page 556
    A. Nocturnal dysrhythmias
    B. Diurnal hypertension
    C. Pulmonary hypertension
    D. Right or left ventricular failure
    E. Myocardial infarction, stroke

17. Box 27-1, page 556
    A. Excessive daytime sleepiness
    B. Diminished quality of life
    C. Adverse personality change
    D. Motor vehicle accidents

18. Pages 554, 556
    A. Gender—3x more common in males
    B. Age—>40
    C. Craniofacial configuration (genetics)
    D. Upper body obesity (neck >16.5 inches)

19. Pages 556, 557
    A. Hypertension
    B. Oxygen desaturation during sleep
    C. Upper body obesity
    D. Habitual snoring
    E. Complaints of fatigue or daytime sleepiness

20. Full-night polysomnogram monitored in the sleep laboratory by a sleep technologist. (page 557)

21. AHI >40 is considered moderate to severe. Normal is less than 5 per hour. (page 557)

22. Box 27-4, page 560
    A. Eliminate apnea, hypopnea, and snoring
    B. Normalize oxygen saturation and ventilation
    C. Improve sleep architecture and continuity

23. First, patients should know the risks of untreated sleep apnea. Behavioral interventions include: weight loss in obese patients, avoidance of alcohol, sedatives, and hypnotic drugs, and avoidance of sleep deprivation. (page 560)

24. CPAP is noninvasive. There are multiple studies that document its effectiveness. (page 560)

25. CPAP splints the upper airway open by raising the pressure inside the airway. (page 560)

26. CPAP works in the lab. About 80% of patients accept their CPAP, but less than 50% may use it most of the time. Compliance with therapy is not related to how sick the patient is. Perceived benefit is a better predictor of compliance. Finally, compliance at 1 month may be a good predictor of more long-term cooperation. Masks may be a factor in compliance as well. (page 563)

27. IPAP and EPAP are titrated separately in bilevel ventilation. IPAP is always higher than EPAP, and is increased in 2.5 cm H_2O increments. IPAP is also raised to improve nonapneic desaturations. (page 564)

28. Page 564
    A. Claustrophobia—Try changing the mask
    B. Nasal congestion—Antihistamines or topical nasal steroids
    C. Rhinorrhea—Same as congestion
    D. Skin irritation—Try a different mask
    E. Nasal dryness—Nasal saline sprays, humidifiers
    F. Pressure—Try a system that ramps up the pressure gradually
    G. Pressure leaks—Try a chin strap or full face mask

29. Tracheostomy was the primary treatment at one time. Now it is reserved for severe cases where all other therapy has been exhausted. (page 565)

30. UPPP has a success rate of less than 50% overall, less with obese patients. It is not recommended. (page 565)

Chapter Highlights
31. Central, mixed

32. Narrow, unstable

33. Daytime, cardiovascular

34. Male, 40, obesity, snoring

35. CPAP

36. Bilevel

37. Surgical

What Does the NBRC Say?

38. C. Obstructive sleep apnea (page 563)

39. D. Central sleep apnea (pages 554, 556)

40. D. III only (page 564)

Food for Thought

41. Positional therapy helps some patients who only snore when they are supine. Sewing a tennis ball into the back of the pajamas keeps the individual from rolling onto their back while asleep. (page 560)

Chapter 28

Better Living Through Chemistry

1. D

2. P

3. F

4. I

5. J

6. C

7. L

8. E

9. B

10. S

11. K

12. G

13. T

14. H

15. Q

16. R

17. N

18. M

19. O

20. A

Just Say Yes

21. Inhalational (usually via aerosol) (page 572)

22. Page 572
   A. Smaller doses
   B. Rapid onset
   C. Target organ delivery
   D. Minimal systemic side effects

23. A. Delivered dose varies
   B. Lack of knowledge about devices (caregivers and patients)

24. They are swallowed from the oropharynx. (page 572)

25. Page 573

	Division	Other name	Transmitter	Airway muscle effect
A.	Sympathetic	Adrenergic	Norepinephrine	Dilation
B.	Parasympathetic	Cholinergic	Acetylcholine	Constriction

Adrenergic Bronchodilators

26. Page 574

	Receptor	Primary effect
A.	Alpha	Vasoconstriction and vasopressor
B.	$Beta_1$	Increased heart rate and contractility
C.	$Beta_2$	Smooth muscle relaxation, increased ciliary activity, possible inhibitory effect on inflammatory mediator release

27. Table 28-2, page 574

Name	Brand Name	Strength	Dose
A. Racemic epinephrine			
	Vapone-frin (others)	2.25%	.25-.50 ml
B. Metaproterenol			
	Alupent	5%	.3 ml
C. Terbutaline			
(svn)	Brethine	.1 %	.25-.5 mg
(MDI)	Brethaire	0.2mg/puff	2 puffs
D. Albuterol			
(svn)	Proventil, Ventolin	0.5%	0.5 ml (2.5 mg)
(MDI)	Same	90µg/puff	2 puffs
E. Bitolterol			
(svn)	Tornalate	0.2%	1.25 ml
(MDI)		0.37 mg/puff	2 puffs q8
F. Pirbuterol			
(MDI)	Maxair	0.2 mg/puff	2 puffs
G. Salmeterol			
(MDI)	Serevent	25 mg/puff	2 puffs
Salmeterol			
(MDI)	Serevent	25 mg/puff	2 puffs
H. Epinephrine			
(SVN)	Adrenalin	1%	.25-.50 ml

28.

Effect	Clinical Uses
Vasoconstriction	Decongestant for croup, control bleeding during procedures

29. Serevent is a maintenance drug, especially for treatment of nocturnal asthma symptoms. It should be avoided during acute episodes of bronchospasm because the onset and peak effect are delayed. Patients should be taught to use this drug only as prescribed, not to expect any immediate effects, and to use a shorter-acting drug such as Proventil during acute episodes. (page 576)

30. Table 28-3, page 576

Drug	Onset	Peak Effect	Duration
A. Isoetharine	1-6 min	15-60 min	1-3 hrs
B. Brethine	5-30 min	30-60 min	3-6 hrs
C. Ventolin	15 min	30-60 min	3-8 hrs
D. Serevent	20 min	3-5 hrs	12 hrs

31. Page 576
   A. Tremor
   B. Headache
   C. Insomnia
   D. Nervousness

32. Page 576
   A. Dizziness
   B. Nausea
   C. Tolerance
   D. Worsening $\dot{V}/\dot{Q}$ (Decreased PaO_2)
   E. Hypokalemia
   F. Propellant-induced bronchospasm

33. Vital signs, breathing pattern, breath sounds—before and after the treatment. (page 576)

34. Peak flow rates, reversibility of obstruction using pre- and post-bronchodilator studies, ABG or pulse oximetry, blood glucose and potassium if available, blood pressure (depending on medications), pulmonary function studies. (pages 576-577)

Anticholinergic Bronchodilators

35. COPD (page 577) (The nasal form is indicated for allergic and nonallergic rhinitis)

36. Table 28-4, page 578

Name	Brand Name	Strength	Dose
Ipratropium bromide			
MDI	Atrovent	18 mcg/puff	2 puffs
SVN		0.02%	0.5mg (2.5ml)

37. Page 578

Drug	Onset	Peak Effect	Duration
Ipratropium	1-5 minutes	1-2 hours	4-8 hours

38. Combivent is available by MDI with 18 µg of ipratropium and 90 µg of albuterol per puff. The advantage for practitioners and patients is the simplified delivery of both drugs. One disadvantage is cost, since no generic is currently available. The other disadvantage is that Combivent is only available in MDI. (page 578)

39. Dry mouth and cough are local side effects. Nervousness, headache, palpitation, and nausea are other possibilities. (Box 28-1, page 579) Eye pain and urinary retention are possible adverse reactions.

40. Atropine is easily absorbed into the bloodstream and may cause systemic side effects. CNS effects, increased heart rate, increased intraocular pressure and other problems may result. (page 579)

Mucous Controlling Agents

41. Table 28-5, page 580

	Dose	Strength	Indication
A. Acetylcysteine (Mucomyst)	3-5 ml	10%-20%	Thick secretions associated with chronic bronchitis, bronchiectasis, others.
B. Dornase alfa (Pulmozyme)	2.5 ml	1mg/ml	Cystic fibrosis with respiratory infection/ purulent mucus (recently approved for COPD)

42. Give a bronchodilator prior to the mucolytic. Dilute Mucomyst to 10%. (page 580)

43. Monitor the quality and quantity of sputum produced. Monitor airflow changes. Assess adequacy of cough and the need for suctioning. Consider adjunct therapy such as PEP or postural drainage/percussion. Long-term: monitor number and severity of respiratory tract infections and need for antibiotics. (pages 580-581)

Inhaled Corticosteroids

44. Hours to days. (page 582)

45. Patients must be taught to use their inhaled steroid as prescribed and not expect immediate relief. They also need to know that these drugs are not bronchodilators, and don't replace them. They will have to follow the treatment regimen every day to get the desired results. (page 582)

46. Box 28-3, page 583
    A. Oropharyngeal fungal infections
    B. Dysphonia
    C. Cough, bronchospasm
    D. Incorrect use of MDI

47. Reservoirs minimize risk of swallowing the drug and producing systemic side effects. (page 583)

48. NAEPP Guidelines recommend peak flow monitoring and assessment of long-term factors such as missed days of work or school. (page 583)

Mediator Antagonists

49. Prevents degranulation of sensitized mast cells. (page 584)

50. Cromolyn and nedocromil are safe for children. (page 584)

51. Cromolyn and nedocromil. (page 583)

52. Table 28-8, page 585
    A. Cromolyn sodium (Intal)—Cough
    B. Nedocromil (Tilade)—Unpleasant taste
    C. Zafirlukast—Headache
    D. Zileuton—Headache

Treating Infection by the Aerosol Route

54. Pentamidine isethionate (Nebupent, Pentam). (page 586)

55. Discuss how to determine whether to give this drug via the oral, inhalational, or IV route. Inhalation is primarily used for prophylaxis in at-risk HIV patients who have a history of PCP infection or low CD4 lymphocyte counts. IV use is reserved for acute episodes of PCP. The drug is not given orally. (page 586)

56. A special nebulizer with one-way valves and a filter is used. The patient is usually isolated during the treatment. Tuberculosis must be considered as well. (page 586)

57. Cough and bronchospasm are possible, along with shortness of breath, fatigue and others. There are numerous systemic side effects that are difficult to distinguish from the infection itself. Bronchodilators may be used to minimize bronchospasm. Patient teaching is also required. (page 586)

58. Tuberculosis. (page 586)

59. Page 587
    A. Indication—treatment of severe respiratory syncytial virus
    B. Patient population—usually children and infants
    C. Equipment—a SPAG generator is used to deliver the drug

60. Mostly antibiotics to treat gram negative bacterial infections (such as Pseudomonas). Tobramycin is currently approved. (page 587)

Case Studies

61. Beclomethasone (Vanceril, Beclovent); 2 puffs, TID or QID of the 42 µg/puff strength (page 582)

62. Reservoir-spacer, holding chamber (page 583)

63. Rinsing reduces systemic absorption from the mouth and throat.

64. Cromolyn sodium or nedocromil. (page 583)

65. Serevent (page 575)

66. Dornase alfa (Pulmozyme) (page 580)

67. A bronchodilator such as albuterol. (page 580)

68. Ipratropium (Atrovent)

69. You could consider Mucomyst, but it is likely to lead to more bronchospasm, and is less effective when nebulized than when it is instilled. (page 580)

What About Those Board Exams?

70. D. Aerosolized pentamidine isethionate (NebuPent) (page 586)

71. B. Nebulized cromolyn sodium (Intal) (page 584)

72. D. Aerosolized racemic epinephrine (Vaponefrin) (page 575)

73. A. Rinse and gargle with water

74. C. Continue the treatment (see Chapter 32)

75. D. Call the doctor to verify the order (Table 28-2, page 574)

Food for Thought

76. Acetaminophen overdose. (page 579)

77. Epinephrine. Problems include short duration, cardiac side effects, and rapidly developing tolerance.

Chapter 29

Tube Terms

endotracheal, polyvinyl, 15, length, beveled, Murphy, cuff, positive, pilot, valve, radiopaque tracheostomy, silver, outer, cuff, flange, inner, obturator

Intubation Procedures

1. Orotracheal intubation (page 592)

2. Page 592
   A. Physician
   B. RCP
   C. Nurse
   D. Paramedic

3. Vomit or secretions may obscure the pharynx or glottis. (page 594)

4. First, check to see that the bulb is tight. Next, check the batteries or replace the bulb. (page 594)

5. Size is determined by age or weight. (page 594)

6. Inflate the cuff and check for leaks. Ideally, this is done with a manometer or with water. (page 595)

7. The head is flexed moderately. A rolled towel may be placed under the head. (page 595)

8. The patient must be ventilated by bag/mask with 100% oxygen for several minutes. (page 595)

9. Intubation attempts must not exceed 30 seconds. Intubation deprives the patient of oxygen and ventilation. (page 595)

10. The arytenoid cartilages and the epiglottis. (page 595)

11. The MacIntosh blade fits into the vallecula (at the base of the tongue) and lifts the epiglottis indirectly. (page 595)

12. (page 597)
    A. Listen for equal and bilateral breath sounds
    B. Listen for air in the epigastrium
    C. Observe the chest wall for equal and adequate expansion
    D. Check the depth of insertion against the tube markings. Normal depth in males is 21-23 cm for oral intubation.
    E. Use the EDD to check for esophageal intubation
    F. Use a light wand to check for tracheal intubation
    G. Use capnometry or colorimetric CO_2 detection devices

13. Cardiac arrest victims have poor pulmonary blood flow, which may make these devices inaccurate for detecting intubation. (page 598)

14. Page 598
    A. Chest radiographs
    B. Fiberoptic laryngoscope or bronchoscope

15. Page 599
    A. Cervical spine injuries
    B. Maxillofacial injuries

16. Pages 600-601
    A. Blind—Insert the tube through the nose in an upright patient, listening through the tube for breath sounds as you advance the tube.
    B. Direct visualization—Advance the tube while using the laryngoscope and the Magill forceps as needed to advance the tube into the larynx.

17. Table 29-1, page 593

A. Avoids epistaxis and sinusitis	O
B. Greater comfort for longterm use	N
C. Easier to suction	O
D. Larger tube	O
E. Greater risk of extubation	O
F. Improved oral hygiene	N
G. Bronchoscopy more difficult	N
H. Increased salivation	O
I. Reduced risk of kinking	O
J. Decreased laryngeal ulceration	N
K. Increased risk of sinusitis	O

Tracheotomy

18. The primary indication is the need for an artificial airway for a prolonged period of time. (page 601)

19. When the patient has an upper airway obstruction or for long-term care of patients with neuromuscular disease. (page 601)

20. The ET tube should remain in place until just prior to inserting the tracheostomy tube. (page 601)

21. Traditional surgical tracheostomy places the tube in the neck over the second or third tracheal ring. Percutaneous tracheostomies are placed between the cricoid cartilage and the first ring, or between the first and second tracheal rings. (pages 602-603)

22. Page 603
    A. Rapid
    B. Avoids the need for transport to the OR
    C. Lower incidence of intraoperative and postoperative complications

Airway Trauma

23. Page 604

Injury	Symptoms	Treatment
A. Glottic edema	Hoarseness, stridor	racemic epinephrine, steroids
B. Vocal cord inflammation	Hoarseness	Usually resolves quickly
C. Laryngeal ulceration	Hoarseness	No treatment
D. Polyp/ granuloma	Difficulty swallowing, hoarseness, stridor	If symptoms do not resolve, surgical removal is indicated
E. Vocal cord paralysis	Hoarseness, stridor	Tracheostomy may be needed
F. Laryngeal stenosis	Stridor, hoarseness	Surgical correction or tracheostomy

24. Page 604
    A. Granulomas
    B. Tracheomalacia
    C. Tracheal stenosis

25. Page 605

Injury	Cause	Pathology	Treatment
A. Malacia	Softening of rings	Collapse of trachea	Resection
B. Stenosis	Narrowing	Fibrous scarring	Laser, resection

26. T-E fistula is caused by tracheal erosion from cuffs, esophageal erosion from NG tubes, malnutrition, or poor surgical technique. Aspiration may occur. Treatment involves surgical closure of the opening. (page 605)

27. A pulsating tracheostomy tube may be the only clue. Once hemorrhage begins, hyperinflation of the cuff may help, but surgery is needed. 75% of these patients will die. (pages 605-606)

Care and Feeding of Your New Airway

28. ET tubes are secured with tape. Tracheostomy tubes are secured with cloth ties. Commercial harnesses are available. (page 606)

29. Extension (head up) moves the tube up. Flexion moves the tube down. The tube may move as much as 1.9 cm in either direction. (pages 606, 607)

30. Complete obstruction of the tube and asphyxiation. (page 607)

31. 32°-35° C. (page 607)

32. Heat and moisture exchangers. (page 607)

33. Box 29-4, page 608
    A. Bypass upper airway filtration
    B. Increase aspiration from the pharynx
    C. Contaminated equipment
    D. Impaired mucociliary clearance
    E. Mucosal damage from tube or suctioning
    F. Ineffective cough

34. Page 608
    A. Adhering to sterile technique with suctioning
    B. Using aseptic or sterile equipment
    C. Handwashing

35. Retained secretions. (page 608)

36. High residual volume, low pressure (page 609)

37. Safe pressure (according to Egan!) is below the 20-25 mm Hg tracheal mucosal capillary perfusion pressure. If cuff pressure exceeds the mucosal perfusion pressure, ischemia, ulceration, and necrosis may result. (page 609)

38. Pages 609-610
    A. Minimal occluding volume—Slowly inflate the cuff until air heard escaping around the cuff during a positive pressure breath ceases. (Note the volume it takes to make a seal) Adjustments must be made if peak pressure changes.
    B. Minimum leak—Fill the cuff as noted above. Then remove a small amount of air until a slight leak occurs during the positive pressure breath.

39. A methylene blue test is performed by adding methylene blue to the patient's tube feedings, or by adding it to some type of food and having the patient swallow a small amount. Next, the airway is suctioned. If you observe blue dye in the secretions, you know that the patient has aspirated. (page 611)

40. Page 611
    A. Obstruction
    B. Cuff leaks
    C. Accidental extubation

41. Page 611
    A. Kinking or biting on the tube
    B. Herniation of the cuff over the tube tip
    C. Jamming of the tube orifice against the tracheal wall (also mucous plugging)

42. Attempting to pass a suction catheter through the tube. (page 611)

43. Extubation and manual ventilation by bag/mask. (and reintubation) (pages 611-612)

44. Remove the inner cannula and check to see if it is plugged, or if the outer cannula is plugged. (page 611)

45. Loss of delivered volume and decreased inspiratory pressures. (page 612)

46. First, try to reinflate the cuff and determine if the leak is in the pilot tube and valve. Check the pressure and tube position to determine if the tube is too high in the airway (which also makes a leak). If the cuff is really blown, and the patient requires ventilation, you must prepare to reintubate. (page 612)

Extubation

47. Page 612
    A. Deflate the cuff completely and occlude the tube. Check for air moving around the tube during spontaneous breathing.
    B. Deflate the cuff and assess leaking around the tube during positive pressure ventilation.

48. Page 612
    A. Suctioning equipment
    B. Oxygen/aerosol equipment
    C. Manual resuscitator and mask
    D. Aerosol nebulizer and racemic epinephrine (prn)
    E. Intubation equipment

49. You need to suction the ET tube and then the pharynx above the cuff. (page 612)

50. Page 613
    A. Remove the tube during peak inspiration delivered by the resuscitation bag.
    B. Remove the tube as the patient coughs.

51. Cool mist with oxygen as needed. (page 613)

52. Attempt to manually ventilate the patient with the resuscitation bag and mask. If unable to ventilate, the patient should be given a neuromuscular blocking agent and reintubated. (page 614)

53. Stridor indicates glottic edema. Racemic epinephrine can be given to reduce the swelling. Reintubation may be needed. (page 614)

54. Up to 24 hours to avoid the risk of aspiration. Ice chips or cool water can be given. (This probably depends on how long the patient was intubated) (page 614)

55.

Technique	Advantage	Disadvantage
A. Fenestrated tubes	Easy to suction, ventilate	Malposition, granuloma
B. Progressively smaller tube	Stoma healing gradual	Impairs cough, obstructs
C. Tracheostomy button	Low resistance, suction	No cuff

56. Advantage: less hypoxemia, cross-contamination is decreased, and cost may be decreased. Ventilation is not interrupted. Disadvantage: inadvertent triggering, extra weight on the circuit, increased resistance. (page 619)

57. The coude catheter (page 616)

58. Pages 619-620

Complication	Cause	Prevention
A. Hypoxemia	Disconnection from O_2	Give 100% prior to suction
B. Cardiac arrhythmia	Hypoxemia (tachycardia)	Preoxygenate
	Vagal stimulation (bradycardia)	Avoid mouth, observe patient—stop if event occurs
C. Hypotension	Arrhythmia, cough	Oxygenate, monitor patient—stop if event occurs
D. Atelectasis	Removal of air	Hyperventilate, limit vacuum, short suction times
E. Mucosal trauma	Catheter adherence	Limit vacuum, twirl
F. Increased ICP	Coughing	Use lidocaine

59. Sniffing position. (page 620)

60. Water soluble lubricant. (page 620)

61. Nasopharyngeal airway. (page 620)

Bronchoscopy

62. The rigid bronchoscope has a large inside diameter that facilitates surgery and removal of foreign material, mucous plugs. It is very uncomfortable, requires an anesthesiologist in an OR setting, and cannot access smaller airways. (page 621)

63. Page 622

Drug Class	Example	Goal
A. Tranquilizer	Valium, Versed	Decrease anxiety
B. Drying agent	Atropine	Aid visibility, anesthesia
C. Narcotic-analgesic	Morphine, fentanyl	Reduce pain, reflexes
D. Anesthetic	Lidocaine, cocaine	Reduce reflexes
E. Vasocon-strictor	Phenyle-phrine, cocaine	Reduce bleeding

64. Page 623
    A. Pulse oximeter
    B. Blood pressure
    C. ECG

Case Studies

65. 6.5-7.5 mm ID (page 594)

66. Check the cuff for leaks by inflating it. (page 595)

67. Assemble the handle and blade and check the bulb for brightness and tightness. (page 594)

68. There are several methods. Listen for equal, bilateral breath sounds and observe chest motion. Check depth of insertion. Use an EDD or colorimeter. Check with a light wand. (pages 597-598)

69. Effective pulmonary circulation may not be achieved. Technique should be assessed. (page 599)

70. Assess breath sounds and look for secretions in the airway. (pages 616-617)

71. -100 to -120 mm Hg (page 616) (Note the difference from standard values!)

72. 14 French (page 618)

73. At least 30 seconds with 100% oxygen, either from the ventilator or a bag. If the ventilator is used, allow for washout time. (page 619)

74. Less than 20-25 mm Hg or 24-30 cm H_2O. (page 609)

What About Those Board Exams?

75. C. I, III only (pages 609-610)

76. C. One-half the inner diameter of the ET tube (page 618)

77. B. A cuffed tracheostomy tube (page 614)

78. D. Stridor (page 614)

79. B. Stylette (page 595)

80. D. II, III only (page 619)

81. B. I, III only (pages 597-599)

82. D. Remove the inner cannula (page 611)

83. A. Capnometry (page 599)

84. D. Lidocaine (page 623)

Food for Thought

85. Case reports suggest less tube movement, less skin damage, and decreased self-extubation with commercial tube holders. They do cost more than tape, and are not all created equal. (page 606)

Chapter 30

Acres of Acronyms

1. ABC—Airway breathing circulation

2. ACLS—Advanced cardiac life support

3. AED—Automated external defibrillator

4. AHA—American Heart Association

5. ARC—American Red Cross

6. BLS—Basic life support

7. BVM—Bag valve mask

8. CDC—Centers for Disease Control

9. CNS—Central nervous system

10. CPR—Cardiopulmonary resuscitation

11. DNR—Do not resuscitate

12. EMS—Emergency medical system (services)

13. OSHA—Occupational Safety and Health Administration

14. PALS—Pediatric advanced life support

15. PVC—Premature ventricular contraction

16. RCP—Respiratory care practitioner

17. SVT—Supraventricular tachycardia

Causes and Prevention of Sudden Death

18. Coronary heart disease (page 630)

19. 100,000-200,000 (page 630)

20. Page 630
    A. Motor vehicle accidents
    B. Drowning
    C. Electrocution
    D. Burns
    E. Suffocation (and drug intoxication)

21. Foreign body obstruction accounts for over 3,000 deaths annually, most of which occur in children under the age of 5. (page 630)

Basic Life Support

22. Box 30-1, page 631

Action	Description
A. Responsiveness	The first step. "Shake and shout"
B. Activate EMS	For adults—Second step, for kids do the ABCs
C. Airway	Open airway—Head-tilt chin-lift
D. Breathing	Look, listen, feel—If no breathing give 2 slow breaths
E. Circulation	Check pulse—Carotid, for infants check brachial

23. Table 30-1, page 631

Category	Adult	Child	Infant
A. Obstructed			
1. Conscious	Heimlich	Heimlich	Five back blows then chest compressions
2. Unconscious	Finger sweep, ventilate, thrusts	Look in mouth, ventilate, thrusts	Look in mouth, ventilate, back blow
B. Breathing	12/min	20/min	20/min
C. Compress			
1. Hands	finger above xiphod heel—both hands	finger above xiphod heel—one hand	finger below nipple 2 fingers
2. Ratio	15:2 (1 rescuer) 5:1 (2 rescuers)	5:1	5:1
3. Cycles	4 at 15:2	20 at 5:1	20 at 5:1
4. Depth	1.5-2 in.	1-1.5 in.	0.5-1 in.
5. Rate	80-100/min.	100/min.	At least 100/min.

24. Suspected spinal injuries. (page 632)

25. Listen over the mouth and nose while watching for the chest to rise. This should take 3-5 seconds. (page 632)

26. Pages 633-634
    A. Adults—Open airway, pinch nose. Take a deep breath and slowly (1.5-2 seconds) but forcefully exhale. Use mouth-to-nose if necessary. Release and repeat x 1.
    B. Children—Age 1-8. Same as adult but breath should be 1-1.5 seconds and only enough air to make the chest rise.
    C. Infants—Under 1 year. Seal your mouth over the victim's nose and mouth. Extend the head slightly to prevent occlusion of the airway.
    D. Hazard—gastric distension

27. Lockjaw or mouth/jaw injuries. (page 634)

28. Get a resuscitation bag. If no bag is available, you could use a cloth to cover the stoma or tube to create a barrier.

29. The carotid artery is checked in adults, the brachial artery in infants. The femoral artery can be used for both. (page 635)

30. Pages 636-638
    A. Adult—Place 2 fingers on the xiphoid process. Place the heel of one hand on the lower third of the sternum above your fingers. Interlock fingers of both hands and compress 1.5-2 inches.
    B. Children—Same as adults, but only use one hand for compressions, and only compress 1-1.5 inches.
    C. Infant—Place index finger on the imaginary line across the nipples. Place middle and ring fingers next to the index finger. Lift the index finger and compress with two fingers to a depth of 0.5-1 inch. (Newborns—use wrap-around technique and compress with thumbs over intermammary line to a depth of 0.5-0.75 inches)

31. Pages 638-639
    A. Near drowning—Don't try to compress in the water. Get the victim onto a hard surface.
    B. Electrocution—Remove the victim from the electrical source. Turn off the power.
    C. Pacemaker—Essentially the same as for any other adult victim.
    D. Artificial heart valve—External compression can damage the valves, but they'll die without CPR anyway. A surgeon is needed to crack the chest so internal compression can be accomplished.

32. Page 639
    A. Advanced life support is available
    B. Spontaneous pulse and breathing are restored
    C. A physician pronounces the victim dead

33. Ventricular fibrillation (page 639)

34. Electrical defibrillation (page 640)

35. "D" stands for defibrillation using AEDs or standard defibrillators, depending on the setting. (page 640)

36. Page 640
    A. Ventilation—observation of chest motion and exhalation
    B. Compression—presence of a palpable pulse with compressions. Improvement of skin color.

37. Page 640
    A. Worsening of existing spinal injury
    B. Gastric distention and vomiting
    C. Trauma to internal organs during compressions

38. Pages 641-642
    A. When the patient is obviously biologically dead (or resuscitation is futile)
    B. When the patient has expressed (and documentation exists) a desire not to be resuscitated.

39. Clutching at the throat with both hands. (page 643)

40. Don't go there. (page 643)

41. Page 643
   A. Heimlich maneuver
   B. Pregnant women and really obese people

42. Page 644
   A. Confirmed expulsion of the foreign body
   B. Breathing and ability to speak
   C. Return of consciousness
   D. Return of normal color

Advanced Cardiac Life Support

43. The maximum amount available. (page 645) (hopefully close to 100%)

44. Page 645
   A. 3   Bag-valve-mask
   B. 1   Mouth-to-mouth
   C. 2   Mouth-to-mask

45. Page 645
   A. Transparent
   B. Capable of sealing tightly
   C. Oxygen inlet
   D. 15-22 mm connector
   E. Available in sizes

46. Place the flange even with the mouth. Measure along the jaw. The correct airway will measure from the corner of the mouth to the end of the jaw. (page 647)

47. Pages 647-648
   A. Guedel (hollow)
   B. Berman (solid)

48. The airway could cause gagging, vomiting, or laryngospasm. (page 647)

49. The nasopharyngeal airway. (page 648)

50. Page 647
   A. Hold the tongue down with a tongue depressor, and insert the oral airway with the curve over the tongue.
   B. Rotate the airway 180 degrees (upside down) and insert it. Then rotate it again.

51. Page 648
   A. Oral—don't
   B. Nasal—water soluble lubricant

52. The ET tube maintains the airway, prevents aspiration, permits suctioning, facilitates ventilation, and provides a route for drug administration. (page 648)

53. 30 seconds (page 648)

54. Page 650
   A. Use a reservoir
   B. Provide the highest possible flow of oxygen
   C. Deliver an appropriate tidal volume
   D. Ensure the longest possible refill time

55. When an IV access cannot be established. (page 653)

56. Defibrillation. (page 652)

57. Page 653
   A. Epinephrine
   B. Lidocaine
   C. Atropine

58. Larger doses (2-2.5 x), saline bolus (10 ml), and ventilation must accompany the drug. (page 653)

59. In adults, 200 joules, then 200-300, then 360 joules. For children 2 joules /kg, then 4 joules/kg. (page 657)

60. Cardioversion is synchronized to the R wave of the heart to avoid causing fibrillation. Cardioversion is also accomplished at much lower energy levels. (and for different rhythms!) (page 657)

61. Pacing is used to treat unresponsive brady-cardias and heart blocks. (page 657)

62. Page 657
   A. Transcutaneous (transthoracic)
   B. Transvenous

The Return of Just Say Yes
63. Table 30-2, page 654

Event	Drug Therapy
A. Ventricular tachycardia	Lidocaine Procainamide Bretyllium
B. Pulseless electrical activity	Atropine
C. Asystole	Epinephrine Atropine
D. Poor cardiac contractility	Dobutamine
E. Hypotension	Dopamine
F. Hypertension	Nitroprusside
G. Ventricular fibrillation	Lidocaine (and epi)
H. SVT	Adenosine
I. Coronary artery occlusion	t-PA Streptokinase
J. CHF/pulmonary edema (fluid overload)	Lasix

NBRC Highlights
64. C. In cases of suspected neck injury (page 632)

65. D. Give another breath after repositioning the head (page 633)

66. A. Brachial artery (page 635)

67. B. Call for help (pages 630-631)

68. B. 12 breaths per minute (page 631)

69. D. Insert a nasal airway (page 647)

70. C. 1:5 (page 631)

71. D. An oral endotracheal tube (page 648)

72. A. Do nothing but reassure the patient (page 643)

73. D. Electrical countershock (page 652)

74. B. Endotracheal instillation of the medications (page 653)

75. C. II, IV only

76. D. Cardioversion (page 657)

Food for Thought
77. 45% of physicians and 80% of nurses surveyed said they would not do mouth-to-mouth on a stranger for fear of contracting a disease. Barriers such as pocket masks, filters, and valves are an alternative. (pages 642-643)

78. I don't think the answer to this question is in the chapter. A good opportunity to discuss "calling a code" and "code buttons." Most hospitals have a specific number such as "5555" to call a code on the phone.

79. Some hospitals have chaplains. AHA ACLS guidelines call for a post-conference or debriefing for providers after a code. Obviously the physician managing the code must take some responsibility. See the AHA ACLS manual for more details.

Chapter 31

Wet Words
hygrometer, body, inspissated, humidifier, heat, moisture, nebulizers ultrasonic, piezoelectric

Meet the Objectives
1. In the upper respiratory tract, mainly the nose. (page 662)

2. Page 662
   A. Reduced ciliary motility
   B. Increased mucous production
   C. Increased airway irritability
   D. Drying and thickening of secretions

3. 4L/min. (page 662)

4. Patients with artificial airways such as endotracheal tubes. (page 662)

5. Table 31-1, page 662

Primary
A. Humidifying dry medical gases
B. Humidify when upper airway is bypassed

Secondary
A. Managing hypothermia
B. Treat bronchospasm from cold air

6. Page 663
A. Temperature (The most important variable)
B. Surface area
C. Time of contact

7. Oronasal oxygen delivery systems. (page 664)

8. Page 664
A. 15-20 mg/L
B. 33%-50%

9. A pop-off or pressure release (page 664)

10. Passover humidifiers can maintain humidification at high flow rates. They also add little or no resistance to gas flow. (page 665)

11. Pages 665-666
A. Condenser humidifier—On inspiration, air cools the condenser element. On exhalation, water from the warm air condenses onto the cool element. On the next inspiration, the air is warmed and humidified by the element.
B. Hygroscopic condenser humidifier— A low thermal conductivity element is impregnated with hygroscopic salt (calcium or lithium chloride). The salt plus the element capture heat and moisture. During inspiration, the moisture is returned to the gas without cooling.

C. Hydrophobic condenser humidifier— Uses a water-repellent element with a large surface area and low thermal conductivity. The element heats up on exhalation. On inspiration, the condenser element cools considerably, capturing water to add to the next breath. (These last two types are about equally efficient, but condensers can also provide bacterial filtration.)

12. Page 670
A. Presence of copious, thick, or bloody secretions
B. Expired tidal volumes less than 70% of inspired volumes
C. Body temperatures below 32° C
D. Minute volumes greater than 10 L/min.

13. Page 670
A. Hyperthermia (or hypothermia)
B. Burns to patient or caregiver
C. Electrical shock (there are many others)

14. Page 670
A. Aerosolized contaminated condensate during disconnects
B. Inadvertent tracheal lavage from condensate
C. Increased work of breathing or ventilator asynchrony

15. Heated wire circuits. (page 672)

16. 30°-37° C. (page 670)

17. Quantity and consistency of secretions. (page 670) or monitoring the humidity level in the system with a portable hygrometer. (page 673)

18. Visually confirm condensation in the flex tubing. (page 673)

19. Page 674
A. Presence of upper airway edema (cool, bland aerosol)
B. Presence of a bypassed upper airway
C. Need for sputum specimens

20. Page 673
    A. Hypotonic sterile water
    B. Isotonic sterile saline
    C. Hypertonic sterile saline

21. Fig. 31-12, page 675
    A. Radio frequency generator
    B. Shielded cable
    C. Piezoelectric crystal transducer
    D. Couplant water reservoir
    E. Solution chamber (patient solution)
    F. Chamber inlet
    G. Chamber outlet

22. Signal frequency. Particle size is inversely proportional to frequency. (page 675)

23. Amplitude control. (page 675)

24. Sputum induction. (pages 676, 677)

25. Hypertonic (3%-7%) saline solution. (page 677)

26. Page 676
    A. CO_2 buildup (high gas flows will prevent)
    B. Heat retention (refrigeration will prevent)

27. Pages 677-679

Problem	Solution
A. Cross-contamination/infection	Strict adherence to infection control guidelines. Disinfection of USNs
B. Environmental safety	Airborne and standard precautions
C. Inadequate mist	Inadequate flow, obstructed siphon tube, jet orifice misalignment. USN—electrical supply, source of flow, amplitude, and couplant level and type of water
D. Overhydration	Avoid continuous use, especially USNs
E. Bronchospasm	Monitor patient, avoidance, bronchodilators
F. NOISE	Use passover humidifiers with infants

Chapter Highlights

28. Moisture, nose

29. 32°-35° C

30. Humidifier

31. Nebulizer

32. Temperature

33. Microaerosols

34. Condensate, infectious

35. Water, edema

Case Studies

Use the algorithm on page 678 to choose the right humidity or bland aerosol system.

36. Page 670
    A. Body temperature is low.
    B. You haven't assessed secretions yet. A near-drowning victim may have pulmonary edema.

37. Heated passover. (page 670)

38. Unheated bubble humidifier

39. He doesn't have an artificial airway

40. HME-CABG requires short-term ventilation in most cases

What About Those Board Exams?

41. D. There is a kink in the oxygen supply tubing. (page 664)

42. D. 3% NaCl solution (page 677)

43. C. I, III only (page 671)

44. D. Replace the HME (page 670)

45. D. 75 ml

Food for Thought

46. Some adult patients, especially those who require long-term O_2, may need humidification at low flows. You would add humidity if the patient had symptoms of nasal irritation and drying such as pain, bloody nasal secretions.

Chapter 32

Terminology Torture

1. A

2. E

3. D

4. G

5. H

6. F

7. I

8. C

9. J

10. B

Characteristics of Therapeutic Aerosols

11. The ability of aerosols to travel through the air, enter the airways, and deposit in the lung is largely based on particle size. (page 684)

12. Inertial impaction (page 685)

13. ≥ 10 micron deposit in the nose and mouth. 5-10 micron deposit in the upper and large airways. (page 685)

14. In the lower airways. Particles 2-5 microns in size. (page 685)

15. Measure the clinical response. (page 687)

Hazards of Aerosol Therapy

16. Page 687
    A. Sterilize reusable nebulizers between patients.
    B. Frequently replace nebulizers with sterile or disinfected units.
    C. Rinse nebulizers with sterile water every 24 hours.

17. Page 687
    A. Acetylcysteine
    B. Antibiotics
    C. Steroids
    D. Cromolyn sodium
    E. Ribavirin (and distilled water)

18. Administer a bronchodilator prior to giving agents that cause spasm. (page 687)

19. Page 687
    A. Measure peak flow or FEV_1
    B. Auscultate
    C. Observe breathing pattern and overall appearance
    D. Communicate with the patient

20. Infants (and patients who can't mobilize secretions (page 687)

21. Reconcentration is when the strength of the drug in the solution increases. This problem is most likely to occur when medications are nebulized for longer than 10-15 minutes, such as in continuous nebulization.

Aerosol Drug Delivery Systems

22. Up to two thirds. (page 689)

23. CFCs are a problem because they may cause adverse reactions in patients and have adverse environmental effects. (page 689)

24. Dispersal agents such as soy lecithin, sorbitan, and oleic acid. (page 689)

25. It varies because the MDI is technique-dependent. (page 689)

26. Corticosteroids depositing in the mouth can result in oral yeast infections (and systemic absorption). (page 689)

27. Box 32-1, page 689
    A. Hold your breath   5
    B. Breathe out normally   3
    C. Wait 1 minute (between puffs)   6
    D. Shake the canister   1
    E. Hold the MDI two fingers from mouth   2
    F. Slowly inhale as deep as you can   4

28. A spacer is a simple valveless extension device that reduces oropharyngeal deposition and improves particle size. Holding chambers incorporate a valve to prevent the chamber from being cleared on exhalation. Holding chambers improve delivery to patients with small tidal volumes. Holding chambers improve delivery over simple spacers. (page 690)

29. With a holding chamber, it is recommended that you continue to breathe through the device for three breaths. (Box 32-2, page 691)

30. DPI is a dry powder inhaler. DPIs don't use harmful propellants, are breath activated and easier to use, and are inexpensive. Patients prefer them. (page 691)

31. Patients inhale rapidly. (page 691)

32. Children under 5 and patients unable to generate a high air flow. During acute episodes, a patient may not be able to use the DPI effectively. They also may not work as well in high-humidity environments. (page 693)

33. Page 693
    A. Compressed gas such as oxygen from a cylinder
    B. Compressed air from a compressor
    C. A 50 psi wall outlet

34. Atomizers don't have baffles. They are usually powered by a hand-squeezed bulb. Since the particles are larger, the drug deposits in the upper airway. You might deliver a local anesthetic through an atomizer prior to bronchoscopy. (pages 693, 699)

35. Page 694
    A. 6-8 L/min
    B. 4 ml

36. What potential problem exists when you deliver an SVN via mask? How can you deal with this problem? If the patient inhales through their nose, most of the drug will be deposited in the upper airway, not the lung. Instruct the patient to breathe through their mouth. (page 696)

37. Drug reconcentration. Consequently, the patient needs to be monitored closely. (page 697)

38. It incorporates a drying chamber with a separate flow control. It is normally used to deliver Ribavirin. (page 697)

39. Table 32-2, page 699

	Advantages	Disadvantages
A.	Small dead volume	Expensive
B.	Quite	Break down easily
C.	Aerosol is not wasted on exhalation	Can't be used with all medications

Case Studies (Figs. 32-15, 32-16; pages 701, 703)

40. MDI (DPI could be used for his bronchodilator)

41. Holding chamber

42. Proper technique for use of his MDIs

43. Redemonstration. (page 705)

44. You could continue with the MDI by repeating the 4 puff sequence 1-2 more times and check peak flows. Another option is to go to to SVN.

45. I recommend the SVN, since his peak flow rates are low.

46. Give the MDI x 4 puffs and check VS and peak flow. Repeat the sequence as needed. The highest peak flow represents the best dose.

47. This patient will be unable to use an MDI, so SVN is indicated. (page 696)

48. Use a mask.

49. Auscultation.

What About Intubated Patients?

50. Give 2-5 times the normal dose. (page 709)

51. Four puffs. (page 709)

52. Inspiratory side, 18 inches from the wye connector. (page 709)

53. Coordinate firing the MDI with the beginning of the ventilator inspiration. (page 709)

54. Use a total volume of 4-6 ml. (page 709)

55. A. I only (page 689)

56. D. Increase medication delivery (page 685) A 10-second breathhold can increase deposition by 10%.

57. B. Utilizing an aerosol mask for delivery (page 696)

58. D. Remove the HME during delivery of the drug. (page 709)

59. A. Recommend MDI instruction (page 699)

60. B. Small particle aerosol generator (page 697)

Food for Thought

61. Page 709
    A. Ribavirin
    B. Pentamidine

62. Use a private room, tent, booth, or specially designed station. A private room should have negative pressure ventilation with at least six air exchanges per hour. HEPA filters should be used to filter room or tent exhaust, or the aerosol should be scavenged to the outside. Special nebulizers can be used that filter exhausted mist. In addition, therapists can wear protective barrier gear to minimize exposure. (pages 709-710)

63. What do the terms HEPA and PAPR refer to? HEPA refers to a "high efficiency particulate air" filter. PAPRs are powered air purifying respirators. (page 711)

Chapter 33

Gas Powered

```
¹R E ²D U C I N G
    I
   ³C A R B O N
    M           ⁴D                    ⁵V
   ⁶R E G U L A T O R                  A
    T           T      ⁷H E  ⁸F L O W
    E                  E      V      ⁹B
   ¹⁰F R ¹¹A ¹²C T I O ¹³N A L  ¹⁴H E L I O X
   ¹⁵F     S  H      I      I      S      U
   ¹⁶D I S S  O      T      U             R
    A       S  R     R    ¹⁷M A ¹⁸N I F O L D
            P         ¹⁹A I R      F      O
        ²⁰Z ²¹O N E         C    ²²P I S S  ²³N I ²⁴T R O U S
   ²⁵D     X                      A         A
    I    ²⁶P I N                           N
    O     D                               K
   ²⁷O X Y G E N
    I
    D
    E
```

Characteristics of Medical Gases

1. Page 716
   A. Nitrogen
   B. Carbon dioxide
   C. Helium

2. Page 716
   A. Oxygen
   B. Nitrous oxide
   C. Air

3. Page 716
   A. Filter—Removes pollutants, water, and carbon dioxide
   B. Compress—To a high pressure to liquefy the air
   C. Cool—Rapid expansion (the Joule-Thompson effect)
   D. Heat—Slow heating in a distillation tower to boiling point of O_2 is reached

4. 99% (Page 716)

5. Page 716
   A. Molecular sieves—Air is forced through sodium aluminum silicate pellets (90%)
   B. Semipermeable membrane—Air is forced through a plastic membrane (40%)

6. Page 717
   A. Hospital—A motor-driven piston compresses the air (filtered) and delivers it to a reservoir tank. Reservoir air is reduced to a working pressure by a reducing valve. Cooling is used to remove water. Teflon piston rings are incorporated to prevent oil contamination.
   B. Home—Diaphragm compressors (or turbine) are used. They don't have a reservoir. Like the hospital system, they are not lubricated with oil.

7. Diagnostic purposes in the laboratory. (page 717)

8. Heliox is a mixture of helium and oxygen. It is used to treat severe large airway obstruction such as life-threatening asthma. (page 717)

9. Nitrous oxide is an anesthetic gas. It takes high levels to achieve true anesthesia, which can cause severe CNS depression, so it is usually mixed with oxygen first, and then used to supplement other anesthetics. Long-term exposure may result in neuropathy. N_2 has been linked with fetal disorders. (page 717-718)

10. Treatment of persistent pulmonary hypertension. (page 718)

11. High concentrations can cause methemoglobinemia. NO and air combine to form a toxic gas. (page 718)

12. Page 716-718

Gas	Symbol
A. Oxygen	O_2
B. Air	AIR
C. Carbon dioxide	CO_2
D. Helium	He
E. Nitrous oxide	N_2O
F. Nitric oxide	NO

13. The cylinder markings on the diagram:
    A. DOT specifications for cylinder construction material
    B. Service (filling) pressure
    C. Original hydrostatic test date
    D. Elastic expansion during testing
    E. Retest dates

14. Page 719
    A. * Indicates DOT approval for ten-year testing
    B. + Indicates that cylinder may be filled to 10% above the service pressure

15. Table 33-2, page 719
A. Oxygen	Green
B. Carbon dioxide	Gray
C. Nitrous oxide	Blue
D. Helium	Brown
E. Nitrogen	Black
F. Air	Yellow

16. Read the label, just like any other drug. (page 719)

17. Oxygen concentrations should be confirmed by analysis. (page 719)

Fill 'er up

18. Page 720
    A. CO_2
    B. N_2O

19. In a gas-filled cylinder, the pressure represents the amount of force required to compress the gas into the smaller space. The pressure in a liquid-filled cylinder represents the vapor pressure above the surface of the liquid. (page 721)

20. Page 721
    A. Gas-filled: The volume of gas is directly proportional to the pressure. If a cylinder is full at 2200 psig, it will be half full when the pressure is 1100 psig.
    B. Liquid-filled: The most accurate way to determine the contents of a liquid-filled cylinder is to weigh the cylinder.

21. Page 722 Cylinder factor = Cubic feet (full) x 28.3 ÷ Pressure (full) in psig (28.3) is the English-metric conversion factor to convert cubic feet to liters.

22. Page 722
    A. E: 0.28
    B. H: 3.14

23. Page 722
    Duration of flow(min) =
    Pressure × Cylinder factor ÷ Flow (L/min)

Bulk Oxygen

24. A manifold is made of many large compressed gas cylinders connected together in series. There are two sides to the manifold. The primary side supplies the gas to the hospital under normal circumstances. If the pressure in the primary side falls too low, a control valve switches over to the reserve bank. You then replace the cylinders in the primary side, and it becomes the new reserve. (page 723)

25. Primarily because large amounts of liquid gas can be stored in a relatively small container. (page 723)

26. Approximately 860 (page 723)

27. The critical temperature of oxygen is -181.1° F, or -118.8° C. Basically, the liquid is stored in a giant "Thermos bottle" that has a vacuum between the inner and outer shells, which eliminates heat conduction. (page 723)

28. 50 psi (page 723)

29. Zone valves are used to shut off the flow of gas to specific areas of the hospital for system maintenance or in case of fire. (page 724)

Safety Systems

30. Page 719
    A. Small cylinder: Fusible plug melts at a specific temperature and releases the gas.
    B. Large cylinder: Frangible disk or spring-loaded valve that opens when pressure in the cylinder gets too high.

31. Page 724

	Abbreviated Name	Full Name
A.	ASSS	American Standard Safety System
B.	DISS	Diameter-Index Safety System
C.	PISS	Pin-Index Safety System

32. This is an ASSS safety system for a large cylinder of oxygen.

CGA refers to the Compressed Gas Association. 540 is the number assigned by the CGA to this connection. The number 14 indicates that there are 14 threads per inch on the connector, and RH means they are right-handed, or that the connecting hex nut is turned clockwise to attach. EXT refers to external threads. (page 725)

33. Small cylinders up to size E. (page 725)

34. Diameter-index safety system. Low pressure in this case means less than 200 psig. (page 726)

35. A variation of the DISS, quick connects make it easier to attach equipment such as flowmeters to the wall station outlets. (page 727)

Regulating Pressure and Flow

36. Page 728
    A. Reducing valve: Reduces gas pressure to a safe/working value
    B. Flowmeter: Controls gas flowrate
    C. Regulator: Controls pressure and flow

37. Pages 728-729
    A. Preset reducing valve: Used with high pressure gas cylinders to reduce pressure to 50 psig for use with respiratory care equipment.
    B. Adjustable reducing valve: Used when you need to adjust the pressure, the most common type is used with a Bourdon-type flowmeter.
    C. Multiple-stage reducing valve: Used to minimize pressure fluctuations during the process of reducing pressure. The most common use is with laboratory and research activities.

38. Page 729
    A. Rapid rise in temperature can cause ignition of combustible materials.
    B. Rapid rise in pressure can cause component failure that produces "high-velocity projectiles."

39. Table 33-7, page 730

	Advantages	Disadvantages
A.	Low cost, simple, reliable	Individual restrictors for each flow
B.	Cannot be set wrong (Gravity independent)	Downstream resistance affects accuracy (Can't use with high-resistance equipment)

40. Fixed-orifice variable-pressure flow metering device. (page 731)

41. It is gravity-independent. (page 731)

42. Indicated flow will be higher than actual flow when there is significant downstream resistance. (page 731)

43. Page 731
    A. Bourdon: Pressure
    B. Thorpe: Flow

44. Compensated Thorpe flowmeters deliver the same flow that is indicated. Uncompensated flowmeters deliver more flow than is indicated when there is downstream resistance. (Figure 33-21, page 733)

45. If the valve is closed, the float will jump, the return to zero as the flow tube is pressurized. (page 733)

Case Studies

51. What type of regulator is most appropriate for transport? Bourdon gauge. (page 731)

52. Page 722

    Formula: Duration = PSI x Factor ÷ Flow

    Calculation: 1000 × 0.28 ÷ 10 L/min = 280 ÷ 10 or 28 minutes.

53. Pages 725-726
    A. Tighten the hand screw (and check the pins and holes).
    B. Check the nylon washer (bushing).

Speaking of Board Exams?

54. C. 10 hours (page 722)

55. A. Replace the flowmeter

56. B. 56 minutes (page 722)

57. C. Plug the flowmeter back into the outlet, CRTT (or CRT in the future). Examinations often ask some type of flowmeter-related troubleshooting problem.

Food for Thought

58. Nitrous could have harmful effects on any pregnant personnel or patients. In a relatively enclosed space personnel could become intoxicated. (page 718)

59. Total failures are reported and major problems occur with up to one third of all bulk systems. First, a protocol should be established to identify and prioritize all affected patients. Next, back-up systems should be used such as portable cylinders and bag-valve-mask resuscitators. Finally, the system should be bypassed and alternate supplies established while the bulk system is repaired. (page 724)

60. We recommend eye protection. Failed components become high-velocity projectiles. (page 729)

Chapter 34

Tank Jockey

1. canulla   *cannula*

2. reservore   *reservoir*

3. lasitude   *lassitude*

4. diaphramatic   *diaphragmatic*

5. retanopathy   *retinopathy*

6. *hypoxemia*   hypoxemea

7. *toxicity*   toxisity

8. *infarction*   infraction

9. displasia   *dysplasia*

10. pendent   *pendant*

11. *concentration*   concintration

12. entranement   *entrainment*

13. *wye*   why

Please Pass the Gas

14. Hypoxemia is a decreased level of oxygen in the blood. *Acute* means sudden. Glossary.

15. Page 739
    A. Adults (and children)
       1. $PaO_2 < 60$ mm Hg
       2. $SaO_2 < 90\%$
    B. Newborns
       1. $PaO_2 < 50$ mm Hg
       2. $SaO_2 < 88\%$

16. Page 738
    A. COPD (and interstitial disease); O_2 decreases dyspnea
    B. Chronic hypoxemia; O_2 improves mental function

17. Page 738
    A. Increased ventilation
    B. Increased cardiac output

18. Myocardial infarction. Because the heart is stressed or damaged, it is especially important to reduce workload. (page 738)

19. Hypoxemia causes vasoconstriction of pulmonary vessels. If prolonged, this results in pulmonary hypertension, increased work of the right heart, and eventually cor pulmonale or right heart failure. (page 738)

20. Page 738
    A. Laboratory evidence
    B. Patient's specific condition or problem
    C. Bedside assessment

21. Page 739
    A. Carbon monoxide poisoning
    B. Cyanide poisoning
    C. Shock
    D. Trauma
    E. Acute myocardial infarction
    F. Postoperative patients

22. Table 34-1, page 739

System	Mild	Severe
A. Respiratory	Tachypnea Dyspnea	Tachypnea Dyspnea
B. Cardiovascular	Tachycardia Mild hypertension	Tachycardia then bradycardia Hypertension then hypotension
C. Neurologic	Restlessness Disorientation	Somnolence Confusion

What Could Go Wrong?

23. Page 740
   A. Lungs
   B. CNS

24. Page 740
   A. PO_2
   B. Exposure time

25. Tracheobronchitis and substernal chest pain develop during the first 12 hours. Next, vital capacity and lung compliance begin to decrease (12-30 hours). A state similar to bronchopneumonia develops. The alveoli and capillaries are damaged, resulting in interstitial edema. Type I cells are destroyed. In the end stages hyaline membranes form, then pulmonary fibrosis and hypertension develop. (pages 740, 741)

26. High FIO_2 causes O_2 toxicity, which causes shunting, which results in lower PO_2 levels, which require higher FIO_2 levels for treatment. (Figure 34-2, page 741)

27. Limit exposure to 100% oxygen to less than 24 hours whenever possible. High FIO_2 levels are acceptable if the concentration can be lowered to 70% within 2 days, and 50% within 5 days. (page 741)

28. Never. (page 742)

29. Patients who are breathing from their hypoxic drive. (page 742)

30. Page 742
   A. Suppression of peripheral receptor drive to breathe increased CO_2
   B. Worsening $\dot{V}/\dot{Q}$ increases CO_2

31. Never. (page 742)

32. Oxygen causes retinal vasoconstriction and vascular necrosis. New blood vessels form and cause hemorrhages and scarring which leads to retinal detachment and blindness. (page 742)

33. Premature infants and neonates up to 1 month. (page 742)

34. Maintain PO_2 levels less than 80 mm Hg. Minimize other factors such as acidosis. (page 742)

35. FIO_2 levels above 0.50 cause atelectasis by washing nitrogen out of poorly ventilated units and depleting nitrogen from tissues. The oxygen is then used up physiologically and the alveoli collapse. (page 742)

36. Patients with low tidal volumes due to sedation, surgical pain, or CNS dysfunction. (page 742)

37. Use lower FIO_2. Encourage deep breathing.

Oxygen Delivery Systems

38. Page 743

Category	Description
A. Low-flow 2	1. Always exceeds patient's inspiratory needs
B. Reservoir 3	2. Provides some of patient's inspiratory needs
C. High-flow 1	3. May meet needs if no leaks occur

39. Well tolerated, simple, easy to use, low-cost, disposable, all ages. (page 745)

40. When flows are greater than 4 L/min (also with infants and children). (page 744)

41. 2 L/min (page 744)

Discuss these answers with your students if you have them perform the exercises.

42. Lowers O_2 usage and cost. (pages 744-745)

43. Many variables affect the FIO_2 delivered by all low-flow systems, including mouth breathing, respiratory rate, tidal volume, inspiratory flowrates, minute ventilation, and so on. Table 34-4, page 748

44. Assess the actual response to the oxygen-physical assessment and pulse oximetry or ABGs. (page 748)

45. Page 745
   A. Advantages: lower O_2 usage and cost, increased mobility, less discomfort
   B. Disadvantages: unattractive, cumbersome, affected by pattern, poor compliance

46. The home. (page 745)

47. Table 34-3, page 745

Mask	FIO_2 Range	Advantage	Disadvantage
A. Simple	35-50%	Cheap, easy	Discomfort, vomitus
B. Partial	35-60%	Moderate FIO_2	See simple mask
C. Non	55-70%	High FIO_2	Suffocation hazard

48. Valves. Particularly between the bag and the mask. (page 750)

49. The bag does not fully deflate on inspiration. (page 751)

50. Table 34-6, page 751

Problem	Solution
A. Confused patient removes mask	Restrain patient
B. Humidifier pop-off activated	Find obstruction, omit humidifier
C. Mask causes claustrophobia	Use another device
D. Bag collapses on inspiration	Increase flow
E. Bag fully inflated on inspiration	Correct leak, fix/replace mask

51. Page 752

Factor	Increased Size	Decreased Size
A. Jet		
1. FIO_2	Increased FIO_2	Decreased FIO_2
2. Flow	Decreased flow	Increased total flow
B. Port		
1. FIO_2	Decreased FIO_2	Increased FIO_2
2. Flow	Increased flow	Decreased total flow

52. Table 34-7, page 754
   A. 100%   0:1
   B. 60%   1:1
   C. 40%   3:1
   D. 35%   5:1
   E. 30%   8:1
   F. 24%   25:1

53. Venti-mask or Venturi mask (page 754)

54. Allows excess flow and patient exhalation to escape (page 755)

55. Little or no effect. (page 752)

56. 35% or less. (page 755)

57. Increase the input flow. (page 756)

58. The small jets limit the oxygen flowrates through the device. (page 756)

59. Page 755

Patient	Aerosol Appliance
A. Tracheostomy tube	T-piece or tracheostomy collar
B. Endotracheal tube	T-piece
C. Intact upper airway	Face tent, aerosol mask

60. Observe the mist on the expiratory side when the patient inhales. Calculate the flow delivered by the device. Measure the patient's minute ventilation and multiply by 3. Compare the two values. (pages 755-756)

61. Page 757
    A. Aerosol: Gas injection nebulizer
    B. Dry: Downs flow generator

62. Downstream resistance increases the FiO_2 and decreases total flow delivered. (page 758)

Mathemagic

63.
    A. Step 1—Compute the ratio
       Formula: $100\% - \% O_2 \div \%O_2 - 21$
       Calculation: $100 - 60 \div 60 - 21$
       Reduce answer to get ratio: $40 \div 39 = 1:1$
    B. Step 2—Add the parts: $1 + 1 = 2$
    C. Step 3—Multiply the sum of the parts times the O_2 flowrate: $10 \times 2 = 20$ L/min

Blenders

64. Page 759
    A. Confirm appropriate air and oxygen inlet pressure
    B. Test alarms by disconnecting each gas source
    C. Analyze at 100%, 21% and one other setting

Put That Child In a Box!

65. Frequent opening and closing causes wide swings in the FiO_2. (page 759)

66. 40%-50% (page 759)

67. It only covers the head and leaves the body free for nursing care. (page 760)

68. 7 L/min to prevent accumulation of CO_2. (page 760)

69. May generate harmful noise levels. (page 760)

70. Increases oxygen consumption and may cause apnea. (page 760)

71. Oxygen hood. (page 760)

72. Helps maintain a neutral thermal environment. (page 760)

HBO

73. Page 763

Chamber	O_2 Delivery	Patient	Staff
A. Monoplace	Cylinder is filled	One only	Outside
B. Multiplace	Patient wears mask	Up to 12	Inside

74. Box 34-6, page 765

Acute	Chronic
A. Decompression sickness	Enhanced wound healing
B. Air or gas embolism	Refractory osteomylitis
C. CO_2 poisoning	Radiation necrosis

75. History of unconsciousness, presence of neuropsychiatric abnormalities, cardiac instability, carboxyhemoglobin 25% in adults (lower in kids and pregnant women). (Box 34-7, page 765)

What Else Could There Be?

76. Pages 766, 767

Gas		Indications
A.	NO	ARDS
		Persistent pulmonary hypertension of the newborn
B.	He	Acute airway obstruction of various causes
		Postextubation stridor in pediatric settings (and croup)

77. O_2. Usually 80% He, 20% O_2. (page 768)

78. Low density. (page 768)

79. Nonrebreathing mask. (page 768)

Case Studies

80. Borderline saturation for a cardiac patient, but meets minimum criteria. Tachycardia may indicate cardiac dysfunction and definitely indicates increased cardiovascular work.

81. In spite of the SpO_2, the patient should be placed on oxygen. The AHA recommends 4 L via nasal cannula. (pages 738, 762)

82. Increased respiratory rate and tidal volume.

83. Increased rate, volume, and minute ventilation decrease the delivered FIO_2. (page 748)

84. Pulse oximeter and clinical signs.

85. The system is not delivering enough flow to meet the patient's needs. The FIO_2 will not be delivered. (page 755)

86. A reservoir on the expiratory side. (page 756)

87. Use two nebulizers in tandem. (page 757)

88. 1:1 (page 754)

89. 24 L/min. (page 753)

Board Exam Broadside

90. D. Inadequate preoxygenation (page 740)

91. D. Reduce the flow to 2 L/min and obtain an ABG (page 742)

92. B. Oxygen hood (page 760)

93. C. Increase the flow to the mask (page 751)

94. D. Nonrebreathing mask (page 768)

95. D. 18 L (page 768)

96. B. 32 L/min (page 753)

97. C. Increased flow rate (page 758)

98. B. 2L/min (pages 753-754)

Food for Thought

99. The device only delivers about 70% oxygen at best. Many clinicians believe that a patient is receiving the maximum amount of oxygen when they are not. A better system when 100% is needed is a nonrebreathing reservoir circuit. (page 751)

100. The AEM produces dry gas without the mist that might produce bronchospasm. (page 745)

Chapter 35

Word Power

1. Atelectasis: "When you don't take deep breaths . . . it's harder for your lungs to work normally. You could develop lung complications."

2. Incentive Spirometer (IS):
   A. "The purpose of this treatment is to . . . help prevent lung complications after your surgery."
   B. "This device will . . . show you how deep a breath you can take."

3. Sustained Maximal Inspiration (SMI):
"I want you to take . . . a slow deep breath until your lungs are full and hold it for three seconds."

4. Intermittent Positive Pressure Breathing (IPPB):
A. "Your doctor has ordered a breathing treatment that will . . . help you take a deep breath."
B. "This machine will . . . help push air into your lungs under pressure."

5. Continuous Positive Airway Pressure (CPAP):
A. "This treatment will . . . help you breathe more easily."
B. "I am going to put a mask on your face . . . with some straps to help make a seal against your face."

Meet the Objectives

6. Abnormal collapse of distal lung parenchyma.

7. Resorption atelectasis occurs when airways are blocked (mucus plugs) and the gas in the alveoli is absorbed into the blood, resulting in alveolar collapse. (page 772)

8. Passive atelectasis is caused by failure to take deep breaths (such as sighs) and fully expand the lungs. It is a common cause of atelectasis in hospital patients. (page 772)

9. General anesthesia, shallow breathing, decreased surfactant production, and pain are all reasons why postoperative patients are at higher risk for atelectasis. (page 772)

10. Decreased FRC is associated with basilar atelectasis. Since perfusion is higher in the dependent portions of the lung, a $\dot{V}/\dot{Q}$ mismatch results. (page 772)

11. Upper abdominal or thoracic surgery. (page 772)

12. Page 772
A. Spinal injury—inability to take deep breaths due to poor muscular function
B. Trauma, or bedridden patients—due to lack of mobility

13. Pages 772-773
A. History—smokers are more likely to have retained secretions and increased mucus production. Postoperative history of upper abdominal or thoracic surgery. History of COPD or other lung disorders.
B. Breaths sounds—presence of fine, late inspiratory crackles and/or bronchial breath sounds heard over the lung parenchyma.
C. Respiratory rate—increases proportionally to the degree of atelectasis.
D. Heart rate—tachycardia may be present if the atelectasis results in hypoxemia.
E. Chest film—confirms atelectasis by the presence of volume loss, air bronchograms, displacement of fissures, elevation of the diaphragm, and shift of the trachea.

14. Pages 773-774
A. Decreasing the surrounding pleural pressure (example, IS)
B. Increasing the alveolar pressure (example, IPPB)

15. Boxes 35-1, 35-2, 35-3, page 775
A. Indications
1. Presence of atelectasis
2. Surgery: upper abdominal, thoracic, or on COPD patients
3. Restrictive defects associated with quadriplegia or diaphragm dysfunction
B. Contraindications
1. Unconscious or uncooperative patients
2. Patients unable to take a deep breath: VC < 10ml/kg, 1C < ⅓ of predicted
C. Hazards
1. Hyperventilation and respiratory alkalosis
2. Discomfort secondary to inadequate pain control

16. Motley, 1947 (page 777)

17. Patients with atelectasis that is unresponsive to IS, and patients who cannot perform IS adequately or cannot cooperate. (page 778)

18. Untreated pneumothorax. (page 779)

19. Box 35-6, page 779
   A. Elevated intracranial pressure
   B. Hemodynamic instability
   C. Active hemoptysis
   D. Tracheoesophageal fistula
   E. Radiographic evidence of blebs (there are several more!)

20. Page 779
   A. Respiratory alkalosis
   B. Gastric distention

21. Collapsed alveoli are recruited as FRC is increased. Increased compliance decreases the work of breathing. Distribution of ventilation is improved via collateral ventilation through the pores of Kohn. Secretions are more efficiently removed. (page 783)

22. Page 783
   A. Hemodynamically unstable patients
   B. Patients who are hypoventilating (there are others . . . pneumothorax, face trauma)

23. Pages 783-784
   A. Hypoventilation—increased work of breathing through the circuit can worsen hypoventilation and hypercapnia.
   B. Barotrauma—most likely to occur in patients with emphysema and blebs.
   C. Gastric distention—occurs when pressures >15 cm H_2O are used and in patients who have poor airway reflexes.

24. A low pressure alarm. (page 784)

Chapter Highlights

25. Ventilation, small

26. Abdominal, thoracic

27. Lung disease, cigarette smoking

28. Fever

29. Rapid shallow

30. Alkalosis, too fast

Case Studies

Use the protocol found in Figure 35-8 on page 787 to help answer the following questions.

31. Smoking, upper abdominal surgery. (page 789)

32. Goal-oriented incentive spirometry (page 787)

33. One third of the predicted IC, or 600 ml for this patient. (page 787)

34. IPPB (CPAP is another possibility) (page 787)

35. They suggest the presence of atelectasis. (page 773)

36. What treatment would you recommend? Why? IPPB. This patient has multiple risk factors for postoperative lung complications and has developed atelectasis. IPPB has been shown to be effective in treating atelectasis. She is unable to perform IS. (page 787)

What About Those Board Exams?

37. A. Breathe more slowly (pages 775, 789)

38. D. Low pressure (page 785)

39. C. "Exhale gently and normally"

40. D. Sensitivity (page 781)

41. A. Pressure limit (page 781)

42. A. Functional residual capacity (page 783)

43. C. There is a leak in the system (page 782)

44. D. "Exhale normally, then inhale slowly and deeply and hold your breath" (page 777)

45. B. 6-10 breaths every hour (page 777)

46. A. IS (pages 779, 783)

47. D. The inspiratory time for a given breath (page 781)

Food for Thought

48. Most IS devices come with a predictive chart for determining IC. A normal young adult male has an IC of 3.6 L and IC is usually about 75% of the VC.

Chapter 36

Acronyms Again?

1. ACB—Active cycle of breathing

2. ARDS—Acute respiratory distress syndrome

3. AD—Autogenic drainage

4. CF—Cystic fibrosis

5 CPT—Chest physical therapy (page 792)

6. CPAP—Continuous positive airway pressure

7. EPAP—Expiratory positive airway pressure (page 807)

8. FET—Forced expiratory technique

9. HFCC—High-frequency chest wall compression

10. HZ—Hertz

11. ICP—Intracranial pressure

12. IPV—Intrapulmonary percussive ventilation

13. MI-E—Mechanical insufflation-exsufflation (page 807)

14. PDPV—Postural drainage percussion and vibration (page 792)

15. PEP—Positive expiratory pressure

16. PIE—Pulmonary interstitial emphysema (page 798)

Airway Clearance

17.

Phase	Impairments
A. Irritation	Anesthesia, CNS depression, narcotics
B. Inspiration	Pain, neuromuscular dysfunction, restriction
C. Compression	Laryngeal damage, artificial airway, abdominal weakness/surgery
D. Expulsion	Airway compression, obstruction, abdominal weakness

18. Full obstruction, like mucus plugging, results in atelectasis and impaired oxygenation through shunting. Partial obstruction results in poor airflow that increases work of breathing, air trapping, and $\dot{V}/\dot{Q}$ mismatch. (page 793)

19. Page 794
    A. Foreign body—external
    B. Tumor—external
    C. Secretions, bronchospasm, inflammation—internal

20. Page 794
    A. Cystic fibrosis
    B. Bronchiectasis

21. Page 794
    A. Muscular dystrophy
    B. ALS
    C. Myasthenia gravis
    D. Poliomyelitis (and cerebral palsy to name a few)

Bronchial Hygiene: Goals and Indications

22. Box 36-2, page 794 and 795
    A. Copious secretions
    B. Acute respiratory failure with retained secretions
    C. Acute lobar atelectasis
    D. Unilateral lung disease

23. Pneumonia may be present without significant sputum production. Uncomplicated asthma also may not have significant sputum clearance problems. (page 795)

24. Bronchial hygiene therapy for chronic conditions is proven to be effective if copious sputum production is present. Examples include cystic fibrosis, bronchiectasis, and some patients with chronic bronchitis. In general, sputum production must exceed 25-30 ml per day for bronchial hygiene therapy to be significantly helpful (page 795)

25. Page 795
    A. Body positioning and patient mobilization may be effective to prevent retained secretions in acutely ill patients.
    B. Exercise and postural drainage, percussion, and vibration have been shown to be effective prophylaxis for patients with cystic fibrosis.

26. (Box 36-3, page 795)

Factor	Significance
A. History	Pulmonary problems known to increase sputum. Also, for patients with upper abdominal or thoracic survey who have high risk due to COPD, obesity, age, and duration of the procedure.
B. Airway	Presence of artificial tracheal airway
C. Chest radiograph	Atelectasis or infiltrates
D. Breath sounds	Decreased, crackles, rhonchi
E. Vital signs	Fever, tachypnea, tachycardia

Bronchial Hygiene: Approaches to Therapy

27. Page 796
    A. Reduced venostasis
    B. Prevention of skin ulcers

28. Page 796
    A. Reduced incidence of atelectasis
    B. Reduced incidence of pneumonia
    C. Shortened ICU stay (in selected patients)
    D. Decreased ventilator days (in selected patients)

29. Page 796
    A. Absolute
       1. Unstable spinal cord injuries
       2. Traction of arm abductors
    B. Relative
       1. Severe diarrhea
       2. Marked agitation (and rise in ICP, drop in BP, hypoxia, arrhythmias)

30. Plumbing problems during turning include ventilator disconnection, accidental extubation, aspiration of circuit condensate, disconnection of vascular lines and urinary catheters. (page 796)

31. Dependent positioning takes advantage of the effects of gravity on pulmonary ventilation and perfusion. In unilateral lung disease, placing the good lung down tends to improve oxygenation by increasing perfusion in well-ventilated parts of the lung. This may be helpful in pneumonia or ARDS. With lung contusion or abscess, the good lung may be placed in the up position. This prevents blood or pus from going into the good lung. This also may be indicated for PIE. Prone positioning has also been suggested for ARDS to improve oxygenation. (pages 796, 798)

32. 1.5 to 2 hours after meals or tube feedings to prevent aspiration and gastroesophageal reflux. (page 799)

33. 3-15 minutes. (page 799)

34. Table 36-2, page 800

Complication	Interventions
A. Hypoxemia	Administer oxygen, or raise the FiO_2. Reposition patient.
B. Increased ICP	Stop. Restore patient position. Consult doctor.
C. Acute hypotension	Stop. Restore patient position. Consult doctor.
D. Pulmonary bleeding	Stop. Restore position. Give O_2. Get doctor immediately!
E. Vomiting	Stop. Suction. O_2. Position. Airway. Physician immediately.
F. Bronchospasm	Stop. Position. O_2. Request bronchodilator from doctor.
G. Cardiac dysrhythmias	Stop. Position. Give/increase O_2 and contact doctor.

35. Coughing should be avoided in head-down positions to avoid increasing ICP. If coughing is necessary, sit the patient up. (page 801)

36. It may take up to 24 hours to see real effectiveness. Therapy should be reevaluated at least every 48 hours for critical care patients, and 72 hours for other patients. (page 801)

37. Page 801
    A. Position(s) used
    B. Duration
    C. Patient tolerance
    D. Subjective and objective indications of effectiveness (amount of sputum)
    E. Adverse reactions

38. Both involve application of mechanical energy to the chest wall. In theory, percussion jars loosen the stuck secretions while vibration moves secretions upward during exhalation. (page 801)

39. The ultimate selection of the best way to percuss or vibrate may be patient preference. Machines do not get tired and deliver very consistent therapy. Manual percussion by a skilled practitioner may be preferred. (pages 801-802)

Coughing Techniques

40. Sitting upright, head slightly flexed, with arms and feet supported. If they can't sit up, at least raise the head of the bed. (page 803)

41. Page 805
    A. Surgical patients
    B. COPD
    C. Neuromuscular disorders

42. What is splinting? Supporting the area of an incision (abdominal or thoracic). (page 805)

43. Manually assisted cough-exerting pressure on the lateral ribs or epigastrium. (page 805)

44. The FET or huff cough has the patient take a moderately large breath then exhale rapidly while saying "huff" to keep the glottis from closing. It helps prevent bronchiolar collapse. It works well with patients who have obstructive lung disease. (pages 805-806)

45. Page 806
    A. Breathing control
    B. Thoracic expansion
    C. FET

46. It is difficult to teach/learn. (page 807)

47. 30-50 cm H_2O is delivered for 1-3 seconds. Pressure is abruptly reversed to -30 to -50 cm H_2O for 2-3 seconds. (page 807)

Positive Airway Pressure

48. Page 808
    A. Reduce air-trapping in asthma and COPD
    B. Mobilize retained secretions in CF and chronic bronchitis
    C. Prevent or reverse atelectasis
    D. Optimize delivery of bronchodilators in patients receiving bronchial hygiene

49. Actual airway pressures—not just set or intended pressures. (page 809)

High-Frequency Compression/Oscillation

50. External—HFCC, or internal-flutter, IPV. (page 810)

51. They are bulky and expensive. (page 810)

52. Page 811
    A. Readily accepted by patients
    B. Inexpensive
    C. Fully portable
    D. Self-administered

Mobilization and Exercise

53. Exercise enhances sputum clearance. It also improves aeration and ventilation perfusion relationships. Finally, exercise may improve fitness, self-esteem, and quality of life. (page 811)

54. Fatigue and oxygen desaturation. (page 811)

Case Studies

Use the algorithm (Figure 36-13) on page 813 to assist you in answering the following questions.

55. Splinting. (page 805)

56. Huff coughing (FET) could be tried if directed cough with splinting is not effective. (pages 805-806)

57. Postural drainage, percussion/vibration. PEP is an alternative. (page 813)

58. What therapy alternatives could you recommend for home use? PEP or flutter. (page 813)

What Does The NBRC Say?

59. A. Decrease the PEP level to 10 cm H_2O (page 809)

60. B. Right middle lobe (page 800)

61. D. Raise the head of the bed (page 801)

62. C. "This will help you cough more effectively" (page 809)

63. D. Notify the doctor and suggest a different secretion management technique (page 800)

64. B. II and IV only

Food for Thought

65. Dehydration or lack of humidification result in thicker secretions. Cool, bland aerosol therapy may enhance clearance in some patients. (pages 793, 801)

66. You should clap over the ribs. You should not clap over incisions, organs (kidney, abdomen) or women's breasts.

Chapter 37

"Look out kid, you're gonna get hit with . . . acronyms!"

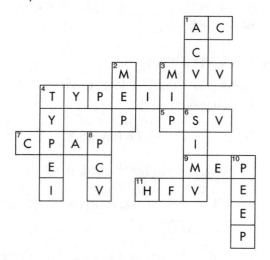

So, What Could Go Wrong?

1. "Inability to maintain either the normal delivery of oxygen to the tissues or the normal removal of carbon dioxide from the tissues." (page 820)

2. Page 820
   A. $PaO_2 < 60$ mm Hg (on room air at sea level)
   B. $PaCO_2 > 50$ mm Hg (in otherwise healthy individuals)

3. When an abnormality of the pulmonary system is the prime determinant of the worsening gas exchange pattern. (page 820)

Let's Review

4. 7.45 33 40 (PaO_2) or acute respiratory alkalosis with hypoxemia. (page 822)

5. $PaCO_2$ and alveolar ventilation vary inversely. (page 821)

6. Page 821 For a complete list see Table 37-1 on page 823. There are many examples.
   A. Decreased ventilatory drive
      1. Drug overdose/sedation
      2. Sleep apnea
   B. Respiratory muscle fatigue/failure
      1. Guillain-Barré
      2. Myasthenia gravis
   C. Increased work of breathing
      1. COPD
      2. Asthma

7. Hypermetabolic states such as severe burns. (page 822)

8. Kidney retention of bicarb or renal compensation. (page 822)

9. These patients are not judged by the simple criterion of increased $PaCO_2$, but by a significant increase above baseline for that patient. (page 823)

10. Page 823
    A. Bacterial or viral infections
    B. CHF
    C. Pulmonary embolus
    D. Chest wall dysfunction
    E. Medical noncompliance

11. Page 823
    A. Normalize pH (and avoiding mechanical ventilation if possible!)
    B. Elevating SaO_2 to $\geq 90\%$
    C. Improving airflow
    D. Treating infection

12. Page 823
    A. Emboli—invasive catheters
    B. Barotrauma—mechanical ventilation
    C. Infection—endotracheal tubes

13. Page 823
    A. Cardiac—arrhythmias, hypotension
    B. Gastrointestinal—hemorrhage, dysmotility
    C. Renal—acute renal failure, positive fluid balance

14. Page 823
    A. Bacteremia
    B. Malnutrition
    C. Psychosis

Mechanical Ventilation

15. Support the patient until the underlying problem is resolved. (page 823)

16. Table 37-2, page 824

Mechanism	Critical Value
A. $PaCO_2$	>55
B. pH	<7.20
C. VC (ml/kg)	<10
D. MIP	≥ -20 mm Hg
E. MVV	$<2 \times V_E$
F. V_E	>10 L/min
G. V_D/V_T	>0.60
H. $P(A\text{-}a)O_2$ on 100%	>350
I. P/F ratio	<200

17. They don't distinguish between readily reversible problems such as pulmonary edema and more complex problems such as acute lung injury. (page 825)

18. Assessment of pH allows you to differentiate acute and chronic hypercapnia. (page 825)

19. Page 825
    A. CNS insults
    B. Drug overdose/oversedation

20. Page 825
    A. Metabolic alkalosis
    B. Malnutrition
    C. Sleep deprivation
    D. Hypothyroidism

21. Neuromuscular disease. (page 825)

22. Page 825
    A. COPD
    B. Kyphoscoliosis
    C. Obesity

23. Page 825
    A. MIP/MEP
    B. FVC
    C. MVV

24. Hypercapnia with acidosis. (page 826)

25. Tachypnea (page 826)

Strategies

26. Table 37-3, page 826

A. Rapidly reversible hypoxemic failure	CPAP
B. Slowly reversible hypoxemic failure	Increased FIO_2, PEEP, IRV
C. Acute alveolar hypoventilation	AC, SIMV with high rates, PS with high pressures
D. Chronic alveolar hypoventilation	Bi-level mask ventilation A/C via tracheostomy
E. Altered mental status	A/C SIMV with adequate back-up rates
F. Acute muscle fatigue	Bi-level mask ventilation A/C, SIMV with adequate rates
G. Chronic muscle fatigue	Nocturnal bi-level mask ventilation A/C/SIMV with tracheostomy

27. Page 827
    A. Use small tidal volumes (6 ml/kg) with pressures ≤ 35 cm H_2O
    B. PCV

28. Volume-cycled assist control (SIMV with high rates and PSV with high pressures can also be used.) (page 827)

29. Avoid respiratory alkalosis and "normalizing" the blood gas. Try to return the patient to a normal pH, not $PaCO_2$. (page 827)

30. These modes require an intact ventilatory drive and the ability to protect the airway via intact reflexes. (page 827)

31. Page 828
    A. Type of support—Full ventilatory support
    B. How long?—24-48 hours

Special Cases

32. Alkalosis and hypocapnia reduce cerebral blood flow. (page 828)

33. 25-30 mm Hg (page 828)

34. PEEP may increase ICP. (page 828)

35. Page 828
    A. Volutrauma
    B. Decreased cardiac output

36. Page 829
    A. Tidal volume—8-10 ml/kg
    B. Flow rate—60-100 L/min

37. Application of extrinsic PEEP. (page 829)

Weird Ways to Ventilate

38. Page 829
    A. Massive hemoptysis
    B. Bronchopleural fistula
    C. Severe unilateral lung disease

39. Page 829
    A. Newborns with risk of volutrauma
    B. Bronchopleural fistula when other methods have failed

40. Weaning patients who do not tolerate PSV (page 830)

41. APRV maintains inspiratory volume, then briefly lowers end-expiratory pressure to promote exhalation (page 830)

42. Proportional assist ventilation is unique because...inspiratory flow, tidal volume, and airway pressure are all patient-effort related. The ventilator determines the appropriate amount of support. (page 830)

Chapter Highlights (page 830)

43. 50, 60

44. Hypoxemic, shunt

45. Hypercapnic, fatigue, breathing

46. Hypercapnia, polycythemia

47. Clinical

48. Work of breathing

49. Noninvasive

50. Minute

Case Studies

51. Acute respiratory alkalosis with hypoxemia (moderate). (page 822)

52. $PA_{O_2} = (760 - 47) .21-32 \div 0.8 =$
    $150 - 40 = 110 (PA_{O_2})$
    $110 - 50 = \textbf{60 mm Hg}$ (page 822)

53. Type I or hypoxemic respiratory failure. (page 822)

54. The textbook recommends administering 100% oxygen to help differentiate $\dot{V}/\dot{Q}$ mismatch from shunting. (page 822)

55. Acute respiratory acidosis with hypoxemia (mild). (page 822) (See also Chapter 12)

56. $PA_{O_2} = (760 - 47) .21 - 60 \div .8 =$
    $150 - 75 = 75$ mm Hg.
    $75 - 65 = \textbf{10 mm Hg.}$ (page 822)

57. Type II or hypercapnic respiratory failure

58. Oxygen therapy is not the issue in this case. The patient is hypoventilating, and this is the cause of the hypoxemia. Intubation and mechanical ventilation are the most likely choices of treatment. (page 822)

59. Partially compensated respiratory acidosis with hypoxemia (moderate). (page 822)

60. $PA_{O_2} = (760 - 47) .21 - 70 \div .8 =$
    $150 - 88 = 62$ mm Hg.
    $62 - 50 = \textbf{12 mm Hg.}$

61. This patient also has hypercapnic respiratory failure, but it is acute respiratory failure superimposed on chronic respiratory failure.

62. The goal for this patient is to normalize the pH while avoiding mechanical ventilation. Bronchodilators would be a simple starting point. Consider bronchial hygiene techniques. He also needs a small amount of oxygen, with the goal to increase the SaO_2 to 90%. 2 L via cannula or 28% by AEM.

What Does the NBRC Say?

63. A. Intubation and mechanical ventilation (page 820)

64. C. Administer oxygen therapy via CPAP (pages 825, 827)

65. C. Increase the rate (page 828)

66. D. Increase the PEEP (page 827)

67. D. Change to synchronized intermittent mandatory ventilation (SIMV) (page 827)

68. B. 28% air entrainment mask (see Chapter 34)

69. A. Respiratory failure secondary to shunting (page 827)

Food for Thought

70. Neuromuscular diseases would be an example of conditions best assessed by VC and MIP. Blood gases are especially useful in patients with COPD, or abnormalities of drive like obesity/hypoventilation.

Chapter 38

Ventilator Verbiage
(Answers to key terms in glossary)

1. B

2. G

3. C

4. I

5. E

6. D

7. H

8. F

9. A

How Ventilators Work

10. What is a ventilator? Simply a machine. A machine is a system designed to alter, transmit, and direct energy to perform useful work. (page 834)

11. Augments or replaces the patient's muscles in performing the work of breathing. (page 834)

12. Page 834
    A. Infant
    B. Transport
    C. Home

13. Pneumatically. (page 834)

14. MRI. (page 835)

15. Page 835
    A. Puritan-Bennett 7200—delivered gas directly inflates the lungs.
    B. Siemens Servo 900C—gas primes a spring-loaded reservoir.
    C. Engstrom Erica IV—gas compresses a reservoir.

16. Proportioning valves can shape the inspiratory flow waveform. (page 836)

17. Page 836
    A. Newport Wave
    B. Puritan-Bennett 7200
    C. Siemens Servo 900C and 300
    D. Bird 8400
    E. Bear 1000 (and Hamilton Veolar)

18. Page 837
    A. Pressure
    B. Volume
    C. Flow

19. There are two forms: pressure is controlled within a breath and volume is controlled between breaths (Siemens 300 volume support) or the ventilator may switch between volume and pressure control within a breath (Bear 1000 pressure augmentation and Bird 8400 VAPS) (page 840)

20. Page 840
    A. Mechanical
    B. Pneumatic
    C. Electric
    D. Electronic
    E. Fluidic

21. Page 840
    A. No moving parts
    B. Immune to electromagnetic interference (such as MRI)

22. Table 38-1, page 841
    A. Trigger variable—determines what causes the breath to begin
    B. Limit variable—determines what parameters are limited
    C. Cycle variable—determines what causes the breath to end
    D. Baseline variable—determines what happens during exhalation

23. Poorly tolerated by conscious patients and often requires sedation or paralysis to be successful. (page 841)

24. Pages 842, 843

Trigger	Advantage	Disadvantage
A. Pressure	Works under most conditions	Increases work of breathing
B. Flow	Decreases work of breathing	Sensitive to leaks, turbulence

25. Pages 841, 843
    A. Pure time triggering—control mode
    B. Pure patient triggering—assist mode
    C. Patient *and* time triggering—assist-control mode

26. A parameter that can reach and maintain a preset level before inspiration ends, but does not terminate inspiration. (Can be pressure, volume or flow). (page 843)

27. Page 844
    A. PSV
    B. PCV

28. Time-cycled, pressure-limited ventilation. (page 844)

29. Monitoring pulmonary mechanics to measure airway resistance and compliance. (page 845)

30. The variable that is measured and used to end inspiration. (page 845)

31. IPPB. (page 845)

32. During true pressure cycling, inspiration ends when a preset pressure is reached. During pressure limiting, the preset peak pressure is reached and held until another parameter such as time, volume, or flow ends the breath. (page 845)

33. Flow. (page 845)

34. The baseline variable is the parameter controlled during exhalation. (page 845)

35. Pressure. (page 845)

36. Pages 845, 846
    A. ZEEP—zero end-expiratory pressure. Normal passive exhalation.
    B. NEEP—negative end-expiratory pressure. Subatmospheric pressure applied to the airway during exhalation.
    C. PEEP—positive end-expiratory pressure. The application of pressure above atmospheric at the airway throughout exhalation.

37. Threshold resistors do not add to exhalation unwanted flow resistance (unaffected by changes in flowrate) that can increase PEEP and work of breathing. (page 846)

38. Box 38-2, page 846
    A. Underwater columns
    B. Spring-loaded diaphragms or disks
    C. Balloon valves
    D. Electromechanical valves

39. Traditionally, PEEP is applying pressure above atmospheric to the airway during exhalation with mechanical breaths. CPAP is applied to both inspiration and exhalation and traditionally applies to spontaneous breaths. (But PEEP can be applied to spontaneous breaths) (page 846) See Figure 38-16.

40. Page 847
    A. Spontaneous—patient breath: triggered and cycled by the patient.
    B. Mandatory—machine breath: either triggered or cycled by the ventilator.

41. A combination of control, phase, and conditional variables that establish a set pattern of mandatory and/or spontaneous breaths. (page 848)

42. Page 848
    A. CMV—all the breaths are mandatory
    B. CSV—all the breaths are spontaneous
    C. IMV—some breaths mandatory, some spontaneous

43. Table 38-3, page 850.

	Acronym	Name	Control variables
A.	CMV	Continuous mandatory ventilation	Pressure, volume, or flow
B.	A/C	Assist-control	Pressure, volume, or flow
C.	AMV	Assisted mechanical ventilation	Pressure, volume, or flow
D.	IMV	Intermittent mandatory ventilation	Pressure, volume, or flow
E.	SIMV	Synchronized IMV	Pressure, volume, or flow
F.	CPAP	Continuous positive airway pressure	Pressure
G.	PCV	Pressure controlled ventilation	Pressure
H.	PC-IMV	Pressure controlled int. mech. vent.	Pressure
I.	PCIRV	Pressure controlled inverse ratio vent.	Pressure
J.	APRV	Airway pressure release ventilation	Pressure
K.	MMV	Mandatory minute ventilation	Volume or flow
L.	VAPS	Volume assisted pressure support	Pressure, volume, or flow
M.	BiPAP	Bi-level positive airway pressure	Pressure

44. Draw these flow patterns. Answers on page 853

   A. Rectangular: Figure 38-24, A-B

   B. Ascending ramp: Figure 38-24, C

   C. Descending ramp: Figure 38-24, D

   D. Sinusoidal: Figure 38-25, E

45. To warn of events that require clinician awareness or action. (page 854)

46. Page 854
   A. Loss of electrical power—power cord pulled from socket
   B. Ventilator inoperative—microprocessor failure
   C. High peak airway pressure—endotracheal tube obstruction
   D. Low peak airway pressure—leak in the patient circuit
   E. High baseline pressure—circuit or exhalation valve obstruction
   F. Low baseline pressure—patient disconnection
   G. Low exhaled tidal volume—leaks, apnea, disconnection
   H. High minute volume—hyperventilation, machine self-triggering
   I. Low minute volume—apnea, leaks, disconnection
   J. Low respiratory rate—apnea

Clinical Application of Ventilator Models

47. When a precise minute ventilation or $PaCO_2$ is required (page 858)

48. Closed-head injury (page 858)

49. Page 858

Control Variable	Volume	Airway Pressure
A. Pressure	Decreases	Remains constant
B. Volume	Constant	Higher airway pressure

50. Controlled ventilation is poorly tolerated. Sedation or paralysis is often necessary to minimize work of breathing. (page 859)

51. A/C is useful in patients with stable ventilatory drives who are unable to generate sufficient spontaneous inspiratory volumes. (page 859)

52. Worsening of air-trapping. (page 859)

53. Use the formulas in Table 38-8 on page 860 to calculate these I:E ratios.
   A. Rate of 10, Inspiratory time 1 second.
      1. Total cycle time: 6 seconds
      2. I:E ratio   1:5
   B. Rate of 15, Inspiratory time 1 second
      1. Total cycle time: 4 seconds
      2. I:E ratio   1:3
   C. Rate of 20, Inspiratory time 2 seconds
      1. Total cycle time: 3 seconds
      2. I:E ratio   2:1

54. Page 860
   A. Weaning
   B. Primary mode of support

55. IMV results in a lower mean airway (and pleural) pressure than CMV because spontaneous breaths during IMV lower pleural pressures. (page 861)

56. Pages 861-862
   A. Continuous flow IMV with external gas source
   B. Demand flow IMV via the ventilator valves

57. Expired volume monitoring is difficult. (page 862)

58. Low-resistance wick-type (page 862)

59. Flow-triggering is preferred when internal demand valves are used. (page 863)

60. Tachypnea with small tidal volumes (page 863)

61. Page 864
   A. Spontaneously breathing patients with respiratory rates above 20 and minute volumes in excess of 10 L/min
   B. COPD patients with muscle weakness who need ventilation for more than 48 hours
   C. Spontaneously breathing patients with muscle weakness or COPD patients who cannot tolerate IMV at low rates or CPAP

62. Page 864
   A. CPAP mode
   B. PSV as the sole mode of support

63. Patients who have adequate spontaneous ventilation, but persistent hypoxemia due to shunting (page 865)

64. Page 865
   A. Continuous flow CPAP systems via mask or artificial airway
   B. Ventilator demand flow CPAP systems

65. Both are spontaneous breathing modes. CPAP applies an elevated baseline on inspiration and exhalation, but bilevel ventilation applies a different level of IPAP and EPAP. (page 866)

66. Page 866
   A. Sleep apnea
   B. Noninvasive ventilatory support for chronic restrictive and obstructive disorders

Case Studies

67. Sensitivity must be set to prevent patient triggering if that is possible with the ventilator being used (page 859)

68. Sedation or paralysis (page 859)

69. What is the most likely cause of the excess ventilator triggering? Anxiety resulting in excess patient triggering. (page 843)

70. First check to make sure that the machine is not autocycling or overtriggering due to an inappropriate sensitivity setting. IMV or SIMV is appropriate for patients able to take spontaneous breaths. Pressure support may be applied as needed.

What Does the NBRC Say?

71. C. Initiate PCIRV (page 860)

72. B. Initiate PSV (page 864)

73. A. SIMV (page 859)

74. D. PCV (page 858)

75. D. Decreased tidal volume (page 858)

Chapter 39

Word Power

1. Physical injury sustained as a result of exposure to ambient pressures above normal

2. The volume of gas compressed in the ventilator circuit and not delivered to the patient during a positive pressure breath

3. The inadvertent build-up of positive pressure in the alveoli due to incomplete exhalation of the inhaled volume; also called auto-PEEP

4. The pressure differential between the mouth and the alveoli that causes gas to flow in and out of the lung

5. A complication of mechanical ventilation in which a patient's spontaneous pattern of breathing is not synchronous with the pattern offered by the ventilator

6. The amount of force needed to move a given volume into the lung with a relaxed chest wall; mathematically, work is the integral of pressure times volume

Meet the Objectives

7. Positive pressure ventilation applies a greater than atmospheric pressure to the airway during inspiration. (page 870)

8. Page 873
   A. Alveolar ventilation—PPV increases alveolar ventilation by increasing minute ventilation
   B. Acid-base balance—Increased alveolar ventilation reduces hypercarbia and elevates the arterial pH
   C. Work of breathing—The ventilator assumes all or part of the work by providing the necessary energy for ventilation which reduces muscle work

9. Pages 873, 874
   A. Greatly reduced work of breathing
   B. Control over ventilatory pattern and $PaCO_2$

10. Page 874
    A. Cardiovascular complications
    B. Barotrauma (and potential for muscle atrophy)

11. Page 874
    A. Lower mean airway pressure which avoids cardiovascular complications
    B. Prevents muscle atrophy (and lower risk of barotrauma)

12. Page 874
    A. Ventilator with low internal volume
    B. Low volume, low compliance tubing
    C. Low volume humidifier

13. Avoid or decrease alveolar damage caused by excessive pressure (page 875)

14. Page 876
    A. Mechanism—development of intrinsic PEEP
    B. Oxygen delivery—improved through alveolar recruitment

15. Alveolar ventilation, rather than oxygenation (page 876)

16. Overcome airway resistance imposed by the endotracheal tube and other mechanical factors (page 877)

17. Page 878
    A. Decreased respiratory rate
    B. Increased tidal volume
    C. Reduced respiratory muscle activity
    D. Decreased oxygen consumption

18. CPAP does not provide ventilation because it does not generate changes in airway pressure between inspiration and exhalation. The patient must generate a spontaneous transrespiratory pressure gradient (page 878)

19. CPAP recruits alveoli and maintains them at higher inflation volumes, resulting in improved oxygenation (page 877)

20. Page 878
    A. Nocturnal ventilatory support for chronic restrictive and obstructive disorders
    B. Preventing intubation in exacerbation of COPD

21. VC-SIMV with PSV (page 878)

22. Improved gas distribution, reduced peak pressure, inspiratory work, V_D/VT, and $P(A-a)O_2$ (page 879)

23. It may lead to air trapping if expiratory time is too short, particularly in COPD (page 879)

24. Page 879
    A. Benefit—improved gas distribution
    B. Drawback—increased I time and potential for auto-PEEP

25. Page 879
    A. Improved oxygenation
    B. Improved lung compliance
    C. Reduced V_D/V_T ratio

26. PEEP may reduce auto-PEEP and dynamic hyperinflation in COPD patients. (page 880)

27. Table 39-1, page 880
    A. Increased incidence of barotrauma
    B. Decreased venous return and cardiac output
    C. Increased work of breathing (with overdistention)
    D. Increased ICP
    E. Increased pulmonary vascular resistance (and increased deadspace, MAP)

28. Page 880
    A. Dynamic hyperinflation
    B. Auto-PEEP
    C. Intrinsic PEEP (and occult PEEP)

29. Page 881
    A. Emphysema
    B. Asthma

30. Utilize flow triggering (page 882)

31. Bronchial hygiene, bronchodilators (pages 882, 883)

32. Spontaneous ventilation distributes the gas to the dependent portions of the lung. PPV directs more gas to the nondependent lung. (Figure 39-9, page 883)

33. PPV compresses pulmonary capillaries. This results in increased vascular resistance and helps direct blood away from areas that are ventilated. This lowers the V̇/Q̇ in these areas, and worsens gas exchange. (page 883)

34. Page 884
    A. Impaired oxygen unloading to the tissues
    B. Hypokalemia may result causing arrhythmias and other muscle disturbances
    C. Cerebral vasoconstriction

35. Page 884
    A. Tidal volume: greater than 10 ml/kg
    B. Alveolar pressure: greater than 50 cm H_2O (damage may occur at 30 cm H_2O)

36. Page 885
    5 to 15%

37. Page 885
    A. Pneumothorax
    B. Pulmonary interstitial and subcutaneous emphysema
    C. Pneumomediastinum (and pericardium and peritoneum)

38. Normally, negative pressure on inspiration enhances venous return, cardiac filling, and pulmonary blood flow. PPV impedes pulmonary blood flow, cardiac filling, and venous return to the right heart. (page 885)

39. In patients with left heart failure, PPV reduces afterload. (page 886)

40. They all increase mean airway pressure and mean plural pressure which may have positive or negative consequences. (pages 886-888)

41. Page 888
    A. Compliant lungs—increased cardiovascular effects. Example: emphysema
    B. Non-compliant lungs—decreased transmission of pressure, less effect. Example: ARDS
    C. Non-compliant chest wall—increased cardiovascular effects. Example: Kyphoscoliosis

42. Hypovolemic patients or loss of peripheral venomotor tone. (page 889)

43. Decreased intravascular volume is another possibility. PPV also affects water and sodium-retaining hormonal functions such as increased ADH. Decreased atrial transmural pressure leads to decreases in atrial natriuretic hormone, which lead to sodium retention and water retention. (page 890)

Chapter Highlights (page 890)

44. Oxygenation, work

45. Flow

46. Decelerating, square

47. Flow, pressure

48. FRC, splint

49. FiO_2, oxygen

50. Ventilation, perfused

51. Return, output

52. Perfusion, capillary

Case Studies

53. Take him off the ventilator and manually ventilate.

54. Hypovolemia and shock (page 889)

55. There are two serious problems here. Identify them.
    A. Serious problem no. 1—hypoxemia on a high FiO_2. (page 879)
    B. Serious problem no. 2—elevated airway pressures (page 884)

56. What change(s) in ventilator strategy would you suggest? PEEP could be increased to increase the PaO_2. (page 879) PCV could be initiated to maintain lower airway pressures if permissive hypercapnia is acceptable. PC-IRV is used in some settings. (Pages 876-877) PC-PSV is another possible choice.

Food for Thought

57. Mortality is high with ARDS anyway. Few large studies have been done on the new modes, so we will have to use the more promising methods to find out exactly when they are useful. (page 877)

58. Hydrogen ion blockers and feeding are two suggestions from Chapter 39. (page 890) Sucralfate is another drug used to treat this problem. GI bleeding may lower hemoglobin, resulting in decreased oxygen transport.

Chapter 40

Case Studies

1. C. 7.5 mm inside diameter (page 894) This is the ideal tube for an adult female (page 914)

2. D. I, II, III, IV (See Chapter 29)

3. A. Advance the tube (page 894)

4. B. Respiratory alkalosis with moderate hypoxemia (See Chapters 12 and 16)

5. C. 40% FiO_2 delivered by a heated aerosol T-piece (See Chapters 16 and 31)

6. A. SIMV, V_T 600, 50%, rate 10, PEEP 3 cm H_2O The patient is spontaneously breathing, but needs full support. (page 895) The tidal volume is appropriate. (page 897) PEEP of 3-5 is a good starting point. (page 901)

7. C. Flail chest (page 907)

8. A. Heated wick humidifier set at 32 degrees C. This patient has bloody secretions and is not a candidate for HME at this time. (page 903)

9. C. PSV (page 914)

10. D. 30 minutes (page 908)

11. C. 35 cm H_2O (page 905)

12. C. 55 cm H_2O (page 904)

13. B. 6.0 L (page 904)

14. B. II, III only (pages 900, 914)

15. A. Increase the peak flow (page 905)

16. C. 1:4 (page 900)

17. B. 60 kg (page 1068)

18. A. 500 ml (pages 897, 904)

19. B. Increase the PEEP (pages 902, 904, 911)

20. C. 15 (page 913) (Although some clinicians would still pick 10, since the PaO_2 is adequate and this pressure is safer. So "B" is acceptable (page 912)

21. A. I, III only (page 904)

22. B. II, III only (page 904) (Prone positioning [page 827])

23. A. Normal with moderate hypoxemia (See Chapters 12 and 16)

24. D. Increase the FiO_2 (page 899)

25. A. Increase the rate (The tidal volume is already high . . . CO_2 needs to be reduced.) (page 897)

26. D. New V_E = Current V_E × (Current $PaCO_2$/Desired $PaCO_2$) (page 909)

27. B. 10 (page 909)

Food for Thought

28. Volume-controlled SIMV with pressure support (page 878)

29. This answer will vary depending on what part of the country and what type of hospitals are in your community of interest.

30. Avoid air-trapping and auto-PEEP. High flow rates, and long I:E ratios will help. Allow patients with existing hypercapnia to maintain their normal $PaCO_2$ while trying to optimize pH. Keep plateau pressures below 35 cm H_2O. Consider sedation, especially in the early part of ventilation to avoid asynchrony and barotrauma. Utilize flow-triggering to reduce work of breathing. Use relatively low rates (8-10) and tidal volumes (10 ml/kg). (page 905)

Chapter 41

Monitoring Match

1. A

2. C

3. E

4. D

5. F

6. G

7. B

8. H

9. I

10. J

General Patient Assessment

11. Page 923
    A. Sputum
    B. Blood
    C. Urine

12. Page 923
    A. Head trauma
    B. Elevated airway temperatures

13. Page 923
    A. Positive pressure ventilation
    B. Cardiac tamponade
    C. Severe bronchospasm

14. One reason is to confirm the accuracy of the monitor. Direct assessment also gives information about the quality of the pulse. (page 924)

15. Pages 924, 925
    A. Atelectasis
    B. Pneumonia
    C. CHF
    D. Pneumothorax

16. Page 925
    A. Pain
    B. Anxiety
    C. Medication side effects

17. Daily. (page 926)

18. Page 926
    A. Atelectasis
    B. Pneumothorax (and hyperinflation, effusion, consolidation, and so on)

19. Page 926
    A. Hemoglobin—oxygen-carrying capacity of the blood
    B. WBC and differential—response to infection

20. Page 926
    A. Intake and output measurements
    B. Weighing the patient

21. Pulmonary edema (page 926)

Physiologic Monitoring

22. Blood gas measurement of PaO_2. (page 928)

23. Infants (page 928)

24. Page 928
    A. Laboratory—cooximeter
    B. Bedside—pulse oximeter

25. Pulse oximeters don't measure $PaCO_2$ and thus ventilatory failure. (page 928)

26. Pressure sores and burns may occur. (page 929)

27. Give the general rule for estimating shunt when a patient is breathing 100% oxygen. Every 100 mm Hg difference between PAO_2 and PaO_2 equals a 5% shunt. (page 929)

28. $Q_s/Q_T = CcO_2 - CaO_2 \div CcO_2 - CvO_2$ (page 930)

29. DO_2 is an estimate of delivered oxygen. The formula is: DO_2 = cardiac output $\times$ CaO_2. (page 930)

30. Cardiac output = $VO_2 \div CaO_2 - CvO_2$

31. Pages 930-931

	Normal	Abnormal	Critical
A. PvO_2	38-42 mm Hg	<35 mm Hg	<30 mm Hg
B. SvO_2	68-77%	<50%	<30%

32. Arterial $PaCO_2$ (page 932)

33. At the endotracheal tube (or at the exhalation valve) (page 932)

34. Page 933
    A. Normal—end-tidal is 1-5 mm Hg less than arterial
    B. Ventilated—up to 15 mm Hg

35. Pages 935-936
    A. Detection of esophageal intubation
    B. Assessment of blood flow during cardiac arrest
    C. Determination of PEEP levels
    D. Measuring expired CO_2 for physiologic deadspace determination

36. $VDS_{phs} = [V_T \times PaCO_2 - PECO_2 \div PaCO_2] - VDS_{mec}$ (page 935)

37. Page 936

Normal	Vent Pt.	Critical
0.33-0.45	0.4-0.6	>0.6

38. 5-10 L/min at rest (page 932)

39. Dynamic compliance—the pressure change needed to overcome total impedance including resistance. Effective compliance separates out the resistance and only includes the pressure needed to inflate the lung. (page 937)

40. Normal compliance is 60-100 cm H_2O/L (page 937)

41. Square wave, or constant flow (page 938)

42. Page 938

Normal	Vent Pt.	Abnormal
0.5-2.5 cm H_2O/L/sec	4.5-8.5 cm H_2O/L/sec	>15 cm H_2O/L/sec

43. Page 939
    A. Pressure—transpulmonary pressure (or pleural or esophageal)
    B. Device—esophageal balloon

44. NIF can be performed on unconscious or uncooperative patients (assuming they are intubated!). Vital capacity requires both coordination and cooperation. (page 940)

45. 20 seconds. (page 940)

46. Page 940
    A. Technique 1: Occlude the airway for 20 seconds
       1. Advantage—simpler
       2. Disadvantage—doesn't achieve maximum results in all patients
    B. Technique 2: Use one-way valves to allow exhalation but not inspiration
       1. Advantage—generates a larger negative pressure
       2. Disadvantage—requires more equipment, lung reinflation needed

Mathemagic

Shunt

47. A patient is breathing 100% oxygen. Pb is 747 (conveniently), $PaCO_2$ is 47 (goodie?) and PaO_2 is 300. Estimate the shunt.
    A. PAO_2 = 700 – 47 = 653 mm Hg
    B. A – a = 653 – 300 = 353 mm Hg
    C. Shunt = 353 ÷ 100 × 5 = 18% (17.67) (page 929)

Fick

48. What is cardiac output for a patient who has an oxygen consumption of 200 ml/min, an arterial content of 20 volumes percent, and a venous content of 16 volumes percent?
    A. Formula: CO (Q_T) = VO_2 ÷ CaO_2 – CvO_2 × 10
    B. Calculation: CO = 200 ÷ 20 – 16 × 10
    C. Answer: 5 L/min (page 930)

Minute ventilation

49. What is the V_E for a patient who has a respiratory rate of 8 and a tidal volume of 400?
    A. Formula: V_E = f × V_T
    B. Calculation: V_E = 8 × 400
    C. Answer: 3.2 L or 3200 ml (page 932)

Bohr

50. Your turn. Calculate V_D/V_T for a patient who has an arterial CO_2 of 40 and an exhaled CO_2 of 20.
    A. Formula: V_D/V_T = $PaCO_2$ – $PECO_2$ ÷ $PaCO_2$
    B. Calculation: V_D/V_T = 40 – 20/40
    C. Answer: 0.5 or 50%

51. Calculate alveolar minute ventilation for a patient who has a rate of 10, tidal volume of 500, arterial CO_2 of 40, and end-tidal CO_2 of 28.
    A. Formula: V_A = f (V_T – V_D)
       V_D/V_T = $PaCO_2$ – $PECO_2$ ÷ $PaCO_2$
    B. Calculation: V_D/V_T = 40 – 28 ÷ 40 or 12 ÷ 40 = 0.3. 0.3 × 500 = 150 (V_D)
    C. Answer: V_A = 10 × (500 – 150) = 3500 ml or 3.5 L

V_D/V_T Nomogram

52. 75% (page 936)

Compliance

53. Page 937
    A. Formula: $Ceff = V_T \div Plateau - PEEP$
    B. Calculation: $1000 \div 35 - 10$
    C. Compliance: $1000 \div 25 = 40$ cm H_2O/ml

54. Page 937
    A. Formula: $Ceff = V_T - (PIP \times Factor) \div Plateau - PEEP$
    B. Calculation: $Ceff = 800 - (4 \times 50) \div 35 - 5$
    C. Compliance: $Ceff = 600 \div 30 = 20$ cm H_2O/ml

Resistance

55. Page 938
    A. Convert flow to liters per second: 30 L/min = 0.5 L/sec
    B. Resistance formula: $Raw = PIP - Plateau \div Flow$
    C. Calculation: $50 - 40 \div 0.5$
    D. Airway resistance is 20 cm H_2O/L/sec

The Art Line

56. Page 942
    A. Radial
    B. Brachial
    C. Femoral

Assessment of Hemodynamics

57. Page 942
    A. Continuous hemodynamic monitoring of systemic arterial pressures
    B. Repeated ABG sampling

58. Page 943
    A. Systolic—90-140 mm Hg
    B. Diastolic—60-90 mm Hg
    C. Mean—70-105 mm Hg
    D. Pulse pressure—35-40 mm Hg

59. 72-96 hours (page 945)

60. Withdraw blood then try to flush the catheter. (page 945)

61. Page 945
    A. Catheter tip against vessel wall (move the catheter)
    B. Partial occlusion by clot (withdraw blood, then flush)
    C. Air bubbles in system (disconnect and reflush system)
    D. Compliant tubing (use short, stiff tubing)

62. Placement of the transducer above or below the phlebostatic axis (mid-chest) (page 945)

Flow-directed, balloon tipped, pulmonary artery catheter.

63. Page 943
    A. Subclavian vein
    B. Internal jugular vein

64. Box 41-2, page 946
    A. Shock
    B. Myocardial infarction with hemodynamic instability
    C. Pulmonary vascular disease
    D. Pulmonary edema
    E. ARDS

65. Figure 41-14, page 946
    A. Injection port
    B. Distal injection port
    C. Balloon inflation valve
    D. Thermistor connector
    E. Proximal injection port
    F. Distal lumen
    G. Balloon
    H. Thermistor
    I. Proximal lumen

66. Figure 41-15, page 947
    A. Right atrial pressure
    B. Right ventricular pressure
    C. Pulmonary artery pressure
    D. Pulmonary artery wedge pressure

67. Table 41-10, page 947
    A. Central venous pressure (CVP) <6 mm Hg
    B. Right atrial pressure (RA) 2-6 mm Hg
    C. Pulmonary artery
       1. Systolic 20-30 mm Hg
       2. Diastolic 6-15 mm Hg
    D. Pulmonary artery wedge pressure (PWP, PCWP, PAWP) 4-12 mm Hg

What Does it All Mean?

68. Table 41-11, page 949
    A. Cardiac output (CO) 4-8 L/min
    B. Cardiac index (CI) 2.5-4.0 L/min/m^2
    C. Systemic vascular resistance (SVR) 15-20 mm Hg/L/min
    D. Pulmonary vascular resistance (PVR) 1.5-3.0 mm Hg/L/min

69. Alveolar hypoxemia (Chapter 34)

70. Calculate PVR for a patient who has a mean pulmonary artery pressure of 15 mm Hg, PAWP of 5 mm Hg, and CO of 5 L/min.
    PVR = MPAP − PAWP ÷ Qt so . . .
    15 − 5 ÷ 5 = 2 mm Hg/L/min (page 949)

71. 25 + (2 × 10) ÷ 3 = 45 ÷ 3 = 15 mm Hg (page 943)

Management of the Patient-Ventilator System

72. Page 951
    A. Verification of patient data and ventilator settings
    B. Documentation of physician orders
    C. Verification of proper ventilator function
    D. Clinical observation of the patient response to ventilatory support

73. Pages 951-952
    A. Visual inspection of the expiratory flow tracing
    B. Measurement of end-expiratory pressure during an expiratory hold

74. OVP stands for operational verification procedure. On a third-generation ventilator this may be a self-test, or it may be an operator test of circuit integrity and ventilator function prior to placing the patient on the ventilator. (page 953)

75. Preoxygenating and hyperventilating the patient before disconnection. (page 954)

76. Exposure to contaminated tubing condensate. (page 954)

77. Box 41-7, page 955
    A. Breath sounds
    B. Spontaneous parameters
    C. Observation of the patient-chest motion, skin color, LOC, and so on.
    D. ET tube stability, position, cuff pressure, etc.
    E. Secretions (There are many other possibilities)

78. Pages 955-959
    A. *Pressure* waveform when inadequate flow is present: Erratic waveform with pressure sinking during inspiration then rising rapidly. (Figure 41-22, pages 955, 956,)
    B. *Pressure-volume loop* when overdistention occurs: Rapid rise in pressure with little change in volume at the end of inspiration giving a "beaked" appearance. (Figure 41-25, page 958)
    C. *Flow-volume loop* when a bronchodilator is needed: peak flow is lower and there is a rapid, early decline in expiratory flow. (Figure 41-27, page 958, page 959)

79. Page 959
    A. Patient
    B. Ventilator
    C. Patient-ventilator interface (airway and tubing)

80. Table 41-13, page 960.

Possible Problem	Corrective Action
A. Sudden increase in PIP	
1. Airway secretions	Suction patient
2. Pneumothorax	Insert chest tube
B. Gradual increase in PIP	
1. Diffuse restrictive or obstructive	Evaluate atelectasis, bronchospasm
C. Sudden decrease in PIP	
1. Volume loss from leaks	Check for leaks, assess patient
D. Decreased minute/tidal volume	
1. Leaks around ET or chest tube	Check cuff, connections
2. Decreased patient triggering	Evaluate patient, check sensitivity
E. Increased respiratory rate	
1. Increased patient triggering	Check rate, sensitivity, evaluate patient
2. Hypoxia	Consider ABG, SpO_2 findings

81. Box 41-9, page 962
   A. Artificial airway problems
   B. Pneumothorax
   C. Bronchospasm
   D. Pulmonary edema

82. Box 41-9, page 962
   A. System leak
   B. Circuit malfunction
   C. Improper sensitivity
   D. Improper flow setting

83. Ensure that the patient is adequately ventilated and oxygenated! (page 961)

84. Disconnect the patient and manually ventilate with a resuscitation bag with 100% oxygen until the problem is resolved! (page 961)

85. Box 41-11, page 962
   A. Tranquilizing agents
     1. Diazepam (Valium)
     2. Chlordiazepoxide (Librium)
     3. Midazolam (Versed)
   B. Narcotic analgesics
     1. Morphine
     2. Fentanyl (Sublimaze)
   C. Neuromuscular blocking agents
     1. Long-term: Pancuronium (Pavulon)
     2. Short-acting: Succinylcholine (Anectine)

Bohred Exams

86. A. Manually ventilate the patient with the resuscitation bag (page 961)

87. D. Recommend a chest tube (page 950, Chapter 22)

88. D. Suction the patient (page 960 Chapter 14, 36)

89. A. Administer Valium (page 961 and Box 40-4, page 905)

90. B. Cardiogenic pulmonary edema (page 946)

91. D. Pulmonary artery (pages 943, 947)

92. D. 80% (page 935)

93. C. 16.0 L (page 932)

94. A. 3.2 L

95. D. 5.0 L/min (page 930)

96. A. Hypovolemia (page 949, 950)

97. C. The transducer elevated above the heart (page 945)

Chapter 42

First Things First

1. Support the patient until the disease state or condition that caused the need for support is improved or resolved. (page 968)

2. Ventilators can sustain life but they can't cure disease. (page 968)

3. Page 968
   A. Drug overdose
   B. Asthma
   C. Postoperative anesthesia recovery (also patients on ventilator <72 hours)

4. Page 968
   A. Chronic lung disease
   B. Neuromuscular disorders
   C. Multiple organ system failure
   D. Patients who have been ventilated for an extended period

5. Page 968
   A. Quick routine removal
   B. Gradual reduction (weaning)
   C. Ventilator-dependent

Reasons for Ventilator Dependence

6. Page 968
   A. Apnea
   B. Acute or impending ventilatory failure
   C. Severe oxygenation problems

7. Page 969
   A. Level of ventilation required
   B. Compliance of lung and thorax
   C. Resistance to gas flow through airways
   D. Mechanically imposed work of breathing

8. They increase demand for ventilation by increasing CO_2 production. (page 969)

9. Page 969
   A. Pulmonary emboli
   B. COPD

10. Table 42-1, page 969
    A. Atelectasis
    B. Pneumonia
    C. ARDS (and pulmonary edema)
    D. Fibrosis

11. Page 969
    A. Obesity
    B. Ascites
    C. Abdominal distention
    D. Pregnancy

12. Table 42-1, page 969
    A. Bronchospasm
    B. Mucosal edema
    C. Secretions

13. Remember that a typical patient has an 8 mm ID endotracheal tube, but the normal trachea is approximately 1 inch (25 mm) in diameter.

14. Box 42-1, page 969
    A. CNS drive
       1. Respiratory alkalosis (or metabolic alkalosis)
       2. Pharmacologic depressants
       3. Sleep deprivation
       4. Hypothyroidism
    B. Muscle strength
       1. Malnutrition or starvation
       2. Electrolyte imbalances (especially calcium, magnesium, potassium)
       3. Muscle atrophy from prolonged controlled ventilation
       4. Neuromuscular disorders

15. At least 24 hours. (page 970)

Patient Evaluation

16. The most important criterion is whether there has been significant improvement or reversal of the condition that caused the patient to be put on the ventilator in the first place. (page 971)

17. Page 971
    A. Is the patient getting better?
    B. Is the initial reason for ventilatory support resolved or improved?
    C. Is the patient clinically stable?

18. Table 42-2, page 971

Measurement	Critical Value
A. $PaCO_2$	<50 mm Hg
B. pH	>7.35
C. VC (ml/kg)	>10-15 ml/kg
D. Spont V_T	>5 ml/kg
E. Spont rate	<30, > 6
F. V_E	<10 L/min
G. MVV	>20 L/min, at least $2 \times V_E$
H. MIF (NIF, MIP)	<−20 cm H_2O
I. V_D/V_T	<0.55-0.60
J. $P(A-a)O_2$ on 100%	<350 mm Hg
K. P/F ratio	>200
L. PaO_2	> 60 mm Hg
M. Q_s/Q_T	<15-20%
N. FiO_2	≤ 0.40-0.50

19. Tachypnea is a sensitive sign of distress, but not a sole criteria. Asynchronous chest wall to diaphragm movement leads to fatigue. These signs suggest early decompensation. Irregular spontaneous breathing or periods of apnea are not good signs of weaning success. (page 971)

20. You can palpate the scalenes (inspiration) or the abdominal muscles (exhalation) for tensing. (page 972)

21. PO.1 is the inspiratory pressure measured 100 milliseconds after airway occlusion. PO.1 is effort independent and correlates well with central respiratory drive. (page 972)

22. Page 972
    A. Calculation: 25/0.35 = 71
    B. Criteria: > 105 breaths/min/L

23. Page 973
    A. PaO_2: At least 60 mm Hg (at least 50 in COPD patients with CO_2 retention)
    B. FiO_2: ≤ 0.40-0.50 (assuming normal Hb, CO, and perfusion)

24. Increased CO_2 production and potential respiratory failure. (page 973)

25. Table 42-3, page 973

Measurement	Values Inconsistent With Weaning
A. Heart rate	<60, >100
B. Systolic pressure	<90, >180
C. Diastolic pressure	<60, >110
D. Hemoglobin	<10
E. Cardiac Index (CI)	<2.1

26. Page 973
    A. Electrolyte disorders impair muscle function (acidosis decreases drive)
    B. Fluid overload may cause edema and impaired gas exchange

27. Awake, alert, free of seizures and able to follow instructions (ideally). Obtunded patients should have cough and gag reflexes (at least). (page 974)

28. The inability to protect the natural airway should be a contraindication to extubation, but the patient may possess adequate drive to breathe and muscle strength. A tracheostomy may be indicated. Other patients may be able to protect the airway but lack muscle strength. They are potential candidates for noninvasive positive or negative pressure ventilation. (page 974)

Preparing the Patient

29. Page 974
    A. Bronchodilators
    B. Antiinflammatory agents

30. Suctioning, adequate humidification, bronchial hygiene techniques (page 974)

31. During the day and evening to avoid sleep deprivation (among other reasons) (page 975)

32. Up to 47%. (page 975)

33. Allow the patient to sleep and increase the nocturnal level of ventilator support. (page 975)

34. Noise reduction, clocks and calendars, radio and television, mobility, and devising methods for communication. (page 976)

35. Page 976
    A. Writing tablets
    B. Picture boards
    C. Alphabet boards

Weaning Methods

36. Low levels of PSV help overcome resistance in the circuit, valves, and airway. (page 976)

37. CPAP helps maintain lung volumes and overcome intrinsic PEEP. (page 976)

38. Alarm settings are maintained. (page 976)

39. 30 minutes (page 976)

40. Semi-Fowler's or head-elevated position. (page 976)

41. The patient is taken off the ventilator for 5-30 minutes on a T-piece. The patient is then put back on full ventilatory support for 1-4 hours. This process is repeated, with the time off the ventilator gradually increasing. (See Box 42-7, page 977 for a more detailed description) (page 966)

42. 10% above the set FiO_2 on the ventilator. (page 977)

43. The patient is placed back on the ventilator at night until they are ready for extubation. (page 977)

44. The same exact method is used but the patient is put into CPAP mode (with a slightly elevated baseline or PSV as needed). (page 977)

45. It is labor and time intensive and offers no alarms. (page 977)

46. T piece is more labor intensive, but is probably faster than IMV or PSV weaning. T-piece doesn't offer alarms. T-piece may be more effective in certain patient populations. T-piece seems to require more assessment skills. (page 977)

47. It is very easy to initiate. (page 977)

48. Use pressure support and/or flow-by (page 978)

49. Page 978
    A. Tidal volume 10-12 ml/kg
    B. Respiratory rate 10-12

50. Rate is usually adjusted by 2 breaths per minute. (page 978)

51. When significant ventilatory muscle fatigue is present. (page 978)

52. Pressure support is a mode of ventilation that assists the patient's spontaneous inspiratory effort with a clinician-selected level of positive airway pressure. (page 979)

53. PSV adjusted to a pressure that provides tidal volumes of 10-12 ml/kg. (page 978)

54. Typically 5 cm H_2O. (page 979)

55. Page 980
    A. Formula:
       $PSV = [(PIP - P_{plat}) \div V_{mech}] \times VI_{max}$
    B. Calculation:
       $PSV = [(50 - 30) \div 1L/sec] \times 0.5 L/sec$
    C. Answer: 10 cm H_2O

56. Alarm systems are still available. (page 980)

57. There is no universal recommendation. Different patients may respond to different methods. (page 982)

58. MMV provides a set level of minute ventilation. The amount of mechanical support varies as the patient increases (or decreases) their spontaneous ventilation. (page 980)

59. Patients with rapid shallow breathing. (page 980)

60. Most ventilators increase the rate, but the Hamilton Veolar increases the level of PSV. (page 981)

61. Decreased work of breathing through demand flow systems. (page 981)

62. These methods automatically adjust pressure support to maintain a preset tidal volume. VAPS adjusts the pressure during the breath, volume support adjusts between breaths. (page 982)

63. NIPPV is primarily used in patients who have been weaned and extubated, can maintain a natural airway, but are doing poorly in terms of maintaining minute ventilation. (page 982)

Monitoring the Patient

64. Page 984
   A. Respiratory rate
   B. Respiratory pattern

65. $PaCO_2$ (page 984)

66. Continuous pulse oximetry. (page 985)

67. Table 42-6, page 986

	Parameter	Expected	Deleterious
A.	Respiratory rate	Increase up to 14	>30
B.	PaO_2	5-10 mm Hg	<60 mm Hg
C.	$PaCO_2$	5-10 mm Hg	>50 mm Hg
D.	Heart rate	Increase up to 20	Persistent tachycardia
E.	Blood pressure	Increase up to 15	Hypotension

Extubation

68. The artificial airway may cause a threefold increase in airway resistance resulting in increased work of breathing. PSV will help decrease work of breathing. (pages 986-987)

69. Ability to manage the airway and provide ventilatory support. (page 987)

70. Ability to reintubate. (page 987)

71. Hoarseness and sore throat. (page 987)

72. After making sure the patient can breathe spontaneously, suction the mouth and upper airway. Then deflate the cuff and briefly occlude the ET tube. Check to see if the patient can breathe around the tube. (page 988)

73. Page 988
   A. Mild—cool mist with oxygen (racemic can be given prn)
   B. Moderate—nebulized racemic epinephrine and possibly decadron. Consider heliox.
   C. Severe—reintubate

74. Patients are at risk if they have an impaired gag or cough reflex. Many patients have impaired glottic function after extubation. Marginal muscle strength has been associated with increased risk of aspiration. Withholding feeding for 4-6 hours prior to extubation may reduce the risk of aspiration. (Chapter 29 recommends making the patient NPO after extubation while offering ice chips.) (page 988)

Failure to Wean

75. Box 42-14, page 988
    A. Oxygenation
       1. V/Q mismatch—asthma, emphysema, bronchospasm
       2. Shunt—atelectasis, pneumonia, ARDS, pulmonary edema
    B. Ventilation
       1. Central hypoventilation—drugs, neurologic injury
       2. Increased dead space—embolism, ARDS, emphysema
    C. Cardiovascular
       1. Left ventricular failure
       2. Hemodynamic instability

76. Home, subacute facility, regional weaning centers (page 988)

77. Table 42-8, pages 989-990

A.	Anemia	Transfuse when Hb is ≤10
B.	Tube related WOB	PSV, change tube, shorten tube
C.	Bronchospasm	Bronchodilators Treat cause
D.	Secretions	Hydration and humidity Chest physiotherapy and suction
E.	Dyspnea	Positioning Promote endurance by alternating weaning with rest
F.	Muscle fatigue	Nourish patient (and fix electrolytes) Decrease work of breathing
G.	Hemodynamics	Volume replacement and drugs Lower mean airway pressure (or wait)
H.	Infection	Identify site and treat
I.	Metabolic	Treat cause and postpone weaning with acidosis Avoid excessive carbohydrates
J.	Nutrition	Assess Nourish
K.	Exercise	Range of motion, sitting/ambulating Secure physiotherapy consult
L.	Psychologic	Psychiatric consult Provide communication Decrease stress/teach relaxation
M.	Sleep	Provide uninterrupted sleep Provide quiet environment Avoid weaning at night
N.	Pain	Minimal analgesics Provide alternative methods of pain control

78. Family and physician (page 990)

79. The attending physician (page 990)

Case Studies

80. Her respiratory status is poor. She has acidosis, tachypnea, and abnormal breath sounds. She requires an FiO_2 of 0.5 to maintain minimal oxygenation. She doesn't meet any of the traditional indices for successful weaning. The only good thing is her $PaCO_2$ (page 971)

81. No. Her cardiac index is low, and she has pulmonary and peripheral edema.

82. What is the rapid shallow breathing index? 140 (28 ÷ 0.2) This value suggests weaning would be unsuccessful. (page 972)

83. She is not ready for weaning. Placing her on SIMV with pressure support is an option, without initiating active weaning. This would help maintain synchrony and muscle strength. (page 978)

84. Mr. Ed meets the traditional criteria for weaning or discontinuance; i.e., MIF, VC, ABGs. He is not tachypneic. (page 971)

85. Yes, he has recovered from his anesthesia.

86. 70 (14 ÷ 0.2) This is a value consistent with weaning/discontinuance. (page 972)

87. Weaning is not really necessary for this patient. He could probably be placed on a brief T-piece trial prior to complete discontinuance and extubation. If you were going to rapidly wean him, you could also place him on CPAP mode with a low level of pressure support. (page 976)

88. His ABGs are acceptable. Other values are acceptable but borderline. (page 971)

89. Yes, although his respiratory muscle strength has not fully returned (MIF −20). Guillain-Barré may resolve slowly in many patients. (See Chapter 26).

90. 100 (22 ÷ .22) This is an acceptable value, but borderline. (page 972)

91. Weaning is indicated. Gradual T-piece weaning (page 977) or SIMV weaning is appropriate. Considering his borderline status, I would reduce his SIMV rate by 2, add pressure support to support his spontaneous tidal volumes, and reassess. (page 978)

What Does the NBRC Say?

92. D. I, III, IV only (page 976)

93. A. Initiate a T-piece trial (page 971)

94. D. Minute volume of 8 L/min (page 971)

95. B. Discontinue mechanical ventilation (pages 978-979)

96. C. I, II, III only. This question is not specifically answered in this chapter and includes material from a number of other chapters. The patient is being overventilated and over-oxygenated for his age and condition. It is not surprising he has little drive to breathe. SIMV mode is appropriate for normalizing ABGs and maintaining muscle strength. PEEP of 3 cm H20 is appropriate in COPD (or any ventilator patient).

97. D. Reduce the rate. Adequate oxygenation is present. The patient is capable of increased ventilation as evidenced by the ABG.

98. A. patient on SIMV experiences difficulty each time you try to reduce the rate below 6.
    B. T-piece weaning (pages 975, 986)

Food for Thought

99. The ventilator might not trigger appropriately. (Chapter 40)

100. There is no single best approach. (page 982)

Chapter 43

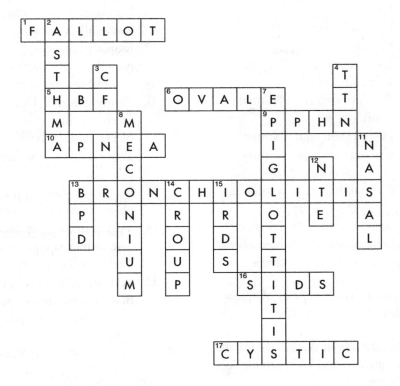

1. Page 995
   A. Stage—Saccule
   B. Week—26-28 weeks

2. The placenta (page 995)

3. There is one umbilical vein that returns blood to the fetus. The two umbilical arteries carry blood to the placenta from the fetus. The vein is larger and thinner-walled. (page 995)

4. Fetal hemoglobin (page 996)

5. The foramen ovale (page 997)

6. Low PO_2 (page 997)

7. 10%. The rest is shunted from the pulmonary artery to the descending aorta via the ductus arteriosus. (page 997)

8. Transpulmonary pressures are very high (-60 cm H_2O). This replaces fluid with air and establishes the FRC. At birth the baby becomes hypoxemic, hypercapnic, and acidotic, which stimulates breathing. As the PO_2 increases, pulmonary vascular resistance decreases and blood flows through the lungs. The ductus arteriosus closes. Systemic blood pressure rises as the placental flow ceases. Increased left heart pressures close the foramen ovale. (pages 997-998)

9. Table 43-2, page 995

	Newborn	Child	Adult
A. Number of alveoli	20 million	300 million	300 million
B. Surface area	3 m^2	32 m^2	70 m^2
C. TLC	0.2 L	3.0 L	6.0 L

Children Aren't "Little Adults"

10. Page 999

	Anatomy	Baby	Adult
A.	Head	Large relative to body	Normal
B.	Tongue	Large relative to mouth	Normal
C.	Nasal passages	Proportionately small	Normal
D.	Larynx	Higher than adult	Normal
E.	Narrow point	Cricoid cartilage	Glottis
F.	Dead space	0.75 ml/lb	1 ml/lb
G.	Airways	Smaller, more compliant	Large, cartilage, elastic fibers

11. Rapid with frequent short periods of apnea and periodic breathing. (page 1000)

12. BMR is 2kcal/kg/hr, about double that of an adult. O_2 consumption and CO_2 production are also double that of the adult. (page 1000)

13. Tidal volume is 6 ml/kg (about 18 ml) and respiratory rate is 35. (page 1000)

14. Small FRC and high oxygen consumption result in severe hypoxemia when oxygenation problems occur. (page 1001)

Assessing the Newborn

15. Table 43-5, page 1001
    A. Pregnancy induced hypertension (preeclampsia)
    B. Alcohol consumption
    C. Smoking

16. Identify five maternal factors likely to lead to premature delivery.
    A. Maternal age <17, >35
    B. Placenta previa
    C. Drug use
    D. Smoking
    E. Pregnancy induced hypertension

17. Diabetes mellitus. (Table 43-5, page 1001)

18. Pages 1001-1002
    A. Ultrasonography: High-frequency sound waves allow viewing the position of the fetus and placenta, measurement of fetal growth, anatomical abnormalities, and amount of amniotic fluid.
    B. Amniocentesis: Direct sampling of the amniotic fluid will show meconium or blood, fetal cells for analysis of genetic abnormalities, and lung maturity via L/S ratios.
    C. Fetal heart rate monitoring: Usually an observation of fetal heart response to contractions. Late decelerations indicate impaired placental blood flow. Tachycardia may indicate hypoxemia.
    D. Fetal blood gas analysis: Scalp blood may be analyzed for pH. A pH below 7.2 may indicate asphyxia.

19. 2:1 at about 34 weeks (page 1001)

20. None. (page 1002)

21. One and five minutes after delivery (page 1002)

22. Table 43-6, page 1003

	Sign	0	1	2
A.	Heart rate	Absent	<100	>100
B.	Respiration	Absent	Slow	Good, crying
C.	Muscle tone	Limp	Flexion	Active motion
D.	Reflex	No response	Grimace	Cough, sneeze, cry
E.	Color	Blue, pale	Blue limbs	Pink all over

23. Page 1003
    A. Before 38 weeks—preterm
    B. 38-42 weeks—term
    C. After 42 weeks—postterm

24. Page 1002
    A. Dubowitz
    B. Ballard

25. Page 1005
    A. VLBW—Very low birth weight <1500
    B. LBW—Low birth weight <2500
    C. AGA—Appropriate for gestational age 10th-90th percentile (about 2600-3700 g)
    D. LGA—Large for gestational age >90th percentile (>3700 g for a term infant)

26. Birth weight and gestational age help identify risk and predict the type of risk. Small preterm infants are at the highest risk. (page 1005)

27. Page 1006
    A. Heart rate—100 to 160
    B. Respiratory rate—40-60
    C. Blood pressure—60/40 (51-72/27-46)

28. Auscultation of the apical pulse. (page 1006) Brachial or femoral can be used.

29. Page 1006
    A. Nasal flaring—increased work of breathing
    B. Cyanosis—Unreliable because it may not be present even when baby is hypoxic
    C. Expiratory grunting—seen in disorders with alveolar collapse
    D. Retractions—increased WOB, poor compliance
    E. Paradoxical breathing—chest wall moves in during inspiration

30. The Silverman Score (page 1007)

31. Page 1006
    A. Radial artery puncture
    B. Arterial line

32. Name two alternate sources.
    A. Umbilical artery
    B. Capillary heel stick

33. Table 43-8, page 1007

Parameter	Preterm	Term	5 Days
A. pH	7.33	7.34	7.38
B. $PaCO_2$	47	35	36
C. PaO_2	60	74	76

What's the Big Idea?

34. When skin temperature is less than 36 degrees C (page 1008)

35. Page 1008
    A. Increased oxygen consumption
    B. Hypoglycemia
    C. Metabolic acidosis
    D. Apnea
    E. Pulmonary hypertension

36. Ambient temperature at which the lowest oxygen consumption occurs while maintaining normal body temperature. (page 1008)

37. 32-35 degrees C (page 1008)

38. Parenterally (page 1008)

39. The hands of caregivers (page 1008)

Respiratory Care Techniques—Basics

40. Page 1009
    A. PaO_2 60-80 mm Hg
    B. FiO_2 0.21-0.50
    C. SpO_2 88%-92%

41. Page 1009 and glossary
    A. ROP—retinopathy of prematurity
    B. BPD—bronchopulmonary dysplasia

42. Box 43-1, page 1009
    A. Prematurity
    B. Blood transfusions (There are many, many others!)

43. When FiO_2 is decreased, the PaO_2 decreases more than expected. When the FiO_2 is returned to the original level, the PaO_2 fails to improve. This is caused by pulmonary vasoconstriction and can be prevented by decreasing the FiO_2 by 1%-2% at a time. (page 1009)

44. Page 1009
    A. FiO_2
    B. Arterial oxygenation (pulse oximetry or transcutaneous)
    C. Temperature

45. Table 43-9, page 1010

Device	Age	Advantage	Disadvantage
A. AEM	≥ 3	Precise, easy	Dry, difficult to fit, maintain
B. Cannula	Any age	Tolerated well	Inaccurate, dry
C. Incubator	<28 days	NTE	Limits access to care
D. Hood	Up to 6 mo.	Warm humid gas, FiO_2	Noise, temp. problems
E. Tent	Up to toddler	Humid, cool, movement care	Isolation, wet, limits care

46. Page 1010
    A. Pneumonia
    B. BPD
    C. CF
    D. Bronchiectasis

47. Management of aspiration of a foreign object (page 1010)

48. Suctioning (page 1010)

49. 1-2 hours (page 1010)

50. Increase the FiO_2 and monitor the SpO_2 (page 1010)

51. Page 1011
    A. Overheating
       1. Tachycardia
       2. Overhydration
       3. Hyperpyrexia
    B. Underheating
       1. Increased O_2 consumption
       2. Hypothermia
       3. Arterial desaturation

52. Bubble humidifiers work well because of the relatively low flow rates. (page 1011)

53. Page 1012
    A. Increased risk of infection
    B. Potential for overhydration
    C. Noise

54. SVN (or MDI via ET tube). (page 1012)

55. Using a spacer with a mask. (page 1012)

56. 0.05 mg/kg, not less than 1.25 mg or more than 2.5 mg. (Table 43-11, page 1013)

57. Table 43-11, page 1013
    A. Dose: 0.25-0.50 ml of a 2.25% solution
    B. Frequency: No more frequently than Q2

58. Table 43-11, page 1013
    A. Dose: 6 g in 300 ml (2% solution)
    B. Treatment schedule: 12-18 hours per day for 3-5 days

59. Table 43-12, page 1014

Age/Weight	ET	Length (oral)	Suction
A. <1000 g	2.5	9-11 cm	6
B. 1000-2000 g	3.0	9-11 cm	6
C. 2000-3000 g	3.5	10-12 cm	6
D. >3000 g	4.0	11-12 cm	8
E. 2 years	4.0-5.0	12-14 cm	8-10
F. 6 years	5.5-6.0	14-16 cm	10

60. Table 43-12, page 1014
    A. Tube ID = (Age + 16) ÷ 4
    B. Tube ID = Height(cm) ÷ 20

61. (4 + 16) ÷ 4 = 5 mm ID

62. $122 \div 20 = 6$ mm ID

63. Miller (page 1014)

64. Infant and pediatric tubes are uncuffed (page 1014)

65. Page 1015
   A. Infants: -60 to -80 mm Hg
   B. Children: -80 to -100 mm Hg

Neonatal Resuscitation

66. In infants less than 1 month old, raise the FIO_2 by 10%-15% for 1 minute (page 1015)

67. Dry and warm the infant. (page 1015)

68. Ideally, the trachea is suctioned through an ET tube. (page 1015)

69. If the heart rate is below 100, bag the baby with 100%. If the heart rate is below 60, start compressions. (page 1015)

More Advanced Questions

70. Refractory hypoxemia. For example, a PaO_2 <50 on ≥50%. (pages 1015, 1016)

71. Box 43-5, page 1016
   A. Tachycardia
   B. Retractions
   C. Grunting
   D. Cyanosis with FIO_2 50%

72. Levels are increased by 1-2 cm H_2O. (page 1016)

73. Nasal prongs (page 1016)

74. Page 1019
   A. Children: 8-10 ml/kg
   B. Term infants: 6-8 ml/kg
   C. Low birth weight infants: 4-6 ml/kg

75. 30 cm H_2O (page 1020)

76. PIP should not exceed their approximate gestational age in weeks. (page 1020)

77. Table 43-14, page 1020
   A. Low birth weight infants: 0.25-0.5 seconds
   B. Term infants: 0.5-0.6 seconds
   C. Toddlers: 0.5-0.75 seconds
   D. Children: 1.0-1.5 seconds

78. Adequate oxygenation. (page 1021)

79. Leaks around the uncuffed tube. (page 1022)

80. Page 1022
   A. FIO_2: Decrease by 2%-5% until below 40%. Preemies require smaller changes.
   B. PEEP: Reduce by 1-2 cm increments down to 3-4 cm H_2O.
   C. Rate: Wean by 2-4 breath increments until <10 per minute.

81. Page 1022
   A. Set rate: <10
   B. PIP: <25 cm H_2O
   C. FIO_2: <0.40
   D. PEEP: +3-4 cm H_2O

82. Measure the amount of inspiratory pressure required to produce a leak. If the pressure is greater than 25 cm H_2O, steroids may be indicated, and postextubation racemic epinephrine. (page 1022)

83. 4-8. This minimizes the work of breathing through the small ET tubes. (page 1022)

84. Box 43-8, page 1023
   A. Severe respiratory failure
   B. Pulmonary barotrauma (PIE, pneumothorax, bronchopleural fistula)
   C. RDS
   D. Air leak syndromes

85. Page 1023
   A. Rates in excess of 150
   B. Tidal volumes of 1-3 ml/kg
   C. Noncompliant tubing

86. Page 1023
   A. HFJV
   B. HFFIV
   C. HFO

87. Page 1024
    A. Mean airway pressure
    B. FIO_2

88. Pressure amplitude or gradient (PIP-PEEP) CO_2 elimination is also frequency dependent. As rate increases, tidal volume drops and so does CO_2 elimination. (page 1024)

89. ECMO is a form of cardiopulmonary bypass that oxygenates blood through an artificial lung or membrane oxygenator. (page 1025)

90. Page 1025
    A. VA—A cannula is placed in the right atrium. Blood is removed, oxygenated, and returned to the aorta by a cannula placed in the right common carotid artery.
    B. VV—A double lumen catheter is placed in the right atrium. Venous drainage flows out through the larger outer cannula and is returned via the smaller inner lumen. Venovenous bypass has fewer complications.

91. Page 1025
    A. PPHN
    B. Meconium aspiration syndrome
    C. Congenital diaphragmatic hernia

New Kids on the Block

92. Meconium is the contents of the fetal bowel and is composed of numerous substances. When it is found in the amniotic fluid it may be a sign of fetal asphyxia. (page 1029)

93. Meconium causes a "ball-valve" type of obstruction. This results in air-trapping and barotrauma (and of course airway obstruction). Meconium also results in lung tissue damage. (page 1029)

94. Page 1029
    A. During delivery: Suction the oropharynx as the head is presented and before the first breath is taken.
    B. After delivery: Intubate the baby and apply suction to the ET tube. Remove the tube and inspect for meconium. If meconium is present, repeat the procedure with a new ET tube until the airway is clear. (Administer O_2 during the procedure)

95. 60-70,000 (page 1030)

96. Inadequate surfactant production secondary to prematurity. (page 1030)

97. Lack of surfactant causes atelectasis and edema which results in severe hypoxemia and acidosis. This increases pulmonary vascular resistance. (page 1030)

98 Definitive diagnosis of RDS is usually made by chest radiograph. Describe the chest film of an infant with RDS. Reticulogranular densities and air bronchograms. There are four stages, but the pattern is diffuse in nature, the lungs are poorly expanded, and a "white out" will appear in severe cases. (pages 1030-1031)

99. CPAP and PEEP to treat the refractory hypoxemia. (page 1031)

100. Surfactant is a liquid that is instilled directly into the endotracheal tube. (page 1031)

101. Page 1031
    A. Exosurf (colfosceril palmitate) is a synthetic preparation.
    B. Survanta (beractant) is a natural bovine extract.

102. Transient tachypnea of the newborn. The cause is thought to be delayed clearance of fetal lung fluid. Preterm infants, and those delivered by C-section, may have delayed clearance, which results in increased airway resistance and decreased compliance. (page 1033)

103. Low levels of O_2 via hood for mild cases. CPAP for more severe cases. Frequent positioning changes. IV antibiotics must be considered since TTN and pneumonia have similar signs. (page 1033)

104. Page 1033
    A. Lasting longer than 20 seconds
    B. Associated with pallor, cyanosis, hypotonia, or bradycardia

105. Table 43-16, page 1033

Cause	Signs	Investigate
A. Infection	Lethargy, unstable temp.	CBC, sepsis
B. Oxygenation	Tachypnea, cyanosis	Monitor O_2, ABG, CXR
C. Maternal	History— especially drugs	Urine drug screen, magnesium
D. Environmental	Lethargy	Temp., baby and environment

106. Methylxanthines such as caffeine or theophylline. (page 1033)

107. Pick baby up, flick the feet, rub the skin. (page 1033)

108. Page 1034
    A. Immaturity
    B. Oxygen toxicity
    C. Positive pressure ventilation (and now malnutrition has been added)

109. Hyaline membrane formation and L-R shunt via PDA or foramen ovale. Pulmonary edema followed by fibrosis and emphysematous changes. (page 1034)

110. Page 1034
    A. O_2
    B. Chest physiotherapy
    C. Bronchodilators

111. Page 1035
    A. Surgical ligation
    B. Pharmacologic (indomethacin)

112. Surgery (page 1035)

Sudden Infant Death Syndrome

113. Etiology is unknown. (page 1035)

114. Describe the typical profile of a baby who dies of SIDS. A preterm black male, born to a poor mother under the age of 20 who received inadequate prenatal care. (page 1035)

115. Prone sleeping. (page 1035)

116. Box 43-14, page 1037
    A. Age <6 months (usually between 1-3 months)
    B. Asleep at night
    C. Mild illness the week before death
    D. History of apparent life-threatening event

117. Teach the family CPR and apnea monitoring. Place the baby supine or side-lying for sleep during the first 6 months. (pages 1035, 1037)

Case Studies

Page 1037
118. Bronchiolitis

119. Immunoflourescent assay of the sputum

120. Humidification and oral decongestants

Page 1038
121. Croup

122. Racemic epinephrine (with or without dexamethasone)

123. In the ED a mask could be used, or blow-by. After admission a tent would be appropriate.

Pages 1039-1040
124. Epiglottitis

125. *Haemophilus influenzae* type B; obtain a culture after the airway is secured

126. Intubation under general anesthesia in the operating room by an expert

127. Don't lie the child down; attempt to intubate outside of the prescribed setting, or otherwise manipulate the airway.

Page 1040
128. Sweat chloride testing

129. Low-fat diet with vitamin supplements and pancreatic enzymes

130.
   A. Humidification
   B. Bronchodilators
   C. Mucolytics
   D. Chest physiotherapy
   E. Airway clearance devices such as PEEP

131. Pulmozyme

132. MDI with a spacer (page 1041)

133. Dad needs some form of parent education. This could be a formal program, such as those offered by the American Lung Association, or a candid discussion of the pros and cons of steroids. (See Chapter 44 for more on effective teaching). Alternatives may have to be offered if the father is adamant.

Pages 1041-1042
134. Pneumonia

135. Bacterial—high fever with rapid onset. The elevated WBCs support this answer.

136. Oxygen, fluids, antibiotics

What Does the NBRC Say?
137. B. L/S ratio (page 1001)

138. D. 9 (page 1003)

139. D. Aminophylline (page 1034)

140. D. Epiglottitis (page 1039)

141. C. Foreign body aspiration

142. A. Sweat chloride (page 334, Chapter 15)

143. B. Narcan

144. A. Nasal prongs (page 1016)

145. C. Lateral neck film (page 1038)

146. B. Racemic epinephrine (page 1038)

Chapter 44

Teacher Talk (Answers in glossary)
1. Affective domain: The area of mood, emotion, or feeling

2. Cognitive domain: The area of mental processes such as memory and reasoning

3. Disease prevention: Activities designed to protect patients or public from health threats

4. Health education: A process of planned learning opportunities designed to enable individuals to make informed decisions about their health

5. Health promotion: Combination of educational, economic, and environmental support necessary for behavior conducive to health including disease prevention and wellness activities

6. Psychomotor domain: The area of observable performance of skills that require some degree of neuromuscular coordination

Patient Education

7. In the eighteenth and nineteenth centuries, as causes of disease such as bacteria were discovered, and risk factors such as poverty, poor nutrition, and contaminated water were discovered. (page 1050)

8. Most major illnesses in the United States have a few central and preventable causes. Public education has the greatest potential for impacting on these diseases. (page 1050)

9. Page 1050
   A. Heart disease
   B. Cancer
   C. Cerebrovascular disease
   D. Accidents
   E. COPD

10. Health promotion and disease prevention. (page 1050)

11. Written objectives help clarify the learning plan and can be used to develop a lesson plan. Objectives make clear what is to be accomplished and give direction for the evaluation process. (page 1050)

12. Begin with a verb and include a single desired behavior. (page 1050)

13. Pages 1050-1051

Domain	Objective
A. Cognitive	Identify the indication for oxygen therapy.
B. Affective	Verbalize willingness to use oxygen appropriately.
C. Psychomotor	Operate an oxygen concentrator.

14. The affective domain. (page 1050)

15. Talk to the patient, listen to concerns, be empathetic, and develop a relationship. (page 1051)

16. Getting the patient to see what's in it for them. (page 1051)

17. Repetition is the key. Redemonstration confirms they can do it. (page 1051)

18. Cleaning equipment can be related to washing dishes. (page 1051)

19. You should use as many of the senses as possible in all teaching situations. With children it is important to present the material at the right level. Rewards may be useful. (page 1052)

20. Lung Association (Mini Clini, page 1052)

21. Stickers or treats (page 1052)

22. Evaluation is the process and it should be started when you develop the objectives before the education begins. (page 1052)

23. One way is to look for evidence that lifestyle changes have taken place. Another way is to engage in frequent discussions with the patient and the family. There are also tests than can be administered to assess attitude and perception. (page 1052)

24. You should take advantage of "teachable moments" when they occur. For example, when a patient brings something up during their treatment at the bedside. (page 1053)

Health Education & Promotion

25. The primary role is to promote behavioral change. (page 1053)

26. Page 1055
    A. High-fat diet
    B. Excessive alcohol use
    C. Use of tobacco products
    D. Inactivity

27. The standard medical approach is to diagnose and treat disease. The public health model attempts to reduce disease through tactics like mass education campaigns such as "drinking and driving." (page 1056)

28. Page 1056

Level	Goal	Example
A. Primary	Prevent disease	Immunization
B. Secondary	Early detection	Mammograms
C. Tertiary	Prevent disease acceleration	Pulmonary rehabilitation

29. Pages 1056-1057
    A. Primary — Nicotine intervention programs
    B. Secondary — Spirometry screening projects
    C. Tertiary — Asthma education programs

30. Page 1057
    A. Worksites
    B. Home
    C. Community
    D. Schools

Case Studies

Examples of objectives are found on pages 1050-1051. Obviously there are many possible "answers" to these questions.

31. Cognitive domain
    A. Identify the indications for peak flow monitoring
    B. State the formula for calculating normal peak flow
    C. Describe the three color zones used in peak flow assessment

32. Affective domain
    A. Agree that peak flow monitoring is important
    B. Verbalize a willingness to teach patients
    C. Follow national guidelines for peak flow monitoring

33. Psychomotor domain
    A. Perform the peak flow maneuver
    B. Clean the peak flowmeter
    C. Set the correct zones

34. How long would your teaching session last? Keep the session short—no more than 20-30 minutes. (pages 1051-1052)

35. Give examples of how you would involve the following senses in your session?
    A. Hearing—hearing the instructor, hearing the sound of exhalation on a good effort
    B. Seeing—watching a video or demonstration
    C. Touching—handling the peak flow meter
    D. Writing—taking notes during the presentation, calculating values
    E. Speaking—giving an instruction to a classmate

36. Pages 1051-1052
    A. Cognitive—give a multiple choice post-test or quiz
    B. Affective—difficult to measure in this setting, observation in clinical is a possibility
    C. Psychomotor—return demonstration

What Does the NBRC Say?

37. C. Ask the patient to demonstrate how to use the inhaler (page 1051)

Food for Thought

38. One reason is that this is a growing area of health care and is a good opportunity for RCPs to expand their scope of practice. Insurance companies and HMOs are now paying for providing this type of service. Another reason would be the satisfaction of making a difference.

39. Caregivers are more educated. Otherwise, the principles are the same. (page 1053)

Chapter 45

Eat Your Words

1. E

2. F

3. A

4. H

5. B

6. I

7. C

8. G

9. J

10. K

11. L

12. D

Meet the Objectives

13. The Food Pyramid is a graphic method developed by the U.S. Department of Agriculture for helping citizens and consumers have a more healthy diet. Fats, oils, and sweets are at the top and should be used sparingly. Grain and cereals are at the bottom and should have the largest number of servings. (Figure 45-1, page 1064)

14. You can achieve half your daily need for protein (about 21 grams) by consuming a 3-ounce portion of meat, fish, poultry or cheese—this is about the size of a deck of cards. (page 1064)

15. Pages 1064-1065

Macro	Calories per gram
A. Protein	4 kcal per gram

   1. Essential amino acids—also called high biologic value proteins
   2. Nonessential

B. Carbohydrates	4 kcal per gram

   1. Simple
   2. Complex

C. Fats	9 kcal per gram

   1. Saturated
   2. Monounsaturated
   3. Polyunsaturated

16. Page 1065
    A. Formula (male) REE kcal/day = 66 + [13.7 × weight(kg)] + [5 × ht (cm)] − 6.8 × age
    B. Calculation (mine) REE = 66 + [13.7 × 83] + [5 × 183] − 6.8 × 43 or 66 + 1137 + 915 − 292 so my REE = 1826 kcal/day

17. 2000-2400 Rule of Thumb, page 1065

18. Page 1066
    A. B_6
    B. Selenium
    C. Fat-soluble vitamins

19. Vitamins are coenzymes in the metabolism of protein, carbohydrates, and fats. (page 1065)

20. Page 1066
    A. Soluble
       1. Regulates cholesterol metabolism
       2. Regulates glucose metabolism
    B. Insoluble
       1. Absorbs water in the GI tract
       2. Prevents constipation

21. Starvation is called marasmus. An RCP might see this in cancer or emphysema patients. Hypercatabolism is called *kwashiorkor*. Septic or burn patients could have hypercatabolism. (Table 45-3, page 1067)

22. Page 1067
    A. Zinc—Impaired clotting, wound heal-
       ing, and immunity
    B. Magnesium—Electrolyte abnormalities,
       cardiac and neuro problems
    C. Hypophosphatemia—Decreased muscle
       strength

23. One third (page 1067)

24. Page 1067
    A. Poor muscle function
    B. Increased likelihood of hypercapnia

25. Increased energy expenditure from work of
    breathing, and inadequate caloric intake
    from dyspnea, psychosocial issues, medica-
    tions, and GI symptoms. (Box 45-3,
    page 1068)

26. Decreased response to hypercapnia and
    hypoxia. Loss of muscle mass and contrac-
    tility in both primary and accessory muscle.
    (Box 45-2, pages 1067-1068)

27. Registered dietitian or clinical nutritionist.
    (page 1067)

28. Page 1068
    A. Males: 106 + 6 (Height [inches] − 60)
    B. Females: 105 + 5 (Height [inches] − 60)

29. Box 45-5, page 1069
    A. Poor intake: anorexia, NPO
    B. Nutrient loss: renal dialysis, draining
       wounds
    C. Hypermetabolism: sepsis, trauma, burns
    D. Drugs: alcohol, steroids, antitumor drugs

30. Box 45-6, page 1070
    A. Patients with morbid obesity
    B. Difficult to wean patients
    C. Patients with severe malnutrition

31. Patient is hemodynamically unstable to the
    point that any disconnections result in
    bradycardia or hypoxemia. Otherwise there
    are no real contraindications. (page 1071)

32. Page 1071
    A. Decreased alveolar volume—increased
       compressible circuit volume
    B. Increased WOB—decreased trigger
       sensitivity

33. Box 45-7, page 1072
    A. 4 hours before the test—rest and avoid
       physical activity
    B. 2 hours before the test—suction patient
       and avoid ventilator changes
    C. 1 hour before the test—supine, com-
       plete rest, sedation PRN

34. Presence of any leaks will invalidate the
    test. (page 1073)

35. Table 45-5, page 1074

	Value	Interpretation	Strategy
A.	>1.0	Overfeeding	Decrease total kcal
B.	0.9-1.0	Carbohydrate oxidation	Decrease carbs, increase lipids
C.	0.7-0.8	Fat and protein oxidation	Increase total kcal

36. REE (kcal/day) = cardiac output $\times$
    hemoglobin $\times$ (SaO_2 − SvO_2) $\times$ 95.18
    (page 1074)

37. Activity and stress levels need to be
    included to adjust REE derived from the
    Harris-Benedict equation. The predicted
    REE $\times$ stress factor $\times$ activity factor will
    give the new actual energy needs. Example:
    bone fracture-factor is 1.2. (page 1074)

38. Page 1075
    A. Protein—increased oxygen consump-
       tion, minute ventilation, and dyspnea
    B. Carbohydrates—increased CO_2 produc-
       tion and work of breathing
    C. Fat—decreased diffusion capacity and
       increased A-a gradient

39. Page 1075
    A. Enteral—oral and tube feedings
    B. Parenteral—intravenous feedings

40. Page 1076
    A. Bolus—rapid infusion of 250-500 ml of feeding several times a day
    B. Intermittent—infusion of feeding over 30 minutes several times a day
    C. Drip—constant flow of formula over 12-24 hours

41. Aspiration is confirmed by suctioning feeding from the lungs. Adding dye to the feeding makes it easy to see. Raising the head of the bed, delivering the feeding past the stomach, and special ET tubes may help prevent this problem. (page 1076)

42. Page 1078
    A. Fatigue
    B. Dyspnea—especially after or during eating
    C. Medication side effects such as nausea, diarrhea, vomiting
    D. Depression

43. A low carbohydrate, high fat diet is desirable. Ideally the diet is individually tailored to provide the lowest amount of fat that produces an acceptable $PaCO_2$. Getting calories in is usually more important. (page 1079)

44. COPD patients should frequently eat small amounts of high calorie, high protein foods. These include peanut butter, dried fruits, nutritional supplements, and more. (Box 45-12, page 1079)

Chapter Highlights (pages 1079-1080)

45. Grains, vegetables

46. Macronutrients

47. Micro

48. Harris-Benedict

49. Malnutrition

50. Predicted

51. Enterally, parenterally, enteral

52. Aspiration, raising, 45 degrees

Case Studies

53. Eat smaller meals more often. (page 1079)

54. Try eating dried fruits, whole milk, ice cream or puddings, rich desserts, adding butter or cheese to vegetables, eating eggs, or trying nutritional supplements.

55. Pulmocare (page 1077)

Food for Thought

56. Besides a carefully tailored nutrition plan to provide necessary nutrients, a high-fat, low-carbohydrate diet may help. (pages 1078-1079)

57. The oral feeding tube may be accidentally placed in the lungs. (page 1076)

Chapter 46

Cerebral Muscle Training

1. B

2. D

3. G

4. H

5. I

6. C

7. A

8. F

9. E

Definitions and Goals

10. "The restoration of the individual to the fullest medical, mental, emotional, social, and vocational potential of which he/she is capable." (page 1084)

11. Pulmonary rehab is a multidisciplinary program designed to stabilize or reverse the harmful effects of pulmonary diseases and help people return to the highest possible function allowed by their pulmonary handicap and overall situation. (page 1084)

12. Page 1084
    A. Control and alleviate symptoms and complications of respiratory impairment
    B. Teach patients how to achieve the capability to carry out their ADLs

Scientific Basis for Pulmonary Rehabilitation

13. Social sciences help determine the psychological, social and vocational impact of disability on the patient and family and help find ways to improve quality of life. (page 1084)

14. MVV is an indicator of ability to handle increased level of physical activity. It may help determine whether the respiratory system is the primary limiting factor for exercise. (page 1085)

15. $FEV_1 \times 35$ (page 1085)

16. Page 1085
    A. Strengthens muscle groups
    B. Improves overall oxygen utilization
    C. Enhances cardiovascular response to physical activity

17. Psychosocial indicators are generally better predictors of hospitalization and whether or not a patient will complete the rehabilitation program. (page 1085)

18. Emotional tension can lead to physical fatigue. Emotional states can aggravate physical problems. Physical manifestations of disease, such as dyspnea, can worsen stress. (page 1086)

Pulmonary Rehabilitation Programs

19. Specific objectives help in development of strategies for success. Demonstration of effectiveness then leads to better acceptance by the medical community. (pages 1088, 1089)

20. Table 46-1, page 1089
    A. Increased physical endurance
    B. Increased maximum O_2 consumption
    C. Increased activity levels
    D. Decreased VO_2
    E. Decreased heart rate (and others)

21. Page 1089
    A. Does not improve PFTs or ABGs
    B. Does not halt the progression of the disease

22. Box 46-2, Page 1090
    A. Before and after 12-minute walking distance
    B. Weight loss or gain
    C. Changes in ADLs

23. Pages 1090-1091
    A. Cardiac arrhythmias
    B. Arterial desaturation
    C. Functional or structural injuries

24. Complete medical history (page 1090)

25. Page 1090
    A. Chest xray
    B. ECG
    C. CBC
    D. Electrolytes

26. Page 1090
    A. Exercise evaluation
       1. Quantifies initial exercise capacity (and degree of desaturation)
       2. Basis for exercise prescription and target heart rate
    B. Pulmonary function testing
       1. Pre- and postbronchodilator information
       2. Overall lung function